Food,
We Need to Talk

Food, We Need to Talk

The Science-Based, Humor-Laced Last Word on Eating, Diet, and Making Peace with Your Body

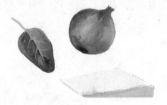

Juna Gjata

and

Edward M. Phillips, MD

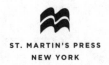

ST. MARTIN'S PRESS
NEW YORK

First published in the United States by St. Martin's Press,
an imprint of St. Martin's Publishing Group

FOOD, WE NEED TO TALK. Copyright © 2023 by Juna Gjata and Edward M. Phillips. All rights reserved. Printed in the United States of America. For information, address St. Martin's Publishing Group, 120 Broadway, New York, NY 10271.

www.stmartins.com

Designed by Devan Norman

The Library of Congress Cataloging-in Publication Data
is available upon request.

ISBN 978-1-250-28368-9 (hardcover)
ISBN 978-1-250-28369-6 (ebook)

Our books may be purchased in bulk for promotional, educational, or business use. Please contact your local bookseller or the Macmillan Corporate and Premium Sales Department at 1-800-221-7945, extension 5442, or by email at MacmillanSpecialMarkets@macmillan.com.

First Edition: 2023

10 9 8 7 6 5 4 3 2 1

Juna would like to dedicate this book to her parents, Irma and Arqile, in the hopes that they now have something to brag about to Albanian relatives—I love you guys.

Also to her grandma—Nena, I know you'll probably never understand this book because it's all in English, and the fam is far too lazy to translate it, but the fact that you're so proud of it without having the slightest clue what the hell it says shows what I've always known to be true: you're a real one. Te dua shume.

Eddie dedicates this book to Alison for joyously sharing our life, our love, and ten thousand home-cooked dinners. Let's grow old together with gratitude and grace.

Contents

The Book Ahead

Before we get started, we thought we would create a little road map to guide you through the book. Although we recommend reading the book in order, because every chapter builds on the knowledge of the ones preceding it, we understand that sometimes the thirst for knowledge is too overwhelming and you just *need to know* the benefits of a good night's sleep or the fundamentals of an awesome gym routine. Take a look at what lies ahead, or, if you're a cheeky little devil, determine where to jump to if you want to read ahead.

1.

From the Victorians to the Kardashians
A Brief History of Dieting

Contrary to popular belief, we do not exist in a low-carb, keto vacuum as the only generation to experience the societal pressures of body image and dieting. Alert: Slim has not always been in! This chapter is a look at dieting and body "ideals" in recent human history.

2.

Before we talk about the fuel that goes into your "car," we're going to spend a bit of time talking about the "engine": how it runs, if you can make it run faster or slower, and that age-old question: "Is [insert arch nemesis's name]'s metabolism truly just faster than mine?" All shall be revealed. (Note: This chapter introduces the terminology and concepts referred to throughout the rest of the book.)

3.

Yes, it's true, we're surrounded by diet culture and a persistent obsession with losing weight. This is what keeps the world of fitspos, diet books, and supplements going around. Here's how and why all diets work, why we keep getting sucked in, and then a (much longer) discussion of the science behind why diets fail . . . at least most of the time.

4.

Should we even care about our weight? Or is it a scheme by Big Pharma, protein-shake companies, and the fitness industry to get you to spend the rest of your life on a treadmill chewing on leaves? Scientific considerations on the link between weight and health are offered in this chapter.

5.

Oh boy . . . here's the big one. At the risk of infuriating every diet camp out there, here is the good, bad, and ugly of what to put into your mouth. Bon appétit!

6.

Exercise is so awesome that we couldn't resist; we both had to talk about it in our own chapters. In this one, Eddie shares the science of cardiovascular exercise, how he built his career around it, and how modest changes to your physical activity will create profound changes to your quality of life.

7.

Not to be *that* person, but this is the story of how Juna fell in love with the gym and how it changed her life and her body. All your questions about "toning," "sculpting," lifting, getting stronger, and overall becoming a boss in the gym are answered. Includes an "I Can't Go to the Gym Because . . ." excuse buster.

8.

Yes, even someone who majored in psychology can have an eating disorder. This chapter explores disordered eating, eating disorders, and whom they can affect. (Hint: It's everyone.)

9.

What was supposed to be a short conversation between Eddie and his daughter to "add a few paragraphs to the book" turned into a whole chapter (in the book as well as their lives). This heartfelt conversation considers how a parent's best intentions to instill healthy food choices can perversely manifest in a life-threatening eating disorder.

10.

Stress, Eating, and Weight

The stress response is what keeps us alive and thriving, but as with everything, too much of a good thing becomes . . . well . . . chronic disease, an expanding waistline, and a very unpleasant mental state. Here are the scientific reasons to chill.

11.

Why You Shouldn't Sleep on Sleep

There's a reason why we evolved to spend a third of our lives completely incapacitated in an unconscious stupor of eerily realistic dreams. This may be shocking, but sleep is important—in fact, crucial. And falling asleep to *Seinfeld* reruns is not ideal. Find out why.

12.

What Matters Most and Making Lasting Change

Time to actually do something with all this information! We go into the science of creating new habits and figuring out what matters most.

Epilogue
To the Reader

We offer some final thoughts in letters from us to you before you go on your merry way, newly armed with your kick-ass science-backed knowledge of the human body.

A Note to You, the Reader

Do you want to know what's absolutely terrifying? Writing a book all about diets, food, exercise, weight, health, fitness, and what science has to say about all of it . . . in the 2020s.

I ask you: Is there anything more personal than the meat suit we walk around in all day long? Is there anything closer to a physical representation of yourself in the world than your body? Honestly, I don't think so.

The deeper you dive into the realms of health, fitness, and the research behind them, the more you realize how complicated all of this can be. Something can be absolutely, unequivocally true in the lab but, at the exact same time, be almost unachievable (i.e., for all practical purposes untrue) in real life. The same behavior can be highly beneficial to your physical health and at the same time debilitating for your mental health. Health advice for one person might be "Consider swapping out some desserts for fruit," and for another person might be "Dude, it's your birthday; live a little and have a freaking piece of cake."

This is because health doesn't just refer to your physical body; it's your quality of life, how you feel, your psychological, emotional, mental, spiritual, and social well-being. But this, too, just like anything else, can be taken to an extreme. Does counting every calorie and eating only "unprocessed food" truly lead to good health? Does not putting any thought into what you put into your body translate as healthy? Does asking rhetorical questions distract you from the fact that I have no idea what the answer is? Shh . . . don't tell anyone.

Let's first get some things clear:

1. Every person is different, so I don't see why being "healthy" wouldn't also be different for every person. Everyone should have the freedom to decide for themselves what "healthy" means *for them*, without fear of judgment, punishment, or being made to feel ashamed. I feel especially strongly about this point be-

cause I see tribalism and irrationality on every part of the "ideal diet" spectrum. If you talk about certain foods being associated with certain health outcomes, you are seen to be promoting diet culture and eating disorders (EDs). If you talk about people being able to live healthy lives in bigger bodies, you are letting people off the hook for eating like slobs and being lazy. If it's not obvious to everyone at this point, the extreme, by its very nature and by definition, is almost never the case. Just like in politics, the opposing ideologies often have remarkably more in common than what separates them. I'm not really interested in being part of any faction, and this book is not meant to be used as ammunition for any faction.

2. Science is messy, complicated, and always biased by whomever is interpreting it. Two people can look at the same data and the same results and come to entirely different conclusions. You can take the same set of studies and tell a story that is completely different from someone else's. Many books in this genre use the same research, and yet every single one comes up with a unique narrative, through line, and thesis. Just because scientific language has statistical methods and conventions that act as guardrails to keep it "objective" and "unbiased" does not mean that, at the end of the day, studies aren't conducted by humans, on humans, and then reported by humans. We come into every topic with a history, an experience, a lens through which we view the world, and anyone who tells us otherwise is lying. So, yeah, I want to be up front that I'm not coming into this book blindly (figuratively, of course, because I actually am *literally* legally blind; but you know what I mean). I have made a conscious effort to look at things as objectively as I can and to consider and understand all sides of any topic. But Eddie (my coauthor) and I are not perfect.

All that said, we can promise you some things: we did our absolute best in researching every topic in this book in its entirety. We tried to not let preconceived notions of subjects cloud our judgment. When we saw a study that went against what we felt was the truth, we tried to understand why, and if we couldn't, we kept researching to find out what *really* was the truth. Eddie and I have asked several experts in the fields we cover to read our chapters, providing us corrections and overall impressions. This is the best we could do, given the research we've read, the experts we've spoken to, and the thought we've put in at the time of publication. Does this mean everything is 100 percent foolproof? *Hell to the no.* To some extent, we are all responsible for our own decisions, so read the book, look up the sources, come to your own conclusions, and for God's sake, *give us a good rating!* (I'm kidding.)

Secondly, we will not be ignoring science to please any faction, or—perhaps more accurately—to avoid being attacked by a certain faction. This is very hard, because I am a people pleaser, and I want to write a book that everybody loves and no one disagrees with or hates on . . . but it seems more and more like that's going to be impossible because people just *care so much* about this topic. And I don't blame them; it's deeply personal, and painful, and, for many, associated with long-held traumas. (PS: I know some of y'all reading this are like, "Girl, it's just a fitness book, chiiiilllll," but I'm telling you, people on all sides of this can get *really mad.*) Either way, there are some indisputable things, at least with the research we have so far, and it doesn't matter how much you may not like the findings—science is science.

The success of this book hinges on *you*, the reader, knowing *yourself.* Which type of person are you? Are you confused and just needing some guidance on navigating the never-ending diet wars? Maybe you just want to learn more about the topic, possibly implement some new habits, see how you feel, and so forth. There are others of you, however, and you'll know who you are, my type A's out there, who can get carried away with things. This is the group I feel I fit in with. I hear, "Ultra-processed food is associated with earlier death," and I go, "No more cake for the rest of my life." So, in this way, I need your help: I need you to know which person you are, and to read the book with that knowledge in mind.

If you're picking up this book, you obviously care about improving your health, whether you're thinking of it as "weight loss," or just eating better, or even feeling better. But if you're the type of person to take things to extremes, I am begging you to take your mental health just as seriously as your physical health. What is the point of living a perfectly "healthy" life (according to science) if you're anxious, obsessed, alone, and miserable?

This is the world I want to live in: A world where we can read books about health and fitness and not use them for self-punishment or judgment. A world where we can hold two opposing ideas in our heads at the same time: this food might not be promoting optimal health, but right now, I want to eat it because I like it. A world where every mention of calories, bodies, or weight does not automatically equate to hating people in bigger bodies. I don't believe that sharing one idea with one group or another means you ascribe to all that group's ideas. So . . . I guess this is all to say, this book does talk about topics that may be triggering for some people—we didn't choose to censor mentions of weight, calories, or words like "obesity," "fat," and so on. In the ideal world, these words would be neutral, simple descriptors or quantifiable entities, but I know for some people, they are not. I trust you to know yourself, and if it's upsetting to you, feel free to throw this out and find something more suitable to you.

I am writing this book for *me,* for my eighteen-year-old self. That's why, although the point of the book is not weight loss, we do discuss weight loss . . . because I know that's what eighteen-year-old Juna was desperate to understand. Do I think I would have been better off never intentionally trying to lose weight? Yes. Do I think it should be the first and only goal of changing eating or movement behaviors? No. But I am not here to dictate people's goals, desires, attitudes toward themselves, or health decisions. I just want to provide the most up-to-date and accurate information possible on the topics that I obsessed over from adolescence on, in the hopes that those reading this book won't do the same things I did. I don't think shaming people, *for anything,* whether it's a desire to lose weight or the opposite, a refusal to assign any value judgments to any food or behavior, is a good way to communicate. So if you're down for it, then we can get started. First, let me tell you a little about myself, since we'll be getting pretty damn close over the next few hundred pages.

Introductions

Who Is This Girl, Anyway?

Let's just get this out of the way: my name is pronounced "Yoo-nah," like with a soft "J." If you call me "Joo-nah" with a hard "J," I will get horrible flashbacks to roll call on the first days of school for seventeen years of my life. Please don't do this to me. The reminder of outfit choices alone is enough to make me want to crawl into a hole in the ground like a human gopher. I was born in Albania, and at age four I had a really severe allergic reaction to a common cold medication, which basically left my vision severely impaired. Before you freak out—it's OK!! I'm fine! My eyes are the reason my family and I left Albania and came to America. They're the reason I have gotten to do all the awesome things I've done and to meet all the awesome people I've met. If it weren't for that allergic reaction, I'd be married with sixteen kids, raising goats and chickens in a rural eastern European village! Plus, I get to cut lines at Disney World now.

I'm joking, I don't. *But wouldn't that be awesome?!* My vision is largely irrelevant to this book and this story, but I need you to know so that when I make blind jokes, you'll chuckle to yourself instead of thinking I'm a callous oaf. To give you a sense of what I can see, imagine looking through a very, very foggy window twenty-four seven. Faces are usually blurry blobs, text on my computer has to be an inch high for me to read it, and glass revolving doors are the bane of my existence—but back to our main topic at hand.

I was never technically "overweight" but also never "skinny." I grew up with two very thin sisters and two very Albanian parents. This meant that I got a lot of comments: "You have such a beautiful body; if only your stomach wasn't so chubby." "You and your sisters just have *different* body types; you're much more like *me* and your grandfather . . . doughy." "Juna, I have a great idea! Your sister could be a model. . . . and you could be her agent!!!"

As we all know, every little girl grows up dreaming of being her sister's modeling agent.

Like any good immigrant child, I took these comments to heart and started doing crunches at age eleven during commercial breaks in my Saturday morning cartoons. I knew what "mountain climbers" were at age twelve. I knew that I could not eat two pieces of pizza at piano recital receptions. I knew to say no or "only a little" when offered cake at birthday parties. And I was acutely aware that my sisters could wear tank tops and shorts with no commentary from our parents, but when I did, it was as if I were making my debut as a porn star.

To be fair to my incredibly hardworking parents and beautiful, loving sisters, a lot of my attitudes about bodies, food, and exercise came from places far outside my family (and I'm not just saying that because I know they'll be reading this, hee-hee). Among my friends, we religiously talked about how we could lose weight. As prom approached, Akirah bought a waist trainer and wore it every day, telling me how it "must be working" because she could barely breathe, while chomping on her favorite lunchtime delicacy: two bags of Hot Fries. Julia, another friend, would update me weekly on what new comment her mom had casually made to her that week: one time it was "cottage cheese knees"; another it was "thunder thighs." Pretty creative stuff.

Even the adult women I knew—piano teachers, family friends, mentors—always seemed to be on diets and practically bursting to tell me about them. I remember thinking that rice cakes and dry salads must just be "acquired" tastes that came with maturity, the same as black coffee or alcohol. It was only when I started my own calorie counting that I realized these were common "diet" foods. It pains me to look back and realize that none of my friends were "overweight"—not that that would make the behaviors any more condonable. But just the thought that all these fifteen-year-old girls, regardless of body size and shape, were even at that age trying to be thinner is particularly sad to me after reviewing all the research on intentional weight loss.

All the women in my life talked constantly about how much they hated their bodies and how I would "understand when I was their age." Oh, what a future to look forward to: condemned to a life of salmon and sparkling water, and a body that stayed the same slightly squishy mass, hovering approximately fifteen pounds above an "acceptable" weight, no matter what you did. Desserts were out of the question, unless you spent the entire time making sure everyone knew how "bad" this was and how you "really shouldn't." Truly inspiring.

My parents were insistent on my losing weight, and I was insistent on never giving them the slightest inkling that I was listening to them. So I hid all of my "weight-loss" behaviors as much as possible. But the truth was that I was dying to order supplements online, weigh myself without hiding the scale, and openly eat leaves and drink gallons of water without being judged by anyone. And college was my chance.

When I got into college, everything went into overdrive. Firstly, I had fulfilled every immigrant parents' wildest dreams and gotten into not just any Ivy, but *the* Ivy: Harvard College. This did make me feel like the shit for approximately 2.5 seconds, until I realized the minute I set foot on campus that every single person there was infinitely more accomplished than I was. I lived in a dorm, where no one watched how much or how often I ate. No one saw what packages I received. No one monitored my exercise. I could do whatever the hell I wanted. And for me, that wasn't partying or drinking alcohol; it was crash dieting and obsessive exercising. As you can tell, I was *obviously* one of the cool kids.

Freshman year was an absolute blast; I made almost no friends, spent all my time alone practicing piano (I wanted to be a pianist once upon a time), and went hard core into operation Finally Be Hot for Once.

For breakfast: fruit.

Lunch: salads and Greek yogurt.

Afternoon snack: a run on the treadmill.

I was a rewards member at the GNC. I got my first bottle of garcinia cambogia weight-loss pills and quickly hid the bottles at the back of my underwear drawer so my roommates wouldn't see them. This would be the magic thing I had been waiting for. I had seen Dr. Oz rave about it in YouTube clips, and he's a doctor, right? This secret mission of losing weight gave me a purpose: it made me feel like there was something I was actively working on, which, once achieved, would solve all my other problems along with it. It was certainly easier than facing the fact that I was not really making friends the way I thought I would, and I had no idea what I wanted to major in.

At the end of freshman year, I looked amazing: I could see my abs, was constantly showered in compliments, received heartfelt apologies from my family and enemies for their past digressions, and had so many guys hitting me up that I created a separate calendar on my phone called "Date Nights." My sister even became *my* modeling agent!

Not.

I was the heaviest I had ever been and gained the "freshman twenty." Ever heard of it? It's when you gain the oh-so-familiar "freshman fifteen," but being the overachiever you are, you decide to go the extra five miles. "How did this happen?" you may be asking yourself. "Weren't you not eating? And exercising? And in general, not going out because of your mild yet potent social anxiety?" Yes, yes, you are very right, my wise and insightful reader, but I have not told you about my snack drawer.

The bottom drawer of my desk in my freshman dorm was gigantic. Almost a foot and a half tall. And every two weeks, my dear mother, bless her heart, would bring me gifts from the utopian wonderland of the Costco snack aisle. Single-serving peanut bags and granola bars, all in big bulk boxes that fit perfectly in the black chasm at the bottom of my desk. They were all "healthy" snacks, and the perfect size for a little pick-me-up mid-homework or between classes. The problem was, I never ate them "as a snack": I would starve all day long and run until those little numbers on the treadmill *finally* read "400 kcals," and then come home to work. By the time it was getting dark outside (at the ripe New England time of 2 P.M.), I was hungry.

I would be working on some economics or psych paper, clock ticking away, music thumping around me from down the hall, and I would reach down and eat one 300-calorie pack of peanuts. The second the fatty nut touched my tongue, it was like heaven. I was eating so little dietary fat at this point, even the slightest morsel would make my mouth water. I would blink and, next thing I knew, had eaten four packs, my lips puckered from the salt. Four packs . . . four packs . . . I would frantically do math and feel my face getting hot and my heart thumping as I realized I had eaten an entire day's worth of calories in the span of six minutes. Panic would set in. I would do more quick calculations: if I skipped breakfast and lunch the next day and ran extra on the treadmill for two days, I could still make everything work. Needless to say, it did not work. This was the beginning of my eating disorder (more on this in chapter 8).

I hesitate to share some of these details only for the fear that they might be used as proof that I am a proponent of weight stigma, eating disorders, and harmful health behaviors. However, at the time, I truly did feel like the only way to be happy was to be in what I used to think was an attractive, thin body. Trust me when I say I've worked on this almost every day of my life since then, but I am by no means perfect, even today. It would be easy to just omit these details from the book in order to earn some sort of false credibility, but I feel it's important for you to know that yes, at one point, weight loss *was* my life, and *all* I cared about.

That is why you will notice in this book we do not shy away from the topic of weight loss as well as overall health. I know that at eighteen I was desperate to understand, and because I didn't understand, I ate far too little, which inevitably led to overeating, and I exercised far too much, and I swallowed pills of unknown substances bought on the internet. Therefore, I want you, the reader, to have accurate, science-based information on how weight loss happens instead of someone telling you, "You shouldn't want this." I know this would have isolated me, made me feel embarrassed for wanting what I wanted, and only pushed me deeper into the arms of the bullshit-based "fitness" industry. Inherent at the heart of this book is that I trust you to make the best decisions for your body, so long as you are given all relevant information. Your body, your choice.

The remainder of my college days were basically the same story, and probably one you are familiar with: each New Year's, I reached a new high weight. I would stand on the scale, horrified, usually crying. I'd pull out all the stops: new diet, new exercise plan, new supplements. Four to five months later, I'd be down twenty pounds, my lowest weight each year. But I was at an emotional and physical breaking point. My binges would begin again. Four days of the week were spent barely eating, and three days were spent eating until it was painful. Despite going on runs twice a day on top of all this, the overeating was so severe that it would undo all the "hard work" I was putting in. Not only did I regain the lost weight every year, I reached a new high weight every winter. As we'll discuss in the chapter on dieting, this is neither an experience unique to me nor is it rare; in fact, it's actually common when people intentionally try to lose weight too quickly.

By the time I graduated college, I hadn't had a consistent period in years. My hormones were, as my endocrinologist put it, "those of a meno-pausal woman, or someone who is being starved." And I was legitimately concerned for my actual health, not just about looking good in a bikini.

Was this my dramatic rock-bottom moment: in my endocrinologist's office, being told I was in danger of getting osteoporosis from my low estrogen levels—followed by a triumphant scene of me throwing away the scale and the box of small crop tops I had been saving for my debut as a skinny person?

Nope.

The change was infinitely slower, and with all the drama of actual peer-reviewed science. The first thing that changed: I started lifting weights. For my entire life, I wanted to be thinner, smaller, and take up less space in the world. I hated exercise; it was my punishment for eating, my way to undo food. So, when I started lifting, it may have started out with similar inten-tions (to look hot naked), but it soon turned into my lifesaver in an ocean of profound postgrad confusion. I went from being terrified of becoming too muscular or looking "manly" to using the gym almost like a daily injection of self-esteem and confidence. It was the first thing I found in life that didn't make me feel like I needed to lose weight to be better.

Lifting introduced me to the science-based nutrition and training com-munity, and I discovered something truly astonishing: my hours of having to decipher research papers in the library (which had, thus far, seemed ex-actly as useless as it sounds) *actually* helped me with something! I hope you were seated for that; I know the shock factor was a lot. If there was one thing I had learned in my bachelor's in cognitive neuroscience and evolu-tionary psychology (a.k.a. my glorified BA in psych), it was how to read and interpret scientific data. And to my delight, the research on nutrition and exercise was extensive and, for the most part, not contentious. This meant I didn't have to rely on an Instagram model or my hair stylist for "the right fitness advice" anymore. There were actual scientists providing actual information.

Finding the right experts and the right information took years. Looking up papers and googling terms took me only slightly less. Implementing what I've learned is still something I'm mastering, but I want this book to be the book I wish I'd had at eighteen before I started all the crazy diets and plans. I want it to communicate the basics of nutrition, exercise, fat loss, metabolism, and health—all the things that I thought were not well understood and largely out of my control. In fact, these things are understandable and very much in your control (OK, you at least have *some* control).

My greatest wishes are, first, to save you endless hours, dollars, and disappointments over the course of your health and fitness journeys; and, second, to make you a professional bullshit detector when it comes to weight-loss marketing and health marketing. There's a reference section in this book. Your brain may have just turned off at those words, but . . . it's there for a reason. We are in our bodies for *the rest of our lives,* and the amount of abuse we put them through because somebody on Instagram "said so" makes me cringe. Science isn't scary, it just plays hard to get. Every word and research paper is a Google search away, but I'll be trying to explain the science in this book in the most nonscience way possible.

Oh, guys, I almost forgot—I have a coauthor! Luckily for everyone involved, this book is *not* just written by me! Eddie's full name is "Edward M. Phillips, MD," which makes him sound very fancy . . . because he is— he's an associate professor at Harvard Medical School and a pioneer of the field of lifestyle medicine. Basically, the thinking behind lifestyle medicine goes as follows: 80 percent of the diseases that are killing us today can be prevented by changing our habits: nutrition, movement, stress, sleep, and so on. One would think this would be very liberating and empowering to hear, but as it turns out, changing these things is really hard, which is where lifestyle medicine comes in.

Now, I know what you're thinking: *Juna, how did you end up coauthoring a book with Dr. Edward M. Phillips?!* And (a) no need to be so shocked, I'm slightly offended; but (b) I've also been talking *way* too much, so I'm going to let him take over the story now.

When Juna Met Eddie

The story of meeting Juna begins in 2010, when I arranged for the US surgeon general, Regina Benjamin, MD, to speak at my lifestyle-medicine course at Harvard Medical School. We reached out to local media, and Carey Goldberg, a health reporter from WBUR, came to cover the story. After chatting with Carey for a couple of minutes at the event, we determined that we graduated in the same class at Yale. Over the next few years Carey would periodically call me (on a slow news day in the health world) to ask me some version of the question, "Why should I exercise today?" Not only was she getting an update on the latest science on the myriad benefits of exercise, but, as it turns out, Carey was also getting inspiration to get herself moving. This continued for years, until about 2016, when I got a different call from Carey: "Do you know what a podcast is?" Uh . . . no, no I did not.

The Magic Pill started off as an extension of an idea I had been practicing for a while, namely prescribing exercise as medicine. Exercise has so many benefits that if any single pill had even a fraction of the results exercise has been consistently shown to have, it would be hailed as a miracle drug that should be prescribed to everyone. The idea of *The Magic Pill* podcast was simple: Carey and I would talk for around five minutes about why you should exercise. Listeners would get one of these episodes every day in their email inboxes and, over the course of twenty-one days, build the habit of loving exercise. I had previously coauthored a book guiding clinicians on why and how to prescribe exercise to their patients as if it were a medicine. The bigger goal was for this podcast, in its digestible and light audio bites, to also be prescribed to patients to hopefully help them dislike exercise *just a little less* than they did.

The lead-up to and release of the podcast was intoxicating because I got to hear my voice on the airwaves of our local Boston NPR news station. "This is just the beginning" was a phrase tossed around by friends and colleagues at the time, and I have to admit: I was excited. *I would be like the next Bob Oaks,* I thought, WBUR's iconic *Morning Edition* host. *Might as well start printing headshots and writing acknowledgment speeches.*

The launch was thrilling, and we received thanks and acknowledgment for inspiring increased exercise in listeners. *The Magic Pill* even won a prestigious regional Edward R. Murrow Award for Excellence in Innovation. But afterward, slightly to my surprise, everything remained completely normal. I put on my tie, went into the hospital, and saw patients as if nothing had happened. Again, Carey would occasionally call me up, and I would relay the day's findings about physical activity and then get back to patients, paperwork, and prescriptions. Until 2018 . . . when I got *another* call.

"Are you interested in doing another podcast?" I'm happy to report that this time, I knew what a podcast was.

My understanding of what would later become *Food, We Need to Talk* was that it was going to be a podcast hosted by Carey and me—a *Magic Pill, Season 2* in a sense. Carey mentioned there was someone that she wanted me to meet, a young woman, whom I thought might potentially be a third host of some kind. Before I came into the station to meet the young woman (who turned out to be Juna), Carey sent me a podcast that Juna had made for a competition. The podcast featured Juna interviewing her college best friends about their attitudes toward blind people, and I remember hearing it, getting home, and immediately telling my family, "You have to listen to this, it's going to make your life better."

What instantly struck me in that ten-minute podcast, and then later in our first meeting, was Juna's incredible ability to engage with and relate to whomever she was talking to. It was almost like she was saying, "I'm going to connect with you so quickly, and make you laugh so often, that you won't even have a chance to make a preconceived judgment about my vision." I couldn't tell if this was a survival mechanism of growing up legally blind in a world of sighted people constantly imposing their limited views upon her or if it was just how Juna was, regardless, but her personality was delightfully disarming.

When I arrived at WBUR, Carey had ordered us tempeh bowls from a local vegan spot. What became clear in our initial meeting was that this was not meant to be Carey and me doing a podcast and Juna tagging along. The podcast was appropriately centered around Juna's story: her years of navigating body image, nutrition, exercise, and other facets of health that all adolescents grow up negotiating. While the podcast would arch with Juna's story, relaying both her experience and the science that explained it, Carey felt that the story could be best told with a second voice, a person providing a different but still additive perspective.

Two things were immediately clear; Juna and I could not be more different in many respects: age, gender, our knowledge of pop culture (e.g., my not knowing what a podcast was), but we both had a passion and interest for very similar topics—what to eat, how to move, how to improve quality of life (although from seemingly different motivations). Juna also happened to be, almost to the month, the same age as my middle daughter. And so, either because we revert to what we know best, or because it just seemed natural, I found myself feeling not only like "the doctor" on the show but also, in a way, like a quasi father figure. *I can be a doctor on a podcast,* I thought to myself. *I do that all day. Plus, I've been a father for twenty-five-plus years.* I envisioned my role as "Dr. Eddie," guiding and instructing an informed but challenging patient. What I found was a quick friend and confidant, a colleague that brought a wealth of knowledge, exuberance, and a quick wit.

We routinely scheduled our recording time for late afternoons in the time and space between my roles as a physician at the hospital and as a dad and husband at home. The studio sessions were joyously stressful. The stress came from trying to sound cogent, upbeat, and like we belonged on NPR. The joy came from the ability to take the time to delve more deeply into Juna's motivations and behaviors than I can with my patients (whom I see for relatively short visits). I was able to dance on the third rail of emotions, weight, and body image without the fear of getting burned, as I was likely to do in broaching the same subjects with my patients or even my kids. There was a certain honesty and coherence that Juna and I could both bring to our conversations without the twenty years of emotional baggage that often crowded the conversations that I had with my daughter, who had had her own struggles with body image and an eating disorder (see chapter 9).

As we put in hour after hour in the studio, I learned that Juna is intensely curious and driven to learn all that she can about herself and whatever topic we were exploring in the podcast. I would reach out to the world's experts on food and nutrition, but it was Juna who wrote the scripts, conducted the interviews, researched the literature, and pulled together the podcast. Put differently, Juna deeply impresses me. I'm lucky to benefit from her curiosity and be the butt of her jokes. She makes long hours at the studio fly by and offers a fresh perspective on things I've spent years researching and teaching. She's a different kind of expert, the kind we need more of.

Food, We Need to Talk was a great success, reaching more than two million downloads, and the thing that people responded to most was Juna's and my relationship on and off the mics. What I found so exciting about the podcast was its reach. While in my practice, I could see thousands of patients over the course of my career, chatting with them in twenty-minute bursts once or twice a year. Here, I could reach tens of thousands in a single episode with a message I wholeheartedly believed in. So when Juna and I were approached with the opportunity to write this book, it seemed like the natural and befitting extension of our original mission.

Throughout the book, you will get to hear from both Juna and me on a range of topics, from metabolism, dieting, weight loss, and nutrition to exercise, sleep, stress, and so on. This book isn't *just* a literature review of the relevant research in any given field; it's also a look at each subject through two different perspectives: Juna's and mine. The lens through which we view the world lends a different experience of the exact same forces for every person on this planet. While Juna has navigated these issues as a young woman growing up in the late 1990s and early 2000s, I experienced it growing up in the 1960s and 1970s, and then through my roles as a father, husband, and physician. We hope that you will see your own experience through one of these lenses, or maybe multiple lenses, and that our perspectives bring as much to the conversation as the papers and citations do.

1

From the Victorians to the Kardashians

A Brief History of Dieting

Why History Matters

In my deeply ingrained view that the world obviously revolves around me and me alone, I don't often stop to think about the context in which I grew up, or the invisible forces that may have played a role in my preoccupation and dissatisfaction with my body. But unfortunately, it has been broken to me that, yes, a context exists outside of my hastily typed out New Year's resolutions, and a history exists behind that context, and it all relates, no matter how distant or irrelevant it may seem. It all relates.

On the one hand, you may be thinking, *Why does the history of dieting matter?* But it does matter, an awful lot. When I was growing up, being stick thin was the look that everyone was going for. Jeans were low-rise (shudder) and no one wanted a butt or curves. But today, "slim-thick" is all the rage. Although this still perpetuates largely unattainable beauty standards of having a tiny waist with massive boobs, butt, and curvy thighs, I do wonder whether I would have felt differently about my body had I been born even a decade later. "Slim-thick" is still, for most, unreachable, but for some reason, "heroin chic" seemed even more drastically distant.

Anyway, history was my least favorite subject in school, so when I thought about including a "History of Dieting" section in this book, my initial response was "meh." But, OK, fine, I stand corrected: this stuff *is,* in fact, important. Plus, Eddie is apparently super into history and has said that he finds it comforting to know that we don't exist in a vacuum. Like whatever problem we think is *so* important right now, chances are, people have been dealing with that problem for decades, if not centuries. In other words, "No, Juna, you are not the only person on this planet to struggle with body image and weight, so get over yourself."

Lean = Broke

The narrative that we focus on a lot today is how body-image issues and dieting are largely "women's" issues, or that they predominantly affect those who present as female in the world. Before the dudes reading this get their panties in a twist, no, this does not mean that men don't also face unrealistic body standards—we all do—but I think we can agree: society is harder, on average, on women and their bodies than on men. This has led feminist authors, such as Naomi Wolf, to call dieting "the most potent political sedative in women's history" and "something serious being done to us to safeguard political power."[1] Interpretations like this make it especially interesting that dieting started out as a *male* thing. (Bet you didn't see that one coming!)

Oh yes, back in the 1800s, when the first-ever dieting book was published, it was actually aimed exclusively at men. And you know why? Because in ye old days of horse-drawn buggies, it was actually considered *hot* for women to be plump. It is information like this that makes ye old Juna wonder, *Shouldeth I have been borneth two hundred years ago?*

Before the 1800s, thinness was associated with weakness, frailty, poverty, and a susceptibility to disease. If you're poor, you don't have enough food. You have a six-pack? OK, I guess you're broke as hell, then. On the other hand, fat was associated with wealth, health, longevity, and beauty. In the early 1800s, a "stout" man was considered respectable and influential. A plump woman was considered feminine, beautiful, and desirable. To be portly was to look "prosperous." However, while one could perhaps never be too prosperous, there *were* perceived limits of corpulence.

Men, Weight, and the Fitness Craze

As early as the 1700s in modern England, "excessive fatness," particularly in men, was seen as a conspicuous sign of overindulgence and associated with "moral corruption." Overeating was warned against in advice manuals for men as being unmanly and "un-English." By the mid-nineteenth century, there was an acceleration of negative associations with overfatness.

Partially in response to the increasing democratization of wealth and political participation in America, and partially due to increasingly sedentary professions, men in the mid-1800s were suddenly very concerned with, well . . . being more "manly." Translation: Men felt threatened, so they felt the need to go more man mode. Why do I feel like this is *still* the exact same way men respond today to their status being even slightly threatened? Has *anything* changed in the past two hundred years besides the buggies?!

Because there was a growing fear that men were becoming too soft and effeminate, there was somewhat of a fitness craze for men, who all of a sudden wanted to be muscular, lean, strong, and more "masculine"—more like the bodies seen in statues of Greek gods. PS: A "fitness craze" is more my interpretation of the new "fitness culture" that was dominant in this period than a scholarly observation. I just find it very amusing to imagine dudes on horseback strapping on weight vests and doing push-ups. Anyway, this is obviously not what they were actually doing, but sometimes I need to make mental images like this to keep myself entertained.

The First Diet Book

And so we come to our first-ever diet book, enticingly called *A Letter on Corpulence*, published in 1863 by William Banting, a British undertaker. This may make Banting the first person to officially lose a ton of weight and then insist on never shutting up about it by publishing more and more detailed versions of his original pamphlet. Basically, Banting advocated for a low-carb, low-sweets, meat-heavy diet, which begs the question, has diet advice really changed at all in the past 150 or so years? (Except . . . interestingly enough, he also advocated for tons of liquor, presumably because of how hard it was to go number two with all that meat and lack of fiber; these are not my words, they're the words of historical scholars.)[2]

The letter defined obesity as "illness" and also put the ability to undo obesity entirely at the control of the individual. Banting saw his own weight loss as "miraculous," extolling how his body weight had severely impaired his abilities and caused him to be ridiculed. In the letter, he stated, "With thinness comes happiness," spoken like a true Instagram fit-fluencer of today.

Banting's recommendations for activities like rowing, smoking, and alcohol consumption were strictly *nonfemale* activities. Furthermore, the testimonials that Banting added to future editions came exclusively from men. Dieting was now seen as an activity for the "striving middle class," a positive sign of ambition, not necessarily for the rich, but also no longer associated with being broke and hungry. It was now a way of showing the self-restraint and mental fitness of the middle-class white man, even in the face of available excess. As we all know, only the middle-class white man has self-restraint and ambition (cough, cough).

From the mid- to late 1800s, as pressures on the obese man were increasing (overweight men were increasingly being used to portray greed and corruption in political cartoons, and diet advice for men was becoming common in newspapers), the ideal female body was actually at its "softest." Women that were looked up to as beauty and sex icons were praised for having "rounded shoulders" and "ample chests" (ew).[3] Being in a bigger body was not only a sign of fertility and health, it was sexy.

I'm gonna harp on this for a second because, in light of today's context, this is *so* interesting: the protruding belly in women was seen as a sign of fertility (I must be very, *very* fertile!). Untrained muscles were an attractive feature, seen as a sign that the lady was loaded, she didn't need to work or (shudder) do physical labor. One author in *Harper's Weekly*, a popular American magazine, wrote, "Leanness in the fair sex is a dreadful evil."[4] "Meagerness" was seen as a serious health and beauty concern, and women would write in to magazines for advice for how to gain weight. Women in college would send letters home to their parents proudly reporting how much weight they'd gained. Being too thin was seen as a sign of engaging in clearly exclusively "masculine" behaviors, such as too much studying or physical activity.

Ladies Start to Diet

I'm about to disappoint all of us ladies who are mad at the money and time we've wasted on dieting and looking for people to blame for it. . . . It wasn't men, doctors, or even fashion designers that first gave women diet and exercise recommendations, but rather early women's rights activists. In 1886, Anna Kingsford, a women's rights advocate and the second *ever* woman to get a medical degree in England (damn girl, get it), published the first-ever (brief) diet program for women. Interestingly, it sounds a lot like TikTok's "that girl" trope of today, advocating not only a healthy diet and exercise but also waking up early and a generally active lifestyle. Rachel Brook Gleason, one of the first American female doctors, recommended women gain more "muscular fiber" and railed against corsets as being bad for health and strength. Just like dieting was associated with self-control and self-mastery for men, dieting started off as a way for women to show they could exert the same level of control and ownership over their own bodies as men did. Women started to exercise, women's gyms started to open, colleges started to include physical education for women, and women's dress started to change. Goodbye corsets, you vices of death!

It's impossible to discuss dieting and body shape without also discussing race and class. The slender female body became associated not only with strength and self-restraint but also with being white and middle class. Plumpness was increasingly seen as a trait of the unkempt, uncontrollable body of the racial and ethnic "other." Body fat started to be associated with laziness, indulgence, a lack of education, and even vulgarity and pornography. For example, the female Black body was often portrayed as rotund and obese, leading to caricatures in popular culture such as "Mammy" or "Aunt Jemima." These depictions not only ignored the shameful treatment of Black people in America but also completely left the Black woman out of what popular culture had deemed as "beautiful" at the time. We still see the effects of this in the portrayal and body standards of women of color today.

Unlike today, women's dieting in the early twentieth century had some conflicting connotations. On the one hand, the slender figure was being embraced more and more by the fashion and beauty industries. Women were warned that not being a good homemaker could lead to being overweight. While dieting was increasingly starting to turn into a way of controlling women's bodies (for example, through standardized clothing sizes), its origins in being "empowering" were still commonly used to sell it to female consumers. Something along the lines of "Girl, you're just as strong and in control as the men; you can navigate your way around a dinner party and not eat a thousand cookies. You're in charge, dammit!"

At the exact same time, though, thinness in women was seen as breaking from societal norms and expectations. For example, fat was still seen as feminine, plumpness as a sign of motherhood and sexual availability. Dieting books warned that dieting could threaten fertility (apparently the only life's purpose for a woman except cooking and cleaning). A diet manual for 1923 noted that plump girls were more likely to marry than thin girls and stated, "Put fat and flesh under your skin, willowy young lady! Don't try to look like the lean and lank caricatures in the awful fashion plates. Men laugh or shudder at those. They never laugh at a plump girl, even if she overdoes it a little."[5] A consistent through line, though: dieting and thinness were for whites and the middle class; having control of your weight and your body shape was, apparently, a sign of refinement.

POPULAR DIETS OF THE PAST

Here are some unique and innovative ways that people have used throughout the past century to try to "snatch that waist"—or whatever they called it back then. Of course, by "unique and innovative," I mean extremely un-unique and un-innovative, because it's almost exactly the same BS as today. Some things never change.

1. The Banting Diet: Originally created by William Banting, this is

your basic low-carb, high-protein diet. It included limitations on bread, potatoes, milk, butter, and eggs, but not alcohol! Woo!

2. The Hay Diet: Concocted by a physician named William Hay in the 1920s, this popular diet basically broke foods up into three categories (alkaline, acidic, and neutral) and then put rules on what foods could be combined.

3. The Chewing Diet: Popularized by Horace Fletcher in the early 1900s, this diet basically consists of chewing your food until it is liquid, which will apparently stop you from overeating and result in fat loss (along with a very muscular jaw!).

4. Eighteen-Day Diet: This diet can be traced all the way back to 1929 but later became known as the "Grapefruit Diet." It consisted of eating some combination of grapefruit, orange, toast, and vegetables for eighteen days. Later versions of it also included simply eating a grapefruit before each meal.

5. The Master Cleanse Diet: Drink lemon juice, maple syrup, and cayenne pepper, and watch the fat melt away. This ingenious torture system was created in the 1940s and serves as scientific proof of the concept that eating barely anything causes weight loss. Truly groundbreaking stuff.

6. The Apple Cider Vinegar Diet: Originally from the 1950s, this diet calls for drinking a concoction of apple cider vinegar and honey. Shockingly, it's still popular even today (as seen on TikTok), despite having very little scientific backing.

7. The Cabbage Soup Diet: Popularized in the 1960s, this diet consisted of eating nothing but a soup made of cabbage, onions, and other vegetables for a period of seven days. Yum.

8. The Scarsdale Diet: Originating in the 1970s, this was a high-protein, high-fat diet that limited your calories to around one thousand per day. The diet was meant to last around seven to fourteen days

because . . . well, who could eat only 1,000 calories a day for any longer than that?

9. The F-Plan Diet: Popularized in the 1980s, this diet restricts calories while also recommending extremely high amounts of fiber. (Does the "F" stand for "fiber" or "flatulence"? Only time will tell!)

10. The Atkins Diet: All the rage in the late 1990s and early 2000s, this is your stereotypical high-protein, high-fat diet. It promotes eating lots of meat, cheese, butter, and eggs while limiting cereals, breads, sugar, and so on.

Body Standards and Their Impact

Throughout the twentieth century, the "ideal" female form fluctuated with whatever was in vogue at the time, tracking alarmingly close to rates of eating disorders. For example, the bust-to-waist ratios of women featured in magazines like *Vogue* and *Ladies' Home Journal* decreased about 60 percent from 1901 to 1925.[6] Coincidentally (or not), prevalence of disordered eating was at one of its highest rates in the 1920s, the era of the slender, almost boyish-bodied flapper.[7]

The bust-to-waist ratios increased (oh-so generously) by about one-third up until the late 1940s. This is when we started to see the fuller figures of icons like Marilyn Monroe becoming popular and being featured in the first issue of *Playboy* in 1953. (Thank God!!! What would our history be without that national treasure, I ask you?) The reign of the fuller-figured queens did not last too long, though, because by the late 1960s, the ratio had once again dropped to its previous low from the 1920s. At least we had a brief stint where exercising became cool in the 1980s, but then it was a prompt plunge into the "heroin-chic" physiques of the 1990s.

The bust-to-waist-ratio high in 1901 was never again even approached for the remainder of the twentieth century. In fact, the ratio stayed at below a 1.3 consistently from the 1960s to close to the end of the twentieth century, the longest period of time that it stayed so low. At the same time that the thin ideal was pervading magazines, television, and advertisements, obesity in America and across the world was increasing, and so was the public messaging warning against it.[8] A dual campaign was being waged on people's body images: you *should* look thin like these models, and *don't* look fat like these obese people.

The Rise of "Slim-Thick"

However, the 2000s has seen the rise of a new body ideal, often termed "slim-thick," best displayed by our bestie Kim Kardashian.[9] This body shape has the flat stomach and thin waist of the thin ideal, but with the bigger butt and thighs traditionally seen in larger women. The slim-thick ideal seems to have been popular in Latino and Black populations before it reached wider adoption among white audiences. The 2000s has also seen an increase in preference for muscularity, coinciding with the "fitspiration," or "fitspo," movements seen on social-media apps like Instagram and TikTok. Other trends have included the glorification of the "thigh gap" (having space between your thighs), the demonization of "hip dips" (the naturally occurring dips that some people have on their upper legs), and the explosion of procedures like the Brazilian butt lift (a procedure where fat is removed from one part of the body, often the stomach, and injected into the buttocks region).

It's not really that shocking that exposure to media affects our notion of the ideal body, but what is quite disheartening is how profound the implications of seemingly arbitrary shifts can be.

Magazine editors decide super skinny is in, and rates of anorexia nervosa shoot up. Certain celebrities become extremely popular, and the demand for butt-implant surgeries skyrocket. Although some change may be happening as companies try to incorporate more body diversity in their campaigns, the prospects still look grim. Some preliminary research suggests that slim-thick imagery may be even more damaging to women's body image, particularly for women who strive to have a "perfect appearance," than the traditional thin ideal.[10]

The bright side is, as detrimental as social media can be in promoting unrealistic body ideals, it is also a catalyst for the democratization of the imagery we consume. It's no longer just big companies in control of the people we see and look up to; it's us. We have a lot of power when we choose whom to follow, what to like, whom to reshare, and even what to post. When I first started posting on social media, I was terrified and embarrassed. Who would follow me or listen to me when I looked nothing like anybody else online? Why should anybody take me seriously? But as time has gone on, I've seen more and more people with different body types, different journeys, and different goals all sharing their love for health and fitness. And it became pretty clear as soon as I started posting that nobody seemed to really care that I wasn't a size 2, because most people aren't a size 2. I hope social media, and this book, are part of a new era of getting your health and fitness advice from science-based, well-researched experts and sources (ahem, ahem), not from models who don't look anything like the average person and likely never have. (Side note: I am definitely not saying I am in any way, shape, or form an expert, but . . . I am extraordinarily average looking. Does this make me extraordinarily knowledgeable?!)

So, with that in mind, let's start talking about my favorite part—the science!

The Takeaways

- The "ideal" body and what people will do to attain it have fluctuated throughout history.

- Before the 1800s, thinness was associated with poverty and being ill, while excess weight was associated with health, wealth, and status.

- By the mid-1800s, fatness was increasingly being associated with femininity and beauty for women but had started to be associated with laziness and corruption for men. Thus, the first diet book was published in 1863 and was directed at men.

- In the mid- to late 1800s, dieting was a way for men to display their masculinity and self-restraint. Curviness was still seen as the ideal for women.

- Dieting was first championed by *other women* in the late nineteenth century as a way of empowering them to be as "in control" and "self-restrained" as men. At first, it was frowned upon to see women dieting because it was thought to interfere with fertility and be "unfeminine."

- As dieting became more and more of an aesthetic pursuit rather than a political one, the "ideal" female body also shifted from being plump to being thinner and more athletic.

- By the early twentieth century, thinness was associated with whiteness and being middle class, while excess weight was associated with the racial and ethnic "other."

- Body ideals have continued to fluctuate throughout the past century, from the boyish flapper aesthetic in the 1920s to the "slim-thick" aesthetic of the past decade. The shifting body ideals tend to correlate with rates of eating disorders and the popularity of cosmetic surgeries.

2

Metabolism and the Physiology of Weight Loss

"It's My Metabolism"

Metabolism is, for many of us, the perfect way to explain the unexplainable. It has been the scapegoat for years, and often for decades, of frustration concerning the opaque and often confusing tendencies of our bodies.

Your sister can eat whatever she wants and doesn't gain weight, while you can feel your thighs expanding from so much as looking at a donut? She must have a faster metabolism. The fact that your clothes seem to be getting tighter even though you're "going to indoor cycling *all the freaking time!*"—it must be your slowing metabolism. Men, who subsist on a diet entirely made up of pasta, breakfast cereal, and G FUEL (is this just the men my age?), don't give a damn but never seem to gain weight. It must be their metabolism. It's perfect! Because we can't control it, because we are just "dealing with the cards we were dealt," metabolism almost serves as an exoneration. It is at once something to lament, and also a catchall that explains all manner of phenomena.

Right? *Right???*

Growing up, I was always under the impression that there was something genetically different about me versus my sisters. Picture this: You're slightly insecure about the fact that you're a tiny bit bigger than your two very skinny sisters. One of them is also very tall; lots of "You could be a model!" comments from relatives. Like the neurotic, comparison-driven type A you are, you take matters into your own hands and start to say no to cake at birthday parties or eat less at piano recitals. Meanwhile, this sister cannot let a bakery go by without going inside to try every single thing that is labeled "toffee" or "salted caramel." While you try to stick to two slices of pizza, she brags about how she's on slice number five. I ask you: *Is this legal?!* Is there a class of trauma called "growing up with a skinny sister" disorder? If not, can we make it a thing and have monthly GUWASS meetings? I think I'm on to something here . . .

I tried my best to eat less than my sister, never was as thin as my sister, and obviously never got the same comments as my sister. I can even remember my grandmother taking my aunt aside once, when she first came to America after not having seen any of us for more than a decade, and genuinely asking: "How can Juna just eat salads and still be . . . not thin?" My family's explanation? My sister had a fast metabolism. My mom would assure me, "You have much more of my body type." This is *definitely* what a fourteen-year-old wants to hear from her middle-aged mother. Even at a young age, this seemed entirely implausible to me simply because of how incredibly unfair it was. How is it legal that one person gets to eat more but stays thinner? There's just no way, and if there were, there would be riots in the streets.

As time went on, this little piece of indignant righteousness was quickly squashed out of me, as often happens through adolescence. It seemed like the forty-something-year-old women were right: there really seemed to be a certain point at which it was out of our control and we were doomed to have a squishy mass of ten to fifteen pounds stuck around our middles—and for some reason, I had been given this fate at age fourteen (truly ahead of the curve in every way).

Demystifying Metabolism

Metabolism, or "energy expenditure," is one of the most complex and elegant systems of the human body, and many of its mechanisms continue to confound the scientific community. But . . . it has been studied *a lot*, and our understanding today is light-years ahead of where it was even two decades ago. Just a warning: we'll be discussing the ins and outs of energy expenditure in detail in this chapter. Sometimes you may think:

Why is it important for me to know what this annoying acronym means?
Did I accidentally buy a biochemistry textbook?
I specifically dropped human physiology to avoid this very topic!!!

Let's put it this way: when I was able to understand this science at its fundamental level, I felt so much more hopeful about the autonomy I had over my own body. I want you to have that same sense of empowerment. Second, truly understanding how things work makes you more likely to act on what you know. I could just tell you that if you take in more energy than you expend, the excess energy gets stored as body fat. But I'm guessing you've already heard this a million times. And if you're anything like me, it hasn't really helped change anything. But if we go a little deeper so you *actually* understand what the heck is going on with your body and metabolism, you're less likely to be duped by the fake products and false claims that saturate our newsstands and social-media platforms. I'm just trying to save you some cash. If we invest a fraction of the time on understanding our bodies that we do on Netflix or school or TikTok, we'd have such a better chance of taking good care of this meat mobile we walk around in. What is that you say? You're totally convinced and can't wait to get started?! Great!!!

By the end of this chapter you'll know the answers to questions like: Do some people just have the "eat endless donuts and stay thin" gene (the technical term for it, of course)? Is my metabolism actually slowing down? Can I speed it up, and if so, how? *Where can I buy the tea to do so??* Is there free shipping? This and much more will soon be revealed.

What the Heck Is a Calorie, Anyway?

Right off the bat, I need to be upfront with you guys: we will be using the "C" word . . . a lot. And by the "C" word, of course, I'm talking about calories. The mention of calories has been known to induce an uncontrollable onset of sudden rage in some of us (oh, is this just me?), but it is crucial to our discussions for the rest of the book. So, first things first: What is a calorie?

For most of us, calories are just numbers that we see on the backs of packages, on our fitness-tracker app, on the treadmill screen, and so on. And now I need to share something embarrassing. Even though I've been using the word "calorie" since before high school, if you asked me to define it, I would just say, "Oh, you know, it's like, the energy . . . in food . . . or that we burn. . . . Oh, look! Is that Anne Hathaway?!"

A calorie is indeed a measure of energy, equivalent to 4.184 joules.[1] This likely means absolutely nothing to 99 percent of us (the last memory I have of high school physics was rolling marbles down a ramp). However, the "calorie" that is most often talked about today is actually technically called the "large calorie," or kilocalorie (kcal), and is equivalent to 1,000 calories.[2] This slightly confusing name switch is supposed to just make things easier for us: imagine a food package saying, "1 serving = 60,000 calories" versus "1 serving = 60 kcal." Definitely much simpler. From now on, when we say "calorie" in this book, we mean the colloquial "calorie," that is, the kilocalorie or Calorie (with a capital "C"). However, the definition you likely learned in high school biology is that a Calorie is the amount of energy needed to raise one kilogram of water by 1 degree Celsius.[3] Again, *What does this have to do with anything I care about?!*

At its most basic, the calorie is a measure of heat, but how does heat translate to an apple or a bowl of cereal? To illustrate this, I considered sharing here the story of the first animal calorimeter (calorie measurer, as it were) but then decided against it. Long story short, it involves a man named Antoine Lavoisier putting a guinea pig in a bucket of ice, insulated by another bucket of snow, and measuring the runoff from the ice melted by the guinea pig's body.[4] However, three paragraphs in, I found myself pondering, *What on God's green earth am I doing with my life???* (Also, side note: Don't worry about the guinea pig; it did not freeze to death, although it must've been very, very cold.)

Suffice it to say, Lavoisier's observation was that living animals had a lot of similarities with fire. Just like a flame, we take in oxygen, and then just like a flame, we produce carbon dioxide and heat. Therefore, he concluded, breathing is some sort of very low-grade combustion. But where does this energy that we are apparently producing (vis-à-vis ice melted by guinea pig) come from?

The First Law of Thermodynamics

As you may have deduced by now, we get the energy that powers our bodies from food. The number of calories "in a food" is the energy stored in the chemical bonds in that food. As our body breaks down the molecules in that food, the energy is either used for various tasks or stored for later usage. If you think of a piece of food as the log on a fire, digestion is the equivalent of breaking that log into smaller wood chips that are easier to burn. And then the same process that happens when a wood chip bursts into flame is what is happening at a cellular level as our cells absorb the molecules from the food item to produce energy. Pretty freaking cool, right?

Something you will come across a lot when reading about the principles of nutrition, fat loss, metabolism, and so on is the first law of thermodynamics. This law states that energy cannot be destroyed or created, only transformed.[5] It is also often called the law of energy conservation. And while this may seem like a completely unnecessary and slightly philosophical tangent, it's actually a crucial governing principle when it comes to food intake, energy expenditure, and subsequent weight changes.

As we take in food, we transform the energy in the food's chemical bonds into other forms of energy. We use it to run, walk, keep our hearts beating, generate new cells, and heat our bodies, among a million other things. There's no magic that turns food into fuel. The energy in the food does not "disappear" once you eat it. Your body doesn't spontaneously "create" energy when you are taking a spin class. Instead, there is a constant transformation of energy happening from the energy stored in the food to the energy your body can use. The overall amount of energy in the system is always conserved, but the form the energy takes is always changing (hence, "law of energy conservation").

There are two crucial portions to the energy-balance equation: the "energy in" part, that is, the food (more on this in chapter 5); and the "energy out" part, or your "metabolism," as we colloquially call it. That's what this chapter is about.

The rules of energy conservation are a lot like the rules of finance (which honestly explains why I simultaneously have no savings *and* can't seem to portion-control Peanut M&M's). If you are spending exactly as much energy—a.k.a. as many calories—as you are eating, you are eating at your caloric maintenance. This is the number of calories you need to maintain your body weight and fulfill your energy needs. There is no excess, there is no deficit, and your weight remains about the same. In terms of finance, imagine you get paid a certain amount of money each month, and you spend exactly that amount of money; you aren't having to dip into your emergency fund, but you also aren't getting to save any extra. Your income is exactly the same as your expenditures.

If you are eating *more calories* than your body needs, you are in a "caloric surplus," and as is stated in the first law of thermodynamics, you can't just destroy that excess energy. Instead, your body stores the excess in two forms: glycogen in your liver and muscles, and lipids in your fat tissue (a.k.a. body fat). The financial equivalent of this would be all my money-savvy peeps who spend less than they get paid and can deposit into a savings account every pay period. Fat stores are your body's savings account.

If you are eating less than you need, you are in a "calorie deficit," and your body will tap into its energy reserves, its fat cells, to release some of that stored energy. Again, this would be if you're like me and don't look at your credit card statement until the dreaded day you gotta pay it, and you have to dip into your "emergency money" because you just "needed" to have a mango-wood desk from Urban Outfitters. Mhm.

The main point here is that whatever energy you are taking in, *something* has to happen to that energy. It cannot disappear, no matter what juice, special herb, type of vinegar, or pill you take. And if there is a product out there that does indeed violate the laws of physics . . . please let me know ASAP so I can invest.

TDEE: A Fancy Way to Say "Metabolism"

The first thing we need to get out of the way is that when scientists talk about metabolism, they don't call it "metabolism." Instead, they call it total daily energy expenditure (TDEE) or sometimes just energy expenditure. This is partially to keep the peasants like me out of their hair, and partially to clarify exactly what we're talking about. For example, "metabolism" can be applied to carbohydrate metabolism (how your body breaks down and uses carbs), alcohol metabolism, or protein metabolism, and that's just to name a few. You see, "metabolism" technically refers to all the biochemical processes that occur within a cell or organism to sustain life. However, when *we* talk about metabolism in our daily lives, we usually mean how many calories our bodies are using, our energy needs. As you can see, this could lead to confusion, so voilà, TDEE comes to the rescue.

As often happens in science, the acronym TDEE basically defines itself (not a lotta creativity here, people; gotta keep things simple and sharp): total daily energy expenditure is the calories (total energy) that your body burns (expends) in a day (daily) in order to complete all the tasks associated with living.[6,7] So from now on, when I say "TDEE," I want your brain to translate it to "metabolism."

Breaking Down Energy Expenditure

Your TDEE can be broken up into three sections: basal metabolic rate (BMR), thermic effect of food (TEF), and activity thermogenesis. If you haven't closed the book at this point, (a) thank you, and (b) I swear these are complicated ways of saying things that are simple to understand.

BMR is your basal metabolic rate. For most people, BMR makes up the majority of their TDEE.[8,9] It's kind of your base burn rate, the minimum amount of energy your body needs just to do the very difficult task of keeping you alive. If we were to measure your BMR, here's how we would do it. We would have you lie down for twenty-four hours. No moving, no eating, no bathroom breaks, no Instagram scrolling. The calories burned in those twenty-four hours would be your basal metabolic rate. This energy is used for things like keeping your blood pumping, your lungs breathing, your hair growing, your skin cells regenerating, and so forth. It's just the minimum payment on your body's energy credit card—the absolute minimum calories you burn by being alive.

About 60–80 percent of BMR can be predicted by your lean body mass, namely all nonfat tissues in your body: your bones, tendons, and, most importantly, your muscle mass.[10] We'll come back to this fact later because it functions as one of your greatest metabolic control levers. Long story short, muscle is a "high maintenance" tissue compared to fat tissue. Because muscle is calorically expensive (uses so much energy) and makes up 40–50 percent of body weight in normal-weight individuals, lean body mass is the most accurate predictor of your basal metabolic rate.[11] This is largely why bigger humans will often have a higher daily energy expenditure: those people simply have more mass—organs, skeletal muscle, bones, and so on—to keep up, which needs calories.

The thermic effect of food (TEF) is the energy you spend digesting your iced lattes and smoothie bowls.[12,13,14] You know that whole process we talked about, of breaking wood into wood chips and turning the molecules in food into energy, blah, blah, blah? Well, that in itself takes energy. In most people, TEF takes up about 10 percent of our total daily energy expenditure, and this rate does not vary much between people. In general, there's not much we can do to alter our TEF, other than maybe increase protein intake, because protein, as opposed to fat and carbohydrates, takes more energy to break down.[15] However, in the grand scheme of things, TEF makes up such a small portion of the TDEE that it's not worth dwelling on too much.

Activity Thermogenesis

Now let's move on to activity thermogenesis, or the energy you expend through movement. This section of your energy expenditure can be broken up into two subcategories: exercise and nonexercise. The first, exercise activity thermogenesis (EAT) is rather ironically named, proving that scientists do indeed have a sense of humor, since it has nothing to do with eating and very much to do with the opposite. EAT is the number of calories you burn while you are engaging in purposeful forms of exercise. ("Purposeful" is the key word here, as you'll see in the section coming up.)[16,17,18] Here is where I need everyone to buckle in and get a box of tissues ready. First, it is important to note that as of 2015, only about 23 percent of US adults met the federal guidelines for physical activity (150 minutes per week of moderate physical activity, or 75 minutes per week of vigorous physical activity and twice weekly resistance exercise).[19] That's not very good y'all; that's less than a fourth . . . of the *entire population*. And these guidelines aren't asking for much: 75 minutes a week of vigorous exercise is like . . . 11 minutes a day.

But back to the matter at hand: Do you know what this means for exercise's contribution to TDEE? For the vast majority of people who are physically inactive, their EAT contributes zip, zero, nada to their total daily energy expenditure.[20,21,22]

I hear what some of you are screaming at this book right now: "No, no, girl! I go to yoga three times a week!" or "Susie and I go to spin on Sundays!" Even for individuals who do engage in purposeful physical activity, on average, research suggests that exercise contributes about 100 calories a day to TDEE. Keep in mind, this calculation factors in rest days as well, taking an overall average of your entire week. So even for those that do exercise regularly, it still only makes up about 5–10 percent of their total energy expenditure. Again, not exactly thrilling news.[23,24,25]

If you'll excuse me, I need to make an obvious statement about exercise, because this figure is often misconstrued. Just because exercise isn't a huge calorie burner *does not* mean that it is a waste of time. Exercise is one of the most powerful tools we have for promoting optimal health and a healthy metabolism, as you'll see in the rest of this chapter. The benefits of exercise go far beyond its paltry calorie burn, and they include, just to name a few: reduced risk of all-cause mortality, improved cognitive function, decreased depression and anxiety, increased quality of life, and that's just the tip of the iceberg.[26] Even when it comes to weight loss, as we'll discuss in chapters 6 and 7, exercise appears to be crucial to resisting weight regain after a weight-loss phase.[27] And yet people want to fixate on the calories and discount everything else. Not on my watch, pal.

So here is a puzzle: If BMR is mostly about your body size and lean body mass, and if TEF and EAT are relatively small calorie burners and also pretty consistent between the majority of individuals, how on earth can it be true that individuals of a similar size can have metabolisms that vary up to 2,000 calories a day?[28] What is causing all this variation, and how do I get ahold of whatever those hot-metabolism people are on? Well, it's not a pill or a tea; it's the final, critical component of TDEE: nonexercise activity thermogenesis.

NEAT

Nonexercise activity thermogenesis (NEAT) is all the energy you expend doing everything that isn't purposeful exercise: washing the dishes, walking around, standing up, sitting down, waiting in line for your latte, shopping.[29] It turns out, depending on what you do for work, where you live, your age, and even your gender, we all have vastly different habits around movement—so much so that the most active among us compared to the least active burn almost three times the number of calories through NEAT.[30,31]

One of the biggest determinants of NEAT is a person's occupation.[32] This finding makes a lot of sense. Compare my occupation—which, thanks to Uber Eats and remote working, requires me to take approximately sixty-three steps a day (bathroom + trips to the fridge)—to my dad's or grandmother's. As a contractor, my dad, now in his mid-sixties, still spends all day carrying things, bending down, picking them up, hammering, sanding, and so on. My grandmother is absolutely unable to sit still. At any given moment, she is either mopping, washing dishes, cooking, or even sweeping the sidewalks. (If that doesn't scream "raised under communism," I don't know what does.) For many of us, our modern lifestyles require vastly lower activity levels than those of our ancestors, even one or two generations back. Indeed, in the United States today, one-third of all people are considered sedentary (<5,000 steps a day), while an additional 47 percent are considered low to somewhat active (5,000–9,999 steps a day).[33]

I suspect nothing here is too groundbreaking or shocking to you, but I know when I heard suggestions like "Park your car farther from the store" or "Take the stairs," I would kind of scoff: I'd so much rather be given a grueling workout plan called "Ninety Days to Your Dream Body" and go super hard than have to walk an extra forty feet. I mean, how much of a difference could those few extra yards really make? Well, the answer is: a big difference. Studies have shown, for example, that individuals with obesity sit on average 2.5 hours more than lean individuals.[34,35,36]

A natural explanation might be that this is because moving is more uncomfortable and more work in a bigger body; however, studies have shown that lean individuals maintain their movement patterns even after gaining weight, and individuals with obesity maintain their more sedentary patterns even after losing weight.[37] This isn't because people are "just being lazy," which is often how it's portrayed in popular media, but rather it seems like those who are predisposed to obesity may actually experience a lower biological drive to move.[38]

Perhaps one of the greatest advantages to incorporating more nonexercise movement into your day is that it doesn't require as much setup as formal exercise, and it can be easily incorporated into preexisting routines. Picture all that has to happen for you to go to the gym: you have to get a gym membership, get ready at home, drive the car, park the car, get out, swipe in, go to the locker room, stretch, do your workout, cool down, shower, fix your hair, drive back, and so on. How many of those minutes were actually spent exercising? And how many times would you do that in a week? Now average that out to the seven days in the week . . . and it makes sense why EAT, even for those who exercise, contributes very little to energy expenditure. Now, instead, picture converting two meetings a day to "walk and talk" meetings, or converting your desk to a treadmill desk. Just by virtue of the fact that you go to work every weekday, and taking meetings and working are already established routines, you are more likely to incorporate this increased movement into your life.[39]

This framework of energy expenditure was, for a long time, *the* framework. And something important to note is that it's additive: If you work out *more,* you will burn *more* calories. If you start running marathons every day, you will increase your metabolic rate by whatever number of calories you run during that marathon. But . . . it turns out, it may not be that simple.

Things Get Complicated in Tanzania

For a long time, the research on energy expenditure and obesity was focused on a fundamental problem with modern societies: we are not burning enough calories, especially considering all the easily available, calorie-dense, and very yummy foods around us. Looking at the components of energy expenditure, there isn't much we can do about BMR or TEF. And exercise, although a crucial piece of overall health, also seems to have a minimal impact on calorie burn when averaged out over time. So this led researchers to believe that NEAT must be the key: perhaps those with naturally higher metabolisms just move around a lot more. And perhaps creating movement-based interventions is what will help people increase their energy expenditure.[40]

But how much are we supposed to move? How many walks, fitness classes, and standing meetings are we supposed to take? After all, I can't spend all day pacing up and down my block; I got shit ta do. To answer this question, Herman Pontzer and his colleagues from Duke University set out for northern Tanzania to study the Hadza tribe.[41]

A little bit about the Hadza: The Hadza are a people who live a lot like our ancestors did—the men and women hunt and forage for food, walking on average four to seven miles a day (more than the average American walks in a week). Obesity and cardiovascular disease are practically unheard of among the Hadza, despite the fact that no one counts calories, follows a diet, or has a Planet Fitness membership.[42]

Pontzer and colleagues set out to measure the energy expenditure of the Hadza tribe using the "doubly labeled water method," the gold-standard, noninvasive way of measuring energy expenditure in free-living individuals.[43] This method involves measuring total carbon dioxide by giving people water enriched with oxygen and hydrogen isotopes and then taking urine samples. If this sounds like gibberish to you, (a) join the club, and (b) let's just move on with the knowledge that, dis shit works, yo. Of course, the researchers were expecting to find high expenditures; after all, these people are moving more in *a day* than we do in *a week*. Instead . . .

(Pause for dramatic effect.)

Hadza men and women burn almost exactly the same number of calories (on average) as those in modernized Western societies (about 2,500 kcal/day for men, and about 1,900 kcal/day for women).[44]

I know what you're thinking: *Clearly, dis shit does* not *work, and the doubly labeled water method must have been doubly wrong.* Thinking there must have been a mistake, the team went back to Tanzania, this time using a different method. They gave members of the tribe individual heart-rate monitors, calibrated the monitors to each person's individual heart rate and corresponding calorie burn, and conducted the experiment again. The results came out exactly the same.

Are you ripping out your hair and throwing your Apple watch across the room right now? Because I did (metaphorically, of course, because . . . yo girl ain't got money for a new Apple watch). Screw "parking farther away" and "taking the stairs," *I am an escalator queen from now on.*

In all seriousness, this finding is pretty disheartening for all of us who thought a standing desk and nightly walk would solve all our problems. How is it possible that these people move *up to 19,000 steps a day* but still have the same energy expenditure as my sedentary ass?

Metabolic Adaptation

It turns out, the human body is incredibly complex and pretty dang smart. For thousands of years, our body's main job has been to stop us from starving and consequently dying. So the physiological mechanisms that have been developed by our bodies are geared toward keeping us alive, not keeping our waistlines in check. One tool that the body uses to do this is called "metabolic adaptation" or "adaptive thermogenesis." As you can probably tell, the key word in both these terms is the "adapt" part. Although the process by which this adaptation occurs is not completely understood, what is clear is that your body is constantly making adjustments to both your metabolic rate and behaviors in response to the stream of information it receives about current energy availability.[45]

Your body continuously "adapts" to the experiences it is going through in an attempt to maintain homeostasis, which, as you may or may not recall from ninth grade bio, is just a fancier way of saying "balance" in whatever system we happen to be talking about. OK, fine, I may have simplified this definition a bit to save us time, but the real definition is so much more annoying: blah, blah, blah, self-regulating biological system . . . maintaining stability in response to changing external circumstances . . . optimizing survival, so on and so forth. I like my way much better.

Unfortunately, if any of us are trying to lose weight—or gain weight—we are by definition trying *not* to maintain balance. And where can you find a more extreme example of dramatic weight loss and its effects on metabolism than the contestants of one of America's most popular reality shows? Also, where do you find a science-y book that also talks about reality TV? I think I have officially fulfilled my life's mission. Thank you, and good night.

Learning from *The Biggest Loser*

If you had told me that hunter-gatherer tribes and reality-show contestants would both have something fundamental to teach us about human physiology, I might have actually considered taking physiology in college, because . . . what on earth are you talking about? But just stick with me for a second here.

Over a decade ago, the researcher Kevin Hall had the idea to study contestants of the popular reality show *The Biggest Loser* to see what happened when people underwent dramatic weight loss.[46] The show is notorious for putting people on extreme diets and insane exercise regimes with the objective of losing the most weight for a cash prize. It's also unfortunately notorious for poor long-term success rates in terms of permanent weight loss for most contestants, and even winners. In his study, Hall found that six years after the competition, participants had regained an average of two-thirds of the lost weight (more on this in chapter 3).[47] Many contestants had even ended up heavier than when they started.

The tendency for people to regain weight after a dramatic weight loss is not exactly a groundbreaking discovery. We've all heard the adage: "Losing weight is the easy part; keeping it off is hard." What was shocking however, was that Hall found the reduction in total energy expenditure after the weight loss was, on average, 500 calories *more* than you would expect, even accounting for the contestants' new lower weight.[48]

If someone undergoes a dramatic weight loss, we would 100 percent expect to see some reduction in their energy expenditure.[49] Remember when we talked about BMR and how it's primarily determined by lean body mass? Bigger people just burn more calories, so if you're becoming a smaller person, naturally you will need fewer calories.[50,51] But the *Biggest Loser* contestants were not only burning fewer than their previous, larger selves, they were burning 500 calories *fewer* than you would expect even a person of a new, smaller size to be burning.[52]

Said another way, imagine you had two people who both weighed two hundred pounds. One had undergone a drastic and rapid weight loss to get down to two hundred, the other had always been around two hundred. This research suggests that the one who had undergone the weight loss would have a substantially slower metabolism than the one who had always been that weight. As the contestants had gone through their grueling journey to extreme weight loss, something had happened; some adaptation had occurred physiologically to make their bodies more efficient at using calories, even after six years of maintaining or even gaining their weight back.

Your Body: A Tesla

"Becoming more efficient" is a good thing at work or at home, but in energy-expenditure terms, it means that your body is performing the same daily tasks of keeping you alive for fewer calories. It's like your body is going from a big gas-guzzling truck to a sleek Tesla (environmental implications aside). If there is a gas shortage (a.k.a. a famine), the Tesla is a way better option. But if gas were everywhere (a.k.a. plentiful, delicious, and calorie-dense foods), we would want a car that could burn as much gas as possible.

In biological terms, what does "becoming a Tesla" even mean, though? Well, there seem to be a couple of tools in the old evolutionary biology tool belt. One is behavioral: your body could spontaneously reduce movement throughout the day. It could be overt, like, you just don't feel like going on walks as much as you previously did; or it can be incredibly subtle: you start standing and fidgeting less than you previously did. This is a well-documented effect in response to calorie restriction, and we'll explore it more in the next chapter.[53,54] But you probably don't need a study to tell you this, because anyone who's been on a diet knows that if you're on week eight of eating leaves and rice cakes . . . the last thing you want to do is go for a walk.

However, your body seems to have more than just a behavioral shift at its disposal. After all, in both the Hadza tribe and *The Biggest Loser,* movement was not the difference. The Hadza people are closing a whole week's worth of Apple watch rings in one day, for God's sake. And the *Biggest Loser* contestants remained highly physically active (80 percent above their baselines), even six years after leaving the show.[55,56]

Based on earlier models of metabolism, you would think these people must have the highest metabolisms ever. Their cells must be running hotter than my heater in the dead of New England winters (PS: That's *hot*). The classic model of metabolism assumes an additive, linear relationship: as physical activity goes up, so does your metabolism.[57] After all, studies have shown that the more physical activity is increased, the more weight people lose.[58] And yet the Hadza had pretty much the same energy expenditures as the average American, and the *Biggest Loser* contestants had lower ones.[59,60] So how the flippin' heck can both of these things be true? Well, particularly in response to high amounts of physical activity, more and more evidence seems to be mounting for a phenomenon called energy compensation (or metabolic adaptation).[61,62]

The physiological responses that your body implements to compensate for high physical activity are much more subtle and much harder to study than the traditional additive model of energy expenditure would imply. But we're starting to get some ideas about what may be happening. It appears as though high amounts of exercise elicit a wide array of adaptations, including suppressing immunity and reproductive hormones, lowering inflammation, and decreasing the stress response, to name a few.[63,64,65] Ironically, it might be these exact same adaptations that make moderate exercise so freaking amazing for both our mental and physical health (more in chapters 6 and 7). However, the suppression of these physiological processes may also save your body a lot of energy (after all, these tasks cost calories), thereby lowering your BMR.[66]

The Constrained Total-Energy-Expenditure Model

Did you know that if a mouse doesn't have enough food to eat, it will reduce the size of its heart, kidneys, liver, and spleen but maintain the size of its brain and—no other way to say it—its balls? Who needs a normal-sized heart and kidneys when you have perfectly working reproductive organs, right? When it comes down to it, and resources are scarce, mouse biology seems to prioritize reproduction above all else, potentially because of a mouse's relatively short life span.[67]

While humans don't show the same prioritization when resources "become scarce"—which in modern times can be you starting an intense exercise regimen, going on a crash diet, or competing on a weight-loss reality show—what's clear is that *some* sort of prioritization does happen. In an attempt to compensate for the increased energy needs, or lower energy availability, the body stops allocating resources to the processes it deems "inessential" and prioritizes the things it thinks *are* essential.[68]

In humans for example, unlike in mice, one of the first things to go is reproductive hormones and function. Although these changes in physiological processes may be hard to study, we can see concrete examples of them pretty easily if we just look around. For example, elite female athletes will routinely lose their periods in response to the high volume of exercise they endure and low levels of body fat they maintain, even if they are eating enough food to fuel their physical activity.[69] Or you may have noticed, if you've ever trained for a super-high-intensity endurance event, for example, that not only are you tired and hungry, but you also have no libido.[70]

The constrained total-energy-expenditure model basically states that there is a certain range that your metabolism can hover in, and your body will downregulate nonessential processes in response to high amounts of physical activity to keep you within that range. While we see a similar effect with calorie restriction (just wait for the bombshell in chapter 3), it's not entirely understood if it's the exact same physiological compensations that are happening in response to both lowered calories and extreme amounts of physical activity.[71] Either way, though, the point is your energy expenditure, or your metabolism, does not just exist in a vacuum.

"Calories Don't Matter" and "Damaged Metabolisms"

The concept of energy balance can be extremely frustrating. You exercise for months and you feel like you're counting every calorie, and it's just not working. Or it works for a bit and then stops working. This leads to the natural conclusion, "Well, screw this, obviously calories don't matter. . . . This is all BS." Trust me, I get it, I've been there, and it's a tempting line of thinking when you feel like you're trying your hardest and seeing no results. But the oversimplification and misinformation that surround energy expenditure is a huge cause of this frustration.

What is often not considered is that "energy in" and "energy out" are not independent of each other. The amount of food you're eating (or not eating) may impact your energy expenditure. Heck, even subcomponents *within* energy expenditure affect other subcomponents of energy expenditure. Metabolism is complex, hard to measure, and dynamic. Its responsiveness is exactly the quality that would keep you from withering away in times of low food availability or high physical demand.

Think of your body as a good business owner. As costs for certain things go up (we start exercising a ton), it will start saving on other expenses to avoid "going bankrupt." Similarly, if revenue goes down (eating a lot less than we need for a long time), again, the body will find places to save. Experiencing this downregulation in metabolic rate does not mean you have a damaged metabolism or that your metabolism is broken. On the contrary, it's your body working exactly the way it was designed to work—becoming smart with how it's using its calories.

Is It Genetic?

One of the things that I was constantly told growing up was how my metabolism was "just genetic." My mom loved to say that I had "her stomach," which coincidentally was also my grandfather's stomach. Needless to say, this is not exactly what you want to hear when both your sisters have faint ab lines in the morning. But if you'll notice in both the additive model of energy expenditure and the constrained model, there is no component for "genetic influence." Does this mean that there is no genetic component to metabolism? Or, if there is, how much is genetic?

In the constrained energy-expenditure model, the genetic component comes in with how your body is deciding its target TDEE. How does your body decide what energy-expenditure budget to defend? Why are some people hypothetically constrained to 2,500 calories, whereas others seem to be constrained at 3,000, or more, calories a day? *And who do I gotta chat with to get a constraint bonus?*

We know that up to 80 percent of the variation in BMR can be accounted for by lean body mass, but that still leaves a portion that we're just not sure about, suggesting there is indeed some genetic component. Some explanation of the variability among people could be the proportion of their bodies that are taken up by energetically expensive organs, such as the liver, heart, and brain, versus energetically inexpensive organs, like the skin, fat tissue, and skeleton.[72]

Yet another component could be developmental. Picture two scenarios: a body that grows up always having adequate nutrition and being physically active, and a body that grows up in a relatively nutrient-poor environment. Evolutionarily speaking, you would expect that the body that grew up without always having enough food to eat might be a bit thriftier with its calorie expenditure.[73] It's similar to if a kid grew up super rich or relatively poor. . . . Who do you think is going to have more frivolous spending patterns as an adult? Probably the rich kid.

Another way that genes play a role is in the way some people adjust their energy expenditure in response to overeating.[74] The first clue to point to this phenomenon is that even when overfed by the same amount, people seem to gain different amounts of weight.[75] For example, in one study, twelve pairs of identical twins were overfed by 1,000 calories per day for eighty-four days. And while everyone gained weight, some gained as little as ten pounds, while others gained as much as thirty.[76] I'm sorry, can we all stop and just . . . absorb? Like how did some people gain twenty pounds more than others from the same number of extra calories?

Here's the thing: twins are genetically identical, and the variation in weight gain was significantly larger among the sets of twins than within the twin pairs.[77] Translation: You were much more likely to gain a similar amount of weight as your twin as compared to all the other people in the study, so there seems to be some genetic component here.

Since the first law of thermodynamics must hold true, and everyone was being overfed by the same amount, there must be something happening to energy expenditure that is accounting for the difference in weight gain. And one possibility may be in the way people are changing their nonexercise activity thermogenesis (NEAT) in response to overeating.[78,79]

Remember, NEAT is the component of your energy expenditure made up of all the nonexercise movements that you perform throughout the day: standing, walking, chores, fidgeting, and so on. And for those people who don't gain much weight even after increasing their food intake, it may be that, subconsciously, they are moving way more as a compensatory mechanism. In another study, subjects were again overfed by 1,000 calories per day for eight weeks, and again, there was a tenfold difference in weight gain among subjects. Researchers estimate that two-thirds of the increase in energy expenditure after overfeeding was due to increases in NEAT.[80] And the degree of this compensatory response may be part of why certain people are more prone to weight gain than others. Does this mean that I will "spontaneously" be walking around my block in circles like a maniac next time I eat half a jar of peanut butter? Shhh . . . you didn't see me.

So is there a genetic component to metabolism? Undoubtedly. But are there things that we can do to promote a higher metabolism? The answer is also undoubtedly.

Can We Increase Our Metabolism?

One tempting reading of this chapter may be: "Well . . . that proves it. There is no point in trying to do anything, because my body will just compensate for whatever changes I make." But, guys, do you think I would write this whole chapter only to leave you with a sense of doom and hopelessness?! That would be such a bummer and opposite to everything I believe about health. Yes, biology is powerful and interesting and intricate, but the beauty of being a human is that at the end of the day, our choices are ours to make. We choose our behaviors. We choose what to eat. We choose how to move. We have a lot of influence. And while there are factors outside of our control, focusing on the parts you don't influence is a waste of time and emotional headspace.

First, we should mention that *not* doing things that might cause drastic compensations in your metabolism would be a great place to start. As always, prevention is a lot easier than reversal. So avoiding extremely low-calorie crash dieting, avoiding long extended periods of overexercising, and giving your body the nutrients and rest it needs whenever possible—all help maintain a healthy metabolism. For some of us, that ship may have sailed (ahem, ahem), but for others, you may have read this book just in time.

The good news is, if your metabolism can compensate downward, there's no reason to believe it can't also compensate upward. Recently, we've seen an increase in popularity of the process of "reverse dieting."[81] This consists of you slowly increasing calories in a stepwise fashion from week to week at the end of a diet in order to avoid rapid weight gain and help restore your pre-diet hormone profile and possibly metabolic function. This technique has become popular particularly among physique athletes, who have to routinely get down to outrageously low body-fat levels for competitions. Although this process has a lot of anecdotal evidence, more research is needed to validate how effective it is.[82]

And, finally, although it may seem like this is the opposite of everything we've been talking about, exercise is *crucial* to almost all aspects of health, including maintaining a healthy metabolism. Remember that when we talk about how "exercise doesn't increase your metabolic rate," we're talking about the upper extreme of physical activity. If you are not very active, increasing your physical activity will undoubtedly increase your total daily energy expenditure.[83] All we're trying to say is . . . if you're running marathons every day, running two marathons a day may not make that big of a difference.

Also, not to jump the gun and give away all of chapters 6 and 7, but . . . this needs to be said. Exercise has been shown to decrease all-cause mortality, risk of cardiovascular disease, many cancers, diabetes, mental illness, and cognitive decline as we age. Increased sedentary time is associated with all sorts of adverse health outcomes, including increased cardiovascular risk and shortened lifespan.[84] Exercise is one of the most powerful tools we have, and if it were in the form of a pill, it would be universally prescribed as a miracle supplement. And yet, just because it may not be the key to losing that ten extra pounds, people give up on it.

Let me give you another reason to exercise. Remember the study conducted on the *Biggest Loser* contestants and how they had experienced this big drop in energy expenditure? Even though the contestants who moved the most experienced the most metabolic adaptation (meaning they had the slowest metabolism), they were also the most successful in terms of long-term weight loss. Oh yes, this makes my brain hurt as much as yours. You would think having a slower metabolism would set you up for weight gain, and yet these individuals were the most likely to keep the weight off. This is likely due to the other key effects that exercise seems to have on biological processes that often drive weight gain, such as reducing appetite.[85] More on this in chapters 6 and 7.

Metabolism and Aging

"You'll see when you're my age." If I had a dollar for every time an adult in my life said this to me, usually while gingerly tossing a dry salad and turning away a cookie, I'd have enough money to pick up my lavishly expensive daily Starbucks habit again. (Note: This is, in fact, the end goal of my life . . . so thanks for buying this book!) To me, it seemed like middle-aged women, in particular, were fixated on their frustrations with their body and their apparently slowing metabolism. I don't think this means that men don't experience something similar (talk to any washed-up college athletes and they'll tell you) but merely that in our society, women were supposed to be preoccupied by this. The message I got, whether intentionally or not, was this: enjoy your metabolism while you can, because the second you turn thirty, it's all downhill from there. "It used to be so easy when I was your age!" was another common saying. Well, the joke is on them, because I feel like I've had a forty-year-old's supposed metabolism for my entire life; but anyway, that's beside the point.

Luckily for us, recently, one of the largest studies of metabolism over the human lifespan was published, studying energy expenditure using our favorite, the doubly labeled water method, in more than six thousand subjects ranging in age from one week old to ninety-five years old.[86] And the findings were pretty shocking.

You may think of your teens and twenties as times when you have a "roaring metabolism," but scientists found that infancy is actually the time when humans experience the highest pound-for-pound metabolic rate. By their first birthday, infants burn 50 percent more calories than adults, even when accounting for their rapidly growing bodies.[87] Something is happening in infants' cells that make them much more active.

After this initial period, the research showed that our metabolism slows by about 3 percent per year, until we reach age twenty, at which point it basically plateaus . . . *for the next forty years.*[88] Oh yes, you read that right. The researchers found no difference in metabolism, controlled for body size and composition, through basically all of adulthood and middle age, even during pregnancy.

At age sixty, we start to see a gradual decline of about 0.7 percent per year, even when you account for the changes in muscle mass and activity. So a person in his or her nineties needs about 26 percent fewer calories each day than a person who is middle-aged. This may be due to a lower energy cost for very energetically expensive organs, such as the brain and liver, as their function starts to slowly decline.[89] And this decreased organ function may also be why we see a rise in noncommunicable diseases around age sixty as well.

Before you get mad and start throwing this book out the window . . . I know what you are thinking. *There's no way this can be true. . . . I know I could eat more when I was younger and not gain weight.* Or: *I know it was easier to lean down in my twenties. . . .* And you are probably right, but not for the reason you think. In fact, the changes in body composition and physical activity that accompany aging are probably what accounts for this phenomenon we all feel personally victim to.[90]

First, we lose about 3–5 percent of our muscle mass for every decade after thirty. Remember, for the average person, basal metabolic rate, or BMR, makes up about 60–80 percent of your total energy expenditure, and the majority of your BMR is actually determined by your lean body mass.[91] So as we age, and we experience loss of muscle mass, the energetic cost of maintaining our body is becoming less and less.[92] Muscle is a very metabolically expensive tissue, so losing muscle is one of the fastest ways to decrease your BMR.

The other thing that happens as we age is we just start moving a lot less. Some data suggests that from age thirty-nine to seventy-five, we spend about 75 percent less time doing moderate or vigorous activities throughout the day. This decline in energy expenditure from physical activity is actually responsible for the majority of the decline in total energy expenditure that we see as we get older.[93]

It's true, there's nothing we can do about the gradual decline in organ function after age sixty. But there's *a lot* we can do about the loss of muscle mass and lowered physical activity we experience throughout adulthood. And again, the prescription is . . . exercise. An analysis of more than forty-nine studies found that progressive resistance-training interventions, like lifting weights, has been shown to *increase* lean body mass, even in older adults, by more than two pounds.[94] Compare that to the half pound or so you lose per year after age fifty. In some research, older women who engaged in regular exercise appeared to have no decline at all in their BMRs, after adjusting for lean body mass, even into their sixties.[95] Bottom line: exercise, exercise, exercise!

We've spent an awful long time talking about energy expenditure, or the "energy out" portion of the equation. But, equally important, we need to talk about the "energy in." In the next chapter, let's do a deep dive into the four-letter word that coincidentally (or not?) has the word "die" in it: *diet*.

From the Doc

Doctors Have Metabolisms, Too

I have never been very overweight or, for that matter, at all underweight. However, in my mid-thirties, during the stressful first couple of years of professional work as an attending physician, soon after the birth of our first child, I found myself on the path of the average adult American: gaining about two pounds per year. Nonetheless, I was feeling pretty good about myself when I finally scheduled an appointment to see a physician for my checkup. This was already a win because many medical doctors never formally see a personal physician for their care and instead rely on their own training or informal conversations with colleagues if something pops up. When I took the time to see my doctor, I was hoping for congratulations on showing up and taking such good care of myself. Instead, the conversation turned to my progressive weight gain. I asked, "Well, how much should I be gaining each year?" The doctor shot me a look, as if to ask, "Where did you go to medical school?" and held up his hand in the shape of a big, round zero. My doctor gently pushed the issue and determined that I was nearly twenty pounds heavier than my college weight.

I was ready to blame my presumably slowing metabolism, now that I had reached the ripe old age of thirty-five. It looked like I was destined to jettison my "rad bod" as a devoted martial artist only to be overtaken by the flabby "dad bod" of a stressed-out, sleep-deprived new father. But was my weight gain inevitable and just the next stage of life?

Even if I were succumbing to a slowing metabolism, I was determined to get off the weight-gain path. I took stock of my habits: I was mindlessly eating copious amounts of food, washed down with delicious, sugar-sweetened Snapple iced teas. I was spending less time in my martial arts classes and doing less exercise overall. As a new parent, I had become a bit more cautious, and my regular bike commuting on the streets of New York City transformed into subway rides. With limited sleep and increased stress, sweets and chocolate were my regular allies to get through the day.

I looked at what had changed in my life, what I had control over, and what was beyond my control. With some reflection and support, I did my best to evolve from mindlessly eating as much as I *wanted* to more mindfully eating as much as I *needed*. Over time, about half the excess weight came off. In retrospect, I acknowledge the privilege and opportunity I had to be able to choose a different path, modify my eating and exercise, and actively pursue modest weight loss. But, as I continue to witness firsthand both in my practice and personal life, for many others, weight loss is not as simple as it has been for me (even if giving up the Snapples was hard). Moreover, I respect that not everyone wants to lose weight.

Recent research indicates that, other than a rapid acceleration of our metabolic rate in infancy, we largely maintain the same metabolic rate from about age twenty until sixty.[96] So the weight gain I was experiencing in my thirties was more likely due to decreased sleep, increased stress, less exercise, and more calories consumed.

Over the ensuing twenty-five years, I have managed to keep my weight in a fairly narrow range. (OK, so it's about fifteen pounds more than my college weight, but at least I am not gaining more.) I also appreciate that I seem to be making this much easier than it has been (more on this in later chapters). However, for the most part, I have done my best to moderate my weight and improve my health by trying to stay informed about our evolving understanding of metabolism and, in turn, using that knowledge to inform and modify my habits.

When nonexercise activity thermogenesis (NEAT) was becoming a more well-known concept and treadmill desks were described by Dr. James Levine as a way to reduce sedentary behavior while improving productivity, I went out and got a bike desk. I use my desk frequently in my office (e.g., while writing this book), answering emails, and to help maintain my level of alertness during the tenth online meeting of the day. Seeing my gently swaying head on the computer screen, a well-meaning colleague called me after a meeting to see if I was "OK" and whether he might assist in treating my *movement disorder*. While on-screen it might have looked like an essential tremor or Parkinson's disease, I explained to him about my bike desk and that, from my perspective, the others on the call who were sitting still would perhaps be better described as having a *lack of movement disorder*. After getting hooked on the bike desk, I have tried to improve my NEAT by also using a standing desk and doing walking meetings when possible.

I also now realize that I can exert some control over my exercise activity thermogenesis (EAT) by maintaining exercise beyond the office-based slow biking, standing, and walking meetings. When EAT became better characterized, I progressively increased my exercise on a daily basis and managed to reduce injuries and boredom by doing a wide variety of exercise, including swimming, biking, running (put together as a triathlon), as well as yoga and hiking. With information about the expected decline in muscle mass as we age, I have upped my resistance training from an ancillary side dish supporting my swimming, biking, and running to the main entrée, with sessions dedicated to strengthening and maintaining trained muscles that burn up more calories than untrained muscle and many more calories than fat. This has become all the more urgent now that I have reached the true slowing-metabolism stage of life past sixty.

You've Got Q's; We've Got A's

Q: Wait, sorry, I love the stories, but I kind of spaced out on the science part. What do I need to remember about EAT and NEAT? Also, is it on the final exam?

A: Not to worry. It comes down to this: the calories you burn from exercise are not going to "give you a fast metabolism." However, moving throughout the day and having some dedicated time for formal exercise is crucial to maintaining any weight loss, *and* crucial to your overall health and happiness (more in chapters 6 and 7)! Also, this won't be on a written test . . . but if you count your overall life quality as a final exam . . . then *yes!*

Q: Can I blame my mother for my slow metabolism?

A: Kind of . . . As with so many things in the body, there is a genetic component. But also there's a lot we do control, and focusing on that makes for a way more fun time!!! The genetic variability of metabolic rate, for the vast majority of people, is not what is causing your jeans not to fit!

Q: Can I blame my father for my slow metabolism?

A: No. See the previous question about blaming your mother.

Q : What kind of special tea, supplement, cream, or garment is recommended to increase my metabolism? Do you guys have a discount code?

A : Save your money. None of those things have been shown to make a difference. Even something like caffeine, for which there's some evidence for "increasing metabolic rate," only does so by a couple of calories a day . . . a fraction of a fraction of a pound.

Q : If it takes calories to digest our food, what you called our TEF (thermic effect of food), then why can't I eat more food and therefore burn more calories?

A : *Aha!* You smart cookie. Wouldn't it be awesome if things worked that way? Here's the issue: if you eat 1,000 extra calories of food, only about 10–15 percent (100–150 calories, depending on what the foods were), would be used for the digestion of those foods. So you're still eating an extra 800–850 calories. Darn, it would've been such a good plan. . . .

Q : If I can't speed up my metabolism with supplements, special foods, *or* burning more calories during exercise, what *can* I do?

A : Lots . . . See chapters 3–12 for details. ☺

The Takeaways

Energy Expenditure Cheat Sheet

- Metabolism, or total daily energy expenditure (TDEE), can be broken up into four components: BMR (basal metabolic rate), TEF (thermic effect of food), EAT (exercise activity thermogenesis), and NEAT (nonexercise activity thermogenesis).

- BMR makes up more than half of your TDEE and is the number of calories needed to keep your body baseline functioning.

- 60–80 percent of BMR is determined by your lean body mass.

- Exercise, for most people, is the smallest part of their energy expenditure, contributing 0 calories to TDEE, because most people do no formal "exercise," and contributing only 5–10 percent to TDEE, even for those that *do* exercise.

- NEAT is one of the most variable parts of energy expenditure, because some people lead much more active lives, either due to their occupation or their leisure activities.

Physiology of Weight Loss

- Energy balance determines changes in weight: Take in more calories than you burn, you'll gain weight. Burn more calories than you eat, you'll lose weight.

- Energy in and energy out are not independent variables. The calories you eat affect the calories you burn, and even the calories you burn doing physical activity also may impact the calories you burn the rest of the day as well as the calories you eat.

Metabolic Adaptation

- Your metabolism is not static; it is constantly adapting to signals of energy availability.

- Weight loss will always lead to a slower metabolism because you are becoming a smaller person. Smaller person = less tissue = fewer cells = less energy needed to upkeep cells.

Genetic Variability

- A small portion of energy expenditure cannot be explained by body composition or activity and is likely genetic.

- People's bodies respond differently to overfeeding, resulting in a wide variation of weight gain from the same calorie surplus.

What Can You Do About It?

- Behaviors like crash dieting and extreme amounts of physical activity can cause compensatory downregulation of TDEE (even beyond what is expected from weight loss) in an attempt to keep you within a constrained amount of energy expenditure. Avoiding these promotes a healthier metabolism.

- Exercise at moderate levels can help promote a plethora of good health outcomes, including a healthy metabolism through increasing/maintaining muscle mass.

- Most of the decline in metabolism we see with aging is due to a loss in muscle mass and a decrease in physical activity. And this effect can be blunted or even negated with regular exercise, in particular, resistance training.

3

Why All Diets Work . . . Then Don't

Part 1: Why All Diets Work

"Eating a Chicken at a Staff Meeting"

"One day, my friend and I were at a staff meeting eating a huge chicken," Kaye, one of the administrative staff at the music department, sheepishly told me during college. She was describing one of the diets she had tried where "you would eat only one food item each day." But don't worry, you could have "as much as you want." Like one day, you could only eat potatoes; another day, you could only eat tomatoes. I pictured Kaye in the music department lounge, eating a rotisserie chicken while everyone else nibbled on cookies and brownies. Funny, but it's just one example of the million "diet adventure" stories I've heard.

If the world of "dieting" doesn't make you want to rip out your hair, then you, my friend, are a stronger individual than I am. Just spending five minutes in that orbit will soon have you questioning whether or not you have lost your mind or perhaps developed a short-term memory loss problem. Didn't they just say vegetables are good for you? But now proponents of the "carnivore diet" say they're bad? This person says low fat is the only way to go. Over here, someone is saying that he eats butter and bacon all day and he's lost forty pounds. It's absolutely maddening.

The worst part is you probably know someone who has gone on one of these diets and may have *actually* seen results (shocking, I know). Even if it's not someone you know yourself, you can definitely find them online.

Suzie lost thirty pounds with keto. John has "never been so energetic" after starting intermittent fasting. Once someone has experienced even the tiniest benefit from a new diet, something very peculiar happens in that person's brain. Scientifically, we call this "the unbearable high-horseification" of individuals. This is where they (a) won't shut up about their diet, and (b) make it their life's mission to get you on said diet. I have seen this illness take hold of even the best of us, and despite all the advances of modern-day science, which have allowed for putting spaceships on Mars and creating brain-computer interfaces, no one can figure out how to make them stop. Needless to say, there are few things people feel more strongly about than politics, the Patriots, and "the best diet."

A Confusing Definition

The definition of "diet' actually has nothing to do with weight loss or "getting in shape." Instead, it simply means "food and drink regularly provided or consumed" or "habitual nourishment." However, for a lot of us, myself included, diets have always meant something else. I never heard the word "diet" growing up, I heard the words "a diet." It's funny how that tiny addition, just the letter "a," turns something from what you're used to eating to "this thing I'm temporarily suffering through to lose weight."

When I was little, I thought that diets were almost magical. There was something special about putting cayenne pepper, lemon juice, and maple syrup together that would cause people to lose weight. Like, something happened with the molecules of those specific foods that would unlock your fat cells and release all the fatty acids. For some reason, this made sense in my head. However, after learning more about how the human body *actually* works, I found out that this was a load of spicy, lemony, bullshit.

This chapter is not a commentary on the societal, gender, and sociocultural influences of dieting, diet culture, and its implications. It's also not a look at "diet" in the strict definition of the word: not a commentary on what to eat for optimal health and longevity (see "What to Eat," chapter 5). Rather, I want to dive into "diet" as I have known it for most of my life—"a diet" as a way to lose weight. This is a look into why all diets work, and yet why all diets eventually fail. It's to gain an understanding of the underlying mechanism behind every diet to demystify the entire process.

We always hear that "diets don't work," and yet you know, and I know, that they clearly do. We've seen people lose weight, we've seen people post amazing before-and-afters on Instagram. We've seen people "pull it together" for their weddings. But we've probably all had the experience of going on a hard-core diet and having it completely fail, leaving us feeling demoralized, depleted, and defeated. What the hell is going on here?

Because we are looking strictly at the weight-loss side of things, we are going to temporarily ignore the parts of "diet" that are arguably more important: the micronutrients, the *quality* of our food, the things that our bodies need to not only survive but thrive (see chapter 5). In the short term, people can get away with ignoring diet quality: you can eat nonfood (a.k.a. junk food) for a period of weeks, months, *maybe* even years and not notice permanent side effects. But in the long term, this will bite you in the proverbial butt in some really scary ways: deficiencies, poor health, poor quality of life, and even disease. Because my teenage self was so obsessed with strictly the weight-loss aspect of diets, that's what I wanted to break down first. But reading this chapter without reading the "What to Eat" chapter would be like going to Trader Joe's in September without getting anything Pumpkin Spice: you're missing the entire point.

The "Magic" of Diets

Here is a statement that is at once simple but at the same time misunderstood. Every diet that has caused someone to lose weight is doing so by causing that person to be in a calorie deficit (see chapter 2).

It does not matter what the foods were—an all-Twinkies diet, an all-pizza diet, an all-veggie diet, a diet of those little chick-shaped Peeps marshmallows; if people lost weight doing it, they were in a calorie deficit. Meaning they were burning more calories than they were ingesting. This is so simple, and so boring, that it is often ignored entirely when people talk about their results from (insert fancy new diet trend). This is the first law of thermodynamics, and it is inescapable, no matter how much people want to pretend it's not.

Who wants to hear the following?

"Hey, guys, it's me, young hot celebrity X! I lost fifteen pounds *by consistently eating fewer calories than I used to, thereby putting me in a caloric deficit and allowing my body to use up fat stores!!!"*

Even I can admit this is abhorrently underwhelming and I would never read an article about it.

Now let's try this:

"Hey, guys, it's me, young hot celebrity X! I lost fifteen pounds *by following my nutritionist's scientifically backed Tomato Diet! Did you know tomatoes are the most fat-burning food on the planet?! Neither did I, but look at my sexy new bod!" (And for a small payment of $15.99 a month, you, too, can have access to the fat-burning Tomato Diet.)*

I mean . . . hello . . . where do I sign up? This lady looks *this* good, eating *tomatoes*?! I love tomatoes! (Or if I don't, I *can* like tomatoes . . . to get abs.)

The point that I'm trying to make here is that the underlying mechanism of all diets is the same, but the marketing, packaging, and branding are wildly variable. The reason for this is partially because you can sell way more products if you differentiate them (cough, cough—the $72 billion diet industry), and because diets aren't just *how* you eat anymore. They are often a signal of *who you are,* what group you belong to: If you are vegan, you care about the environment and are likely left leaning. If you "eat clean," you love CrossFit. If you drink green juices every day, you do Pilates and yoga and likely live in L.A. But regardless of how "different" they may appear from the outside, every diet is the same.

The O.G. Diet

(Note to Eddie: "O.G." means original.)

The most basic diet, and the least frilly, is a simple calorie target (see "What the Heck Is a Calorie, Anyway?" in chapter 2). This used to be more popular when I was growing up in the early 2000s. There would be some "number" to shoot for, and you could "count" what you were eating by adding up the numbers on the back of packages or looking up the nutrition information. (Psst: The dirty little secret of the diet industry is that these diets are popular today as well, just marketed differently, because it's not "cool" to count calories anymore.) A lot of people do this through programs like Weight Watchers (now known as WW), which would assign "points" instead of calories to make things simpler, or more fun? Who knows? The reason is beyond me. (Interestingly enough, even apps today involve similar food-tracking systems, although they are packaged differently, for example, rating foods with green, yellow, and red categories, or counting macronutrients as well as calories.)

Calorie counting and "point" counting (even macro counting) are all pretty straightforward—and it's easy to see how they could potentially cause weight loss. When Amy eats whatever she wants (in studies, this is called *ad libitum*) without counting anything, she eats, let's say, 2,300 calories a day. All of a sudden, Amy hears you need to eat 1,700 calories a day to lose weight. (PS: These are made-up numbers.) She starts counting what she's eating, which results in her eating less than usual. A calorie deficit is achieved. Amy loses weight . . . at least at first.

Counting macronutrients, or "macros," is an extension of the same concept. It's like counting calories . . . on steroids. "Macros" is shorthand for macronutrients: the three types of nutrients that make up food and that our body needs. We will dive into macros quite a bit in later chapters as well, but roughly speaking, all calories can be further categorized by which of the three macronutrients they come from: carbohydrates, fats, or protein. (We're just going to go ahead and ignore alcohol for the purpose of simplifying things here, but yes, alcohol also does contain calories, usually quite a few.) For optimal health, we all need some combination of the three macronutrients, although the variety of different macro ratios is as diverse as the array of different diets people follow. Macronutrients are a lot more than sources of energy; for example, our bodies need protein to build and repair muscle tissue, we need fats for proper hormone function, and so on. However, in this chapter, which is strictly looking at "diet" in the weight-loss/management sense, we will mostly focus on their caloric values. We should note that different ratios of macronutrients can have profound impacts on overall appetite, hunger signaling, and satiation cues, so . . . it's not *all* about the calories.

Most naturally occurring foods contain all three macronutrients in varying proportions. For example, potatoes are mostly carbohydrates, animal foods are typically a mixture of protein and fats, while nuts are primarily fat, and so on. Ignoring *all* the other important things you need different macronutrients for: one gram of carbohydrates is 4 calories, one gram of protein is also 4 calories, and one gram of fat is 9 calories. "Counting macros" is therefore just counting calories in *way more* detail. It's basically saying, "Not only am I going to count every unit of energy I eat, but I will be categorizing it into one of these three buckets." It's not really important to know the caloric values of each macronutrient, it's more important to know that macros and calories coexist; it's not one or the other. Every food has a caloric value (how much energy it contains), and that energy can be further broken down into three different nutrient types.

So people count calories, count points, or if you want to be super exact, count macros in an attempt to lower food consumption, cause a calorie deficit, and thus lose weight. Every single diet that has ever caused a person to lose weight has done this exact same thing *for that person,* given their individual energy needs, even if the diet hasn't explicitly instructed the person to restrict calories.

You may be asking yourself, *How is a diet making you restrict calories if it's not telling you to eat less?* Some diets will, in fact, seemingly tell you the opposite: eat as much of this food as you want, just make sure it's only chicken. Or: eat whatever you want, just make sure it's not in a package.

Regardless of the messaging, the mechanism underlying the diet is the same: somehow, someway, these instructions, rules, protocols, or rituals are getting you to eat less than you were.

There are no magic foods.

There are no magic times to eat.

There are no magic ratios.

There are just different ways of achieving the same thing.

How Every Diet Is the Same

Let's look at a straightforward example of how diets work, for example, eating "low-fat." (This was all the rage when I was growing up.) If you eat fat, you'll get fat, right? People would get low-fat yogurts, low-fat milks, "skinny" lattes. So how is this diet causing weight loss? If you tell a person to eat low-fat, not only do they make a lot of food swaps, they are also forced to cut out a lot of foods altogether: nuts, oils, avocado, and most importantly, many processed foods. All ultra-processed foods, desserts, chips, candy bars, and so on, are primarily carbohydrates and fats, *and* are extremely calorically dense. Given that the standard American diet (or SAD, as it's aptly nicknamed) consists of more than 50 percent ultra-processed foods (more on this in chapter 5), putting a low-fat restriction on people automatically cuts out a bunch of their sources of calories.[1] And so, oftentimes, a person will be eating a lot less, even if that's not necessarily what the diet called for.

Keto, which is the exact *opposite* of low-fat (for many, a diet of butter, bacon, and coconut oil . . . yum), ironically often does the exact same thing. Because a ketogenic diet mostly involves eating "high-fat" foods, people often cut out entire food groups: no grains, cereals, breads, pastas, sugar, or even fruit. Given that the average American gets 42 percent of their calories from refined carbohydrates, it's no wonder keto so often causes weight loss for people: it's cutting out almost half of their daily food options.[2] Granted, people make up for this by eating a lot more high-fat food, but still . . . take out fries, cereals, and sodas, and what is there left, really?

So far, the two diets we've talked about have mainly imposed caloric restrictions by putting emphasis on or taking it away from a particular macronutrient. However, this isn't the only way diets work. They can put restrictions on types of foods. For example, "eating clean" involves cutting out all ultra-processed foods; for Kaye (see the beginning of this chapter), her diet only allowed her to eat a particular food each day.

Alternatively, diets can simply impose time restrictions on *when* you eat: No eating after 7 P.M. No eating before noon. And again, there's nothing *special* about the calories you eat after 7 . . . except, of course, the fact that they are additional calories. Intermittent fasting, for example, has become a popular technique for losing weight, and while its other benefits may be debatable, simply from a fat-loss perspective, eating in an eight-hour window provides no additional benefits.[3,4] However, when you give people only eight hours to eat, instead of their usual fourteen or fifteen, of course they end up eating a lot less.

Yet other diets can rely on mechanisms such as your body's fullness signals to lower food intake. So, for example, any diet that calls for you to vastly increase your vegetable intake, without putting any other foods off-limits, still often leads to people eating less. Why is this? Because, of course, apart from providing you with a plethora of nutrients, vegetables are very voluminous: they take up a lot of space in your stomach for not that many calories. And so if you are eating a ton of vegetables, there is just way less space in your stomach for other stuff and you feel fuller. In this way, again, the diet is indirectly causing you to eat fewer calories overall, without explicitly telling you to do so.

Low-Carb vs. Low-Fat Diets for Weight Loss

When it comes to weight loss, every low-carb, keto, or clean-eating zealot will swear up and down that there is something "special" about their diet. For example, the low-carb-insulin hypothesis of obesity states that carbohydrates, not overall calorie balance, are responsible for the obesity epidemic. The logic goes (roughly): eating high-glycemic foods (foods that spike your blood sugar) causes hormonal changes that promote fat storage and increase hunger, independent of energy balance. However, study after study has shown that this is simply not the case. When calories and protein are equated, people lose the same amount of weight, regardless of whether their calories are low-carb, low-fat, high-carb, high-fat, all sugar, or all veggies.[5]

PS: The reason protein is important here (as opposed to carbs and fat) is because protein is a bit harder for your body to break down. It takes more energy to digest protein, thus increasing the thermic effect of food (the calories used to break down and absorb nutrients). So, if one diet protocol includes the same number of calories but a higher proportion of those calories come from protein, it may result in more weight loss.

Studying diet protocols is really hard, and there are a lot of poorly designed studies out there. For example, scientists will often put one group on an intermittent-fasting protocol (let's call this the "IF group"), while the control group just eats whatever and whenever they want, as usual. The IF group will often lose weight, and this will lead the people on the intermittent-fasting team to exclaim, "*Aha!* Intermittent fasting is superior for weight loss!" And that would be fine and dandy if it weren't for the fact that . . . nobody was measuring how much either of these two groups was eating. This completely ignores the fact that the IF group likely ate way less than the group that was eating ad lib, around the clock, meaning it wasn't the "fasting" causing weight loss; it was the fact that the intermittent-fasting group ate fewer calories because they had less time to eat. Spread out the same number of calories over the course of their entire day, and they would have most likely seen the exact same results.[6]

Other studies will compare two dietary protocols, like high-fat versus high-carb, and not control for diet quality. This usually means that one diet (the one the researchers probably think is better) is set up to be very high quality (full of veggies and other whole foods), while the other diet is set up as a sort of straw man: a cheap, unhealthy alternative. How are we supposed to decide if low-fat or low-carb is "better" if one was full of veggies and the other was full of bacon? These studies also don't often ensure they're including equal amounts of protein between conditions, which can impact diet success, because high-protein diets are so satiating[7] (i.e., people will eat less when their diets are higher in protein).

Having poor research studies is not necessarily the fault of scientists who are cackling in a back room, plotting for even more ways to confuse us with opposing findings. The fact is: it's just damn hard to conduct good, well-controlled nutrition research.

This is for a couple of reasons:

1. People are not very good at sticking to diet protocols. I mean, come on: you've done it, I've done it, it's freaking hard, and a lot of the time it's miserable.

2. People are not particularly accurate when they have to self-report what they've eaten. Many studies have shown that all people underreport their own energy intake, but certain subgroups, such as overweight individuals or women, underreport intake substantially more (up to 70 percent in some cases).[8]

Just to be clear, this is not because people are coming into the lab, maniacally twirling their mustaches, and thinking, *Muhaha, I will fool these scientists today!! I will* not *tell them about that Snickers bar from last night!* It's actually simply because, a vast majority of the time, people just don't know what the hell they are eating. Food is everywhere, and we eat without even thinking about it. If only we could lock people in some sort of ward where we could monitor every morsel of food they ate and truly compare dietary protocols. . . .

Oh, wait . . . *we can!*

A lot of the gold-standard research that compares dietary protocols has come out of studies conducted in metabolic wards: studies in which people literally live in a lab, and every food item and movement is being monitored, sometimes for weeks on end. As you can imagine, these studies are exorbitantly expensive, but they provide us with really good, solid science to compare dietary protocols (at least in the short term). To put an end to the diet wars, Kevin Hall and his colleagues put seventeen subjects in a metabolic ward for four weeks, first on a high-carbohydrate diet, then four weeks on a high-fat, ketogenic diet with the same number of calories and protein, and guess what they found? There was *no difference* in weight loss between the two protocols.[9] What is that sound, you say? Oh, it's just the deafening crickets from all the people claiming keto or high-carb diets are the best for weight loss.

Another study proved the exact same result, except people were not locked in a lab, they were left out in the wild. The researchers initially set out to find out: Why do some people in weight-loss studies do *super* well on a diet, whereas other people don't?[10] Are there genes that can tell us which diet is best for us?

The short answer? No, or at least, not that we know of yet. But the study showed us something else that is maybe more important. The sub-jects were randomly assigned to either the low-carb or low-fat protocol, but crucially, both groups were instructed on how to eat their assigned diet in the healthiest way possible. The groups were not given calorie targets or quotas, just told to eat whatever they wanted, as long as it followed their new assigned protocol. After a year, on average, the two groups lost basi-cally the same amount of weight.[11] But again, as we always see, the range of responses was huge: some people lost substantial amounts of weight, while other people actually *gained* weight, *in a weight-loss study!!!* Take-away: A healthy low-fat diet or a healthy low-carb diet on average works about the same, but how an individual person responds is totally variable.

You Can Literally Eat Anything and Lose Weight

Let's shatter some more fake-diet weight-loss scams: When time-restricted energy restriction (this sounds horrendous, but in English it translates to intentionally running a calorie deficit while intermittent fasting) has been compared to running a calorie deficit *with no* intermittent fasting, again, there was no difference found in weight loss.[12] Notably, though, the IF group *did* experience a lot more lean-body-mass *loss*, and if you read chap-ter 2, you know that is *no bueno* for the ol' metabolism. The group that was doing the intermittent fasting also experienced a reduction in spontaneous movement. In short: when you don't eat enough and concentrate the little food you *do* get in a fewer number of hours, you're freaking exhausted all day and you don't move as much. Truly shocking, I know. Plus, your body loses not only the stuff you wanted it to (like fat tissue) but also the stuff you *didn't* want it to (lean tissues such as muscle). Hmm . . . not exactly the magic bullet people so often claim it to be.

To really put the nail in the "magic-weight-loss diet" coffin, Mark Haub, a professor of human nutrition at Kansas State University, com-mitted himself to a diet of a Twinkie every three hours, with some Dor-itos, cereals, and Oreos thrown in there for variety. His diet was basically junk—although little enough junk that it was below his caloric require-ments for maintaining his weight. Haub started the diet at 201 pounds, and after ten weeks on this diet, he weighed 174—a pretty dramatic 27-pound weight loss.

Whoa there! Before you go off and start raiding the snack aisle for your next beach-body plan . . . there are implications beyond weight loss that come with Twinkie-eating. We'll talk about this more in chapter 5, "What to Eat." But for now, the important thing to understand is that at a strictly weight-loss level, calories really *do matter.*

Part 2: Why (Almost) All Diets Fail

The Abysmal Success Rate

I'm sure you've heard some sort of adage like "95 percent of diets fail." And if you're like me, you think, *That can't be right, because then why would so many people diet? And also, Then why does it seem like I know so many people who have succeeded? Where does this number even come from? Has anyone taken the time to actually look at this? Or did someone just get fed up with their kale and salmon one day and post a flagrant blog article that took over the blogosphere and has now just become common "knowledge"?*

In reality, this statistic is slightly misleading: it makes it sound like 95 percent of people that go on a diet will not lose any weight, which is certainly not the case. A lot of people are successful at weight loss *at some point* in their lives. However, the story becomes very, very different when you look at how many people have been able to maintain the weight loss. The saying should go something like "95 percent of people will regain the weight they lose on a diet," and it turns out that this actually has been studied . . . *a lot.*

In scientific writing, a meta-analysis is an overview of a bunch of independent studies all looking at the same topic, such as what percentage of people can actually maintain weight loss. It's kind of like a gigantic summary of studies so that we don't just draw conclusions from one random trial from one random lab. It can be pretty handy-dandy when you want to look at a topic's larger trends and conclusions. In regard to the larger trend of weight-loss maintenance? Well, in scientific terms, the conclusions freaking suck.

In a meta-analysis of twenty-nine studies, more than half of the weight lost by subjects was regained within two years, and more than 80 percent was regained within five years.[13] If you are killing yourself trying to eat a chicken at a staff meeting while everybody around you eats cookies . . . this statistic is horrifying. Why put yourself through all the pain of dieting if it's most likely going to fail and you will regain most of the weight and perhaps more? In fact, not only does dieting not predict weight loss, it may predict *weight gain*.[14] This sadistic twist of fate has led some people (me) to conclude with 1,000 percent certainty that, yes, it's true, the universe does indeed have a maddeningly dark sense of humor that I do not find funny in the slightest.

Do Diets Make You Fat?

The association between dieting and weight gain has long been established in scientific literature, particularly when it comes to lean individuals or normal-weight individuals who go on diets.[15] Since the 1990s, more than fifteen prospective studies, conducted in adults, adolescents, and children, have shown an association between dieting to lose weight and future weight gain and obesity. (PS: A prospective cohort study is one in which subjects are enrolled before they exhibit the disease or outcome in question, i.e., before they have gained weight or developed obesity. The subjects are then followed, often for a period of years, and then we can look back at the information collected about them—socioeconomic, biological, environmental, behavioral, and so on—to see if there were any associations between any factors and the outcome being studied.)

The statistics from these studies are dizzying. One study found that adolescents with baseline dieting, compared to nondieters, had three times the risk of developing obesity, even when you control for initial body mass index (BMI).[16] The risk of major weight gain (more than twenty-two pounds) was twice as high in normal-weight subjects who tried to diet compared to nondieters.[17] Interestingly, the same study did not find this association among individuals who were overweight when they tried to diet, suggesting that dieting's association with weight gain may particularly affect lean or normal-weight people.

Whether or not dieting is itself the cause of the weight gain seen in these studies has been contentious. The most obvious interpretation would be: people who report more dieting later are heavier; therefore, dieting causes weight gain. But another way to see it is that perhaps people who are worried about weight gain (i.e., those predisposed to weight gain) are more likely to go on diets. In other words, if you grew up like me: not quite overweight, but also not super skinny (perhaps more predisposed to becoming overweight), you're also the type of individual that would be more likely to go on a diet. It's the classic chicken-and-egg scenario: Is dieting causing weight gain, or is propensity to weight gain causing dieting?

Whenever we have a question like this, the best place to look is twins studies. If we study a set of twins who are genetically identical, we can isolate the effect of just the dieting behavior that is under question. Several studies have shown that there does seem to be a genetic or familial component to dieting, meaning there is something about being predisposed to weight gain that makes people more likely to engage in dieting behaviors.[18,19] However, in a study of more than four thousand individual twins, despite being the exact same weight at the beginning of the study, the twin that engaged in dieting behaviors had gained more weight at age twenty-five than the nondieting twin had.[20] So, the twin that had engaged in intentional weight loss at least once before was on average one pound heavier than the nondieting twin. This may not seem like much, but keep in mind, the study only measured their weight by age twenty-five, and we don't know how much greater the effect would be with chronic dieting versus one or two tries.

In another study of elite Finnish athletes, those who had competed in sports that regularly involved weight cycling, such as wrestling or weightlifting, showed a greater BMI from ages twenty to sixty than those who had engaged in sports that did not require weight cycling.[21] Hmm . . . can a study be done on the "elite" individuals who engage in the sport of "look shredded for summer"? (Asking for a friend, obviously.)

Why Am I Heavier After a Diet?

The phenomenon of "overshooting" lost weight after "starvation" has been well-documented. I'm purposely using the word "starvation" here because, in essence, that is what a diet is: voluntary mini-starvation. In a landmark study meant to shed light on how to help people coming out of extreme food deprivation during World War II, scientists ran a year-long study looking at how humans respond to starvation. Questionable ethically, I know (that shit would not fly today), but . . . nevertheless for a good scientific cause. PS: One of these scientists was Ancel Keys; remember him, because this dude was instrumental in the creation of the Body Mass Index (BMI) and the demonization of dietary fat that ruled nutritional guidelines for the next fifty years. . . . But we'll come back to him later.

Anyway, back to the experiment: In 1944, thirty-six men volunteered to put themselves through semistarvation in the name of science.[22] The study called for the men to spend twelve weeks eating at a weight-maintenance number of calories (~3,200), then six months on a semistarvation diet (~1,570 calories), another three months of somewhat restricted calories for rehabilitation (~2,000–3,000 calories), and a final eight-week phase in which they could eat as much as they wanted. The protocol called for the men to lose 25 percent of their body weight, and by the end, thirty-two of the men were able to complete the study.

While in the "semistarvation" phase, the men became gaunt, lost their sex drives, experienced lower heart rates, body temperatures, strength, stamina, and became obsessed with food, often fantasizing about it during the day and dreaming about it at night. (Coincidentally, this is an alarmingly accurate description of my early twenties.)

None of this is surprising to anyone who has severely underfed themselves for a long time. But the interesting part came *after* the controlled refeeding, the part in which the men were allowed to eat *ad libitum,* however much their hearts desired, no limits, no restrictions. The twelve men who stayed in the lab for the *ad libitum* phase (bless their hearts; the rest skipped outta that hell hole) ate *substantially* more than they had in the initial weight-maintenance phase of the study, *even after* they had regained the lost weight.[23] And so they went from being semistarved to actually significantly overshooting their original weight. Hmm . . . doesn't sound familiar at all. . . . Definitely not what happens to me every single year. . . . Nope. For sure, not.

I have two things to say about this: (1) The fact that twelve people stayed after they were semistarved just so we could "scientifically" confirm that you'll overeat post-diet is astonishing (these dudes were dedicated to science, man); and (2) Can someone please explain to me how popular weight-loss apps are still giving 1,200 as a calorie target when these men were exhibiting signs of "insanity" on 1,570 calories? Hello? I don't want to trivialize at all what these men went through; their suffering is well-documented and prolonged, and it was all so we could better understand starvation. The fact that we see milder versions of this in people purposefully dieting because of the abundance of food we have today is just another sign of the privilege that many of us have of excess food. But it doesn't change the fact that dieting, even if it's less intense than the starvation experiment, can have profound, long-lasting biological and physical effects.

A more recent study of healthy, lean men completing an eight-week Army Ranger training investigated the effects of a more moderate "mini-starvation": a 1,000-calorie deficit.[24] Although the men experienced more moderate weight loss due to the shorter time period and smaller deficit (~12 percent weight loss), the participants' body weights still overshot their original weights by more than ten pounds after five weeks of the post-training recovery period, in which they could eat as much as they wanted. All ten men in the study exhibited higher fat mass at the end of the study than prior to the weight loss.

To sum up: the relationship between dieting and weight gain appears to be bidirectional, meaning it goes both ways. Yes, people who are predisposed to gaining weight, either due to genetic or familial factors, may be more likely to engage in dieting. But, also, dieting itself contributes to risk of future weight gain and the onset of obesity. A possible explanation for this relationship could be the fact that when those who are normal weight or are lean diet, they often overshoot their original weight in the regain phase after the diet.

The Post-Diet Diet

Dieting in the short term *does* work, but the real problem comes in the post-diet. Why do we always seem to regain the weight? Why do we often gain even more weight than we lost? *Why am I asking questions as if someone is going to pop out of my computer screen to answer them as I type this?*

Weight regain is a problem that, if solved, could potentially put an end to the "obesity epidemic." All of us would do some cleanse once a year, shed a quick thirty pounds or more, and then go on with our lives. As trivial as it seems, the simple act of adding the word "a" to "diet" is exactly the problem: "a diet" is by definition temporary; it is only for a period of time; it is not the collective "diet" that is your new pattern of eating. The deep-rooted problem of dieting is that people think they can go on "a diet," lose weight, and go back to what they were doing. And the truth is that whatever weight loss you achieved on that diet can only be maintained by following that diet for the rest of your life.

No one thinks about the diet after the diet, but *that* diet is what's going to put you in the 20 percent that succeed or 80 percent who don't. If continuing your new eating pattern and exercise regime isn't hard enough, there is also a strong biological drive to regain the weight that you have lost—a powerful, complex, and redundant system of physiological changes that prime you to pack on the pounds. Buckle up people, it's going to be a bumpy ride.

The Biological Drive to Regain Weight

Part of why we regain weight is that we don't think of diets as permanent lifestyle changes. Instead, we treat them like two-week "eat nothing but leaves and chicken" torture sessions that are supposed to result in a big slo-mo reveal of your new body as you unwrap your towel at your sister's pool party. But another part of it is that your body probably does not want you to just keep on losing weight forever. My own body?! Working against me?! Alas, it would seem so, my friend.

It can be easy to approach subjects like this with a sense of internal doom. Like, *I try so hard, and my body just doesn't want me to have what I want,* but I think this is not giving your body much credit at all for what it does. Contrary to popular belief, it is not your body's goal to stop you from fitting into your old jeans; your body's main goal, as we discussed in chapter 2, is to maintain homeostasis, or balance. It does this through an intricate system of checks and balances that involve the brain and other organs constantly sending signals back and forth.

Your brain constantly gets signals from the rest of your body. In the context of weight management, it's getting signals about energy stores (how much energy is available in your body through fat stores, glycogen, etc.) and nutrient supply (how much food it's getting). Based on this information, your brain sends out signals to adjust things like energy expenditure, food-seeking behaviors, and so on. Things get more complicated when we consider other factors, like environment, genetic influences, and behavioral motivations, to name a few. But no matter what your New Year's resolution is, the bottom line is that your brain and body are in a constant conversation that we're not even privy to (sorry to go all British on you for a second there).

The Body's Thermostat

First, let's start with a theory called "body-weight set point," which suggests that your body seems to almost work like a thermostat.[25] Imagine you're in your house and you set the temperature to 68 degrees Farenheit. If the rooms of the house are at 65, the thermostat turns on the heat to get the temperature up. If your house is at 72, it turns on the AC to bring the temperature down. The purpose of the thermostat is not to heat or cool; it is to return the house temperature to where you have set it.

The idea that there is one magic number on the scale that your body wants to be at is a bit simplistic and outdated. However, a more plausible framework is that there seems to be an upper and lower threshold, a "set range," in a sense, that your body likes to hover between.[26] Within these two thresholds, your weight can fluctuate with little to no physiological influences. If you lose weight past a certain point, the body turns on its inner biological mechanisms that will promote a return to your set range, that is, mechanisms that promote weight gain. On the other hand, if you gain weight past a certain point, the body will do the opposite, turning up the mechanisms that will help you lose weight. How wide of a range you have is likely influenced by a lot of factors, including your genetics, environment, and behavioral patterns, but . . . getting away from this set range, at either end, is actually extremely difficult.

Of course, a lot of us have experienced the inevitable creep-up of the scale after we have reached a new low weigh-in, but it also happens on the weight-*gain* side. Ask anybody who has had to purposefully put on a substantial amount of weight, such as a Hollywood actor for a role, and that person will tell you it's miserable. You stuff yourself constantly until you're sick of food; everything in your body is telling you to stop eating, and yet you have to force it down to gain weight.

For example, when Charlize Theron had to gain almost fifty pounds for her role in the movie *Tully,* she said, "The first three weeks are always fun because you're just like a kid in a candy store. . . . Then after three weeks, it's not fun anymore. Like, all of a sudden you're just done eating that amount and then it becomes a job. I remember having to set my alarm in the middle of the night in order to just maintain [the weight]. I would literally wake up at two in the morning and I'd have a cup of cold macaroni and cheese just next to me."[27]

(Side note: As a person who has *never* struggled with weight gain, I still find these accounts hard to believe and am often convinced they are part of the conspiracy to make us feel bad for hot people, like Ryan Reynolds, in an attempt to humanize them.)

How does your body regulate its internal weight range? Through a lot of complex biological processes.[28] Your body could upregulate or downregulate hunger signals, making you more or less likely to seek out food or overeat. Or your body could increase heat production (as with people that get really hot anytime they eat a big meal). Or it could downregulate hormones such as those controlling thyroid function, thereby lowering your basal metabolic rate (see chapter 2). Or it could spontaneously increase or decrease your movement throughout the day. It could make you go harder or less hard in a workout. There are so many factors that are able to be manipulated without us even necessarily noticing, which is at once insanely cool and also kind of scary.

A lot of these subtle biological changes are hard to study in humans. This is because our behaviors are driven by so many pressures *other than* our biology: psychological pressures, social pressures, environmental pressures, and so forth. Separating what is your biology from what is because you're feeling sad about some shitty guy on Hinge (oops, is this just me?) is hard. Either way, though, our biology is complex and powerful and often ignored. I spend most of my time operating as if I am in control of all my actions, and I don't care what is going on with my hormones—leptin, ghrelin, insulin, and free T4. While it's true that we are in control of our individual decisions, there are a lot of silent forces at play that influence our decision-making.

One question you may be asking is, If our bodies try to regulate our weight like a thermostat, why is my thermostat stuck at fifteen pounds above where I want it to be? Why would there be a weight problem at all? This appears to have to do mainly with the changes in our environment over the past fifty years, which has become much more "obesogenic": it's an environment that promotes eating in excess of energy needs. This change in the environment actually puts a constant pressure on the thermostat to go up. Meaning that living in an environment full of calorie-dense, delicious, and readily available foods *and* not having to move much throughout the day, combined with living in a society that doesn't promote good sleep habits *and* values work above all else, thus causing constant amounts of low-level stress—well, it matters. All these seem to move that thermostat from being in the sixties to being in the sweltering seventies or even eighties.

We are all subjected to these obesogenic pressures, and for a lot of us, excess energy slowly accumulates in the form of fat. But there are two things to point out here: first, the average American gains only about a pound a year, which roughly means that the body's "thermostat" is off by somewhere between 10 and 20 calories a day.[29] So really, your body is doing an excellent job, just not quite as excellent as you might want.

Second, it is also your body's inner thermostat that stops you from gaining weight infinitely. As your body is built to do, it adapts to the environment by increasing your metabolic rate as you gain weight. Bigger people have more tissues to upkeep, meaning they have a higher metabolism, and so eventually a new equilibrium is reached.[30] This is why we don't all continue gaining weight indefinitely despite continuing to live in the same obesogenic environment. For most of us, our bodies have a weight that they like to settle at, albeit a higher one than we may prefer.

The thing is: the mechanisms that our biology has in place to stop us from *losing* too much weight are likely much stronger and much more redundant than the mechanisms that are in place to stop us from *gaining* too much weight. And this makes sense: How often, in the past few thousand years, has the problem been, "Man, there's just too much yummy food! And I just sit on my butt all day!! What gives?" Much more likely, the problem our bodies evolved to adapt to was, "Bro, where the hell are all the plants and animals? I'm hungry and tired, and I've been looking around for days. . . . Send help!"

My Sister's Thermostat Works Better Than Mine

We are all subject to the same obesogenic environment, and yet some of us feel our thighs expanding if we so much as look at ice cream, and others seem to never give their weight a second thought. I was monitoring my pizza slices at birthdays at age twelve and secretly doing crunches in my bedroom every night. My sister was trying to see if she could finish an entire pizza by herself and was about thirty pounds lighter. My sister and I grew up in the exact same environment, so why did she never have to monitor her intake or movement? Why was her thermostat so dang quick to readjust?

To figure out what was going on, Paul MacLean and colleagues put rats in a similar obesogenic environment—lots of high-fat, high-carb rat chow available and not much movement—and they found a similar effect. Some rats gained weight (the obesity-prone, or OP, group) and some didn't (the obesity-resistant, or OR, group).[31] These groups experienced a positive energy balance, meaning both were consuming more than they were burning, but the OR rats seemed to spontaneously increase energy expenditure and fat oxidation and reestablish energy balance. The obesity-prone rodents, a.k.a. *me*, continued to eat in excess until the new weight they had gained had increased their body size, and consequently their metabolic rate, enough that they were once again at a new "homeostasis." There was nothing magical happening in the OR rats: they were still overeating by the same amount, but for some reason, their brains sensed it and modified behaviors and biology accordingly

Interestingly, it's the same mechanisms that *stopped* the OP rats from gaining weight indefinitely that explain the all-too-common weight regain post-diet. Your body's biological defenses kick into gear the moment your body starts to sense a negative energy balance. You say, "I'm gonna eat less and move more." Your body says, "Ha ha, go ahead and try." The homeostatic voodoo juju starts to take effect, and eventually it stalls all weight loss, even though you are not doing anything differently.

You probably have experienced this: the diet's been going well, you've been getting leaner, you're starting to look a little longer in the mirror, you get a few compliments here and there. All of a sudden, the scale won't freaking budge, even though you are still *busting your ass*. In order to instigate further weight loss, you need to kick all your weight-loss behaviors up a notch: drop calories even lower, increase movement even more. After several cycles of this process—reaching a plateau, eating less, moving more; reaching another plateau, eating even less, moving even more—you may eventually actually reach your goal weight, and guess what? In order to keep whatever weight loss you achieved, you need to not change a single thing you're doing . . . forever.

At the end of a diet, people often think that they can just go back to whatever they were doing before. We see diets as temporary hardships that we can power through until after the wedding, the photo shoot, the vacation. But the biological milieu of the post-weight-loss individual has a very different plan in mind, a plan that makes sticking to your new fitness-guru lifestyle extremely difficult.

Higher Appetite, Lower Movement: The Energy Gap

The first thing to note about losing weight is that it increases your appetite. This could be partially due to a decrease in the hormone leptin during a weight-loss phase. To understand this, we need to take a quick tour of the fat cell. Contrary to what may make intuitive sense, the number of fat cells in your body is fixed from around early adulthood on, meaning that you have the same number of fat cells (more or less) for your entire adult life.[32]

So how do you gain weight if you have the same number of fat cells for your entire life? Simple: your fat cells undergo hypertrophy; in other words, they grow. If you are eating in a calorie surplus and you have excess energy to store, your fat cells will swell up as they store more lipids. As you lose weight, the opposite happens: they shrink down. Think of them like little balloons, except instead of being filled with air, they're filled with lipids. Fat cells in humans can have anywhere from a 20-micrometer diameter to a 300-micrometer diameter, that's a more than a thousandfold difference in terms of volume.[33] So, basically, these suckers can get huge or get tiny.

Back to leptin. Leptin is a hormone that is primarily controlled by the *size* of fat cells. Less fat tissue, or *smaller* fat cells, produce *less* leptin. Bigger fat cells produce more leptin. Who cares? Well, the reason your body has this chemical messenger of fat-cell size is because it needs a way to communicate to your brain, your fatness level, a.k.a. your adiposity. I know what you're thinking: *Why is your brain so nosy, anyway? Why does it need to know your waistline? Isn't that your business alone?* Well, if your fat stores are low, your brain needs to know so that it can do all it can to replenish the ol' energy stores. So leptin tells your brain, "Not enough food! Alert! Alert!" and your brain responds by increasing appetite and lowering your motivation to move.

Once leptin gets to the part of your brain called the hypothalamus, it activates an array of neural peptides that are associated with increased or decreased feeding.[34] Because of this, leptin is often referred to as the "satiety hormone." High leptin usually means you have adequate amounts of fat tissue, which is reflected in a normal appetite. Lower leptin signals lower fat stores, which tells your brain, "We need food," and increases appetite. In fact, humans and rodents that are missing either leptin proteins or the receptors they bind to exhibit "voracious feeding." The increased appetite you may experience at the end of a diet only goes away when fat cells return to their original size, that is, once the lost weight has been regained.[35] Individuals who have maintained weight loss for years *still* experience a higher appetite than they did pre–weight loss.[36] This is another thing you have to be OK with if you want to maintain a lower weight.

(Side note: Reduced leptin leads to a host of other downstream effects, such as lowered energy expenditure, decreased thyroid and reproductive hormones, and decreased immunity.[37] To put it lightly . . . it's a pretty important hormone.)

A brief detour here: if you're wondering why we study these effects in rats instead of in humans, the answer is because humans are wack and interfere with their biology *all the freaking time*. A rat would never maintain a lower weight if it meant being permanently a little hungrier, but humans do it regularly.

When we study people (as opposed to rats), it is really hard to separate biological hunger, or the biological drive to eat, from the psychosocial drivers to eat. Us humans constantly exhibit cognitive restraint to meet goals, comply with societal standards, do better in our sports teams, fit in socially, and so forth. Rodents, on the other hand, do not purposefully eat less lab cheese in order to fit into a rodent bikini. Thus, their behaviors are a reflection of strictly their biology and environment. When we see that rodents, after being put on restricted calories for a period of time, will substantially increase their meal size until they have regained all the lost weight, it's a pretty good indicator that the biological driver to eat does truly change when you have been underfeeding; it's not just you "lacking willpower."[38,39]

Let's be clear: biology does not control our actions. But . . . your body *sure* wants you to eat that cookie—and that's even more true than usual at the end of a diet.

Now let's look at the other side of the energy equation, the energy out, or total daily energy expenditure. *(Yes! TDEE makes a comeback!)*

If you think back to chapter 2, our total daily energy expenditure is the energy that we spend in a day. It is made up of four components: your basal metabolic rate (this is just the energy you need to keep your body baseline functioning), thermic effect of food (the energy you use to digest food), nonexercise activity thermogenesis (the energy you burn doing unplanned movements throughout the day like walking, washing dishes, etc.), and exercise activity thermogenesis (the energy you burn in exercise). Well, it seems like dieting, or losing weight, impacts all of these components.

Starting with the most basic, when you lose weight, you are literally becoming a smaller person, and this affects your TDEE in three ways. First, a smaller person simply requires less fuel to keep alive: there are fewer cells, less tissue, less lean body mass, less fat mass—there's just less of your body that needs calories.[40] Consequently, your basal metabolic rate takes a hit, particularly since so much of BMR is driven by the amount of lean body mass. Even if nothing else was affected by weight loss, just by how metabolism works, you will need to eat less to maintain a smaller body for the rest of your life. A lighter version of you requires fewer calories than a heavier version of you. Given this undeniable reality, seeing a diet as just a "temporary thing" is already setting yourself up for failure.

Secondly, as a smaller person, you also require fewer calories to move around.[41] If you've ever tried doing exercise with a weight vest on, you viscerally understand this. In one of my New Year's resolution frenzies, I bought a twenty-pound vest that I vowed to wear for all my nightly walks. (I had heard a Navy Seal on a podcast say he did this, and I thought . . . *perfect!*) Of course, this lasted all of two walks . . . literally. Even walking to Starbucks with the vest was exhausting, and that's with only twenty pounds of excess weight. Since the same tasks in a larger body require more energy, losing weight also decreases not only the number of calories you would burn during typical exercise sessions, it also decreases all the calories you burn throughout the day just doing regular tasks like standing, walking, cleaning, and so on. So NEAT and EAT both go down, even if you change nothing about your movement patterns.

And finally, the reduced fat mass also seems to lower energy expenditure by changing the metabolic efficiency of homeostatic processes through leptin and insulin reduction. OK, I know that last sentence went in one ear and out the other, so let's break it down. The impact of body mass on your BMR, EAT, and NEAT is pretty straightforward: less person = fewer or smaller cells = less energy needed. But studies have also shown that there is a reduction in basal metabolic rate even *beyond* what you would expect from just the lower body mass. Let's say you get your body weight down to 160 pounds from 180 pounds with weeks of dieting and exercise. Your metabolic rate at the end of this diet would likely be slower than that of an identical 160-pound person who moves and eats the exact same way as you. From the classic understanding of energy expenditure, this would not make sense, because, all things being identical, two people of the same size should have the same metabolic rate. But it appears that the body will increase the efficiency of other metabolic processes in the weight-loss process to conserve energy and thus will actually leave you with a slower metabolism than you would expect given your new lower weight.

This is perhaps a milder version of the same concept of metabolic adaptation that we talked about in chapter 2 with the Hadza tribe and the *Biggest Loser* contestants: Your body is becoming a Tesla, except not in the sense that it's a sexy car to show off that you're cool and have money. . . . More like it requires a lot less gas.[42,43]

Another component of this equation is that people exhibit less unconscious movement when they are on a diet, further lowering their energy expenditure from exercise and nonexercise.[44] Again, in humans this can be a bit harder to study because there are other motivations besides biology that compel us to maintain exercise levels: we go to the gym even if we're tired; we go on a walk to meet our step goals. But in rats, you can see this effect more clearly, because they don't force themselves to ever move if they don't have to, just to "stay fit." The more obesity-prone rats that have lost weight lower their "volitional wheel running" and are less compliant with "daily treadmill exercise" during their weight regain. How the hell you get rats to comply at all with "daily treadmill exercise" is beyond me, but that's not the point: biology, again in an attempt to undo the weight loss and reinstate homeostasis, appears to decrease intrinsic physical activity and the motivation to be active.

Finally, it should be mentioned that the last part of TDEE, the thermic effect of food, is also decreased after weight loss.[45] This is simply because you are eating less food, so there is less food to ingest, absorb, metabolize, store, and so forth. (Yes, this is probably a "smaller" effect, in the grand scheme of things, but I'm just trying to be thorough here, people.)

So, as you can see, at the end of a diet, biology is just not on your side. You experience increased appetite and a suppressed total daily energy expenditure, and these two create a devilishly clever cocktail of circumstances that scientists have dubbed . . . (pause for dramatic effect) "the energy gap."[46] I mean, seriously, can we not come up with a more dramatic title? Like, I'm over here busting my ass, exhausted and hungry, and the best science can do is say, "You're experiencing the energy gap"?! Anyway, I'm not saying that long-term weight loss is impossible, because it clearly isn't (20 percent of people are still able to maintain a 10 percent weight loss after three years).[47] But I *am* saying it's hard.

Primed for Weight Gain

Now let's say you do reach your goal weight at the end of a diet; not only do you experience an energy gap that drives the impetus to regain weight, but your body seems to be better at retaining fat. Oh yes, you guessed it: it doesn't get easier. It turns out that being in a weight-loss phase actually makes your body much more efficient at capturing and holding on to fat, for a variety of reasons.

First, as you lose weight, you are improving your insulin sensitivity (which is actually a good thing healthwise), but improved insulin sensitivity also means that your body will preferentially shuttle fat into fat cells instead of using it for energy.[48] Again, while improved insulin sensitivity is generally a good thing, it also primes your body for weight gain if you overeat. Obviously, if you never overeat after your diet, this isn't really a problem, but if you're like me and get elbow-deep into a six-serving bag of white-chocolate Peppermint Pretzel Slims the second they come out in November . . . let's just say the Trader Joe's market share of holiday snacks is not the only thing expanding.

Energy-restricted weight loss also seems to change gene expression in several areas of the body, including the liver, skeletal muscle, and fat tissue, in a way that facilitates more efficient weight regain.[49] For example, as you lose weight and your fat cells shrink, they experience a global downregulation of several genes, a.k.a. a change in gene "expression." As you transition into weight maintenance and weight regain, your fat cells change to an expression profile that favors fat storage.[50] "How can this be?" I hear you asking. "Your genes are set at birth; what do you mean they're changing their expression?"

Many people think that our genes are static, rigid things that serve as little instruction manuals telling our cells what to do. But in reality, the past few decades of the field of epigenetics have shown us that the way genes are *expressed,* meaning whether they are turned on or off, is actually quite dependent on external factors, such as your environment and behaviors. Weight loss, followed by weight maintenance or weight gain, turns on genes in your fat cells that make them better able to store excess calories as body fat the next time you overeat.[51]

To understand this a little more clearly: imagine a set of twins who have the same total daily energy expenditure and the same DNA. One twin is at the end of a diet, one is not. If they both eat the same size "cheat meal," in which they go way over their calorie budget for the day, the one at the end of the diet would gain more weight after this meal, even though it was just as much of a caloric surplus for that twin as for the other. Your body is just more efficient at storing fat at the end of a prolonged calorie deficit.

Finally (and I swear we will stop here because I'm getting kind of depressed writing this), not only does your body (a) create an energy gap that promotes more eating and less energy expenditure, and (b) capture more of the calories you overeat when you do inevitably overeat, it may also (c) give you a higher capacity for excess weight in the future.[52]

If you recall back to our tour of the fat cell, you'll remember that you pretty much have a fixed number of fat cells for your entire life. Losing weight causes them to shrink; gaining weight causes them to expand. However, some recent research (again in rodents) suggests that in certain metabolic conditions—that is, upon refeeding after weight loss—a small number of new fat cells are created.[53] *Who cares?* you may be thinking. . . . Well, this increased number of fat cells also means an increased capacity for fat storage.

What we've seen in *some* rodents who diet down and then are allowed to refeed is that they stop overeating once they have reached their pre-diet weight and (not coincidentally) once their fat cells return to their pre-diet size. This is obviously the work of the "internal weight thermostat." And you would logically think that your body senses the amount of total fat tissue and basically propels you to overeat until you reach that amount of fat tissue. But it actually seems like this thermostat is controlled by *fat-cell size.* In studies, rats will continue overeating until their fat cells are the exact same size as they were pre-diet, almost to the micrometer.[54]

But here's the rub: the rats that showed increased numbers of fat cells did the same thing as the rats who didn't—that is, they overate until their fat-cell diameter went back to what it was pre–weight loss, except . . . they have *more* fat cells, which means they gain *more* weight than they lost and overshoot their original weight. There is some evidence that this phenomenon of fat-cell hyperplasia (or the creation of new fat cells) also occurs in humans upon rapid refeeding after weight loss, but the exact mechanisms are still not understood, and it's something that likely happens in a small subset of humans. If you think about it, your fat cells are each little pockets of potential fat storage, and if you increase the number of fat cells, you are basically increasing your overall capacity to store fat.[55]

Although it definitely needs further study, the phenomenon of fat-cell hyperplasia may explain why the act of getting leaner and then rapidly regaining weight, over and over again, makes it harder for you to lose weight in the future. Many people will anecdotally report that they were able to easily lose weight on their first diet, but as they went through more and more diet cycles, it took more drastic measures and a longer timescale to achieve the same weight loss. Similarly, you may notice that the more you diet, the more quickly you regain weight *after* each diet. The physiological changes in fat cells may in part explain a lot of the effects we see of yo-yo dieting, particularly how people will often steadily gain weight in the long run even though they are always "on a diet" in the short run. It may be that (through these changes in fat cells) your body has some sort of "diet memory" that makes it more resistant to weight loss in future calorie-restriction phases.

Should Weight Loss Even Be a Goal?

The last thing I want is for this research to make people give up and say, "There's no point, I'm just gonna eat whatever and do whatever because it's impossible." Firstly, we know it's not impossible, because it has been done, even if by a small portion of the population who attempt it. But if you'll indulge me for a second, my real moral dilemma comes with whether it's even a good idea to pursue weight loss in the first place. The biological factors that make it difficult are one thing, but the health implications of multiple weight-loss failures . . . that's another. If there's one thing everyone agrees on, it's that repeated bouts of weight cycling (losing weight, then regaining it) are extremely unhealthy.

Long-term dramatic weight loss is *not* a requirement of a "successful lifestyle change" (see chapter 4, "Weight and Health"). You can 100 percent improve your health and not lose a pound on the scale, and that doesn't mean you've failed. For years, I pursued weight loss as my singular goal, and it made me more and more sick. I ate nutrient-poor foods because they were labeled "low-fat" and "high-protein." I was terrified of avocados because of how many calories they contained. I exercised too much. I lost my period for years, had the hormonal profile of a sixty-year-old woman, and missed out on priceless social experiences that I will never be able to get back, all on top of the mental anguish of constantly hating my body (more on this in the eating-disorders section in chapter 8). Clearly I was not "healthier" even though I was lighter. But at the same time, maintaining even a 5 percent weight loss for those who are overweight does confer health benefits regardless of how the weight loss is achieved.[56]

Living with these two truths is confusing and complex, especially when people want to put you in one extreme or the other. When you talk about the mountains of research saying that diets don't work, you automatically get put in the camp of "weight is entirely out of your control and you shouldn't even bother." On the other hand, if you talk about weight loss, calories, food choices, and exercise, you are accused of promoting eating disorders, overexercising, and an unhealthy relationship with your body.

I fundamentally believe in people's freedom to do whatever they want with their bodies, as long as they are making an informed decision. This book is meant to provide you with the science on both sides: the science of successful weight loss, if that's your goal, and the science of just being healthier and happier, regardless of weight. Choosing to eat more nutrient-dense foods, moving your body, cultivating a healthier mindset, nurturing better relationships, getting a better night's sleep, reducing stress—all impact short- and long-term health. Sometimes weight loss is a by-product of developing better lifestyle habits. Sometimes it's not, and that's OK.

When I was growing up, I did not have the information to go about setting dietary and fitness goals in a responsible way, and I really messed up because of it. So regardless of what you want to pursue—whether it's a bikini bod, or being a badass in the gym, or even just living a longer, happier life—I want you to have scientifically backed information to help you make your decisions.

In the next chapter, we'll explore whether weight and health are truly linked or if it's just a plot by Big Pharma and protein-shake companies to keep you on the treadmill, taking medications, and munching on lettuce leaves for the rest of your life.

From the Doc

Secrets of Those Who "Keep It Off"

Despite the somewhat gloomy prognosis of how most weight-loss efforts fail or even backfire with subsequent weight gain, some of us do succeed in keeping the weight off. You can easily find anecdotal success stories on social media or infomercials, complete with before-and-after photos. But what if we could collect data from large numbers of individuals who have maintained their weight loss? Could we then discern patterns or habits that might be helpful to the rest of us who are not yet quite as successful?

That's what Rena Wing, PhD, of Brown University and James O. Hill, PhD, of the University of Colorado set out to answer when they established the National Weight Control Registry (NWCR) in 1993. Their question: What are people who are successful at long-term weight-loss maintenance doing differently than the rest of us? The NWCR is the largest prospective study of individuals maintaining long-term weight loss, tracking more than ten thousand people who have lost at least thirty pounds and kept it off for more than a year. Although there is tremendous variability within the registry, members have lost an average of sixty-six pounds and kept it off for an average of 5.5 years. The registry members complete an annual survey about their behavioral and psychological strategies, giving us some insights.

Here are some general stats: 98 percent of members report modifying their food intake (no surprises there); 94 percent report increased physical activity, with the most common activity being walking (again, not too shocking); and 78 percent eat breakfast every day. But there's more to be learned from the NWCR.

Exercise

Physical activity appears to be one of the most important commonalities among people who lose weight and successfully keep it off, even though the calories burned in exercise are not sufficient on their own to cause them to lose weight. When it comes to *why* exercise is so crucial for weight-loss maintenance, the exact mechanisms are not fully understood. One plausible theory is that exercise helps diminish some of the biological changes that are associated with weight loss, a.k.a. some of the mechanisms that promote weight gain. That is, exercise may help attenuate the dreaded "energy gap" by decreasing overfeeding while increasing energy expenditure.[57]

In the National Weight Control Registry, more than 85 percent of men and women report using physical activity as a weight-maintenance strategy, and the average NWCR member is markedly more active than the average American, averaging about 60–75 minutes per day of moderate-intensity exercise, like brisk walking, or about 35–45 minutes per day of higher intensity exercise.[58] (For reference, current recommendations from the *Physical Activity Guidelines for Americans* are at least 150 minutes of moderate-intensity exercise or 75 minutes of vigorous-intensity exercise per week.[59]) The data also shows that the more active you are, the lower the incidence of weight regain. So the bottom line is, exercise may not be the silver bullet for losing weight, but it sure is crucial for keeping it off.

Self-Monitoring and Tracking

You may have a love-hate relationship with your scale, but those who successfully maintain weight loss do tend to monitor their weight (44 percent weigh themselves daily, 31 percent weigh themselves about once a week). In fact, reductions in "self-monitoring" are associated with increased weight regain.[60,61] The logic goes, if you see your weight creeping up, you are more likely to make behavior changes to counteract the regain. A 2017 study found that 92 percent of members of the NWCR used some sort of weight-, diet-, or exercise-tracking tool. Participants had 23.1 times greater odds of success by using diet-, food-, or calorie-tracking apps and 15.5 times greater odds by using weight-monitoring apps as compared to the general population.[62] However, for a subset of the population, self-monitoring might be more harmful than helpful, particularly for those individuals who are predisposed to developing an eating disorder or who tie a lot of their self-worth to their body.[63] As always, take study data with a grain of salt: it's true that individuals who weigh themselves exhibit a higher likelihood of maintaining weight loss, but that doesn't mean that you have to weigh yourself or constantly watch the scale to lose weight and keep it off.

Dietary Restraint and Dietary Patterns

This just in: those who are able to successfully maintain weight loss tend to eat a low-calorie and (relatively) low-fat diet.[64] This is not because eating low-fat is beneficial to losing weight but because cutting out calorically dense processed food also often drastically cuts down on fat consumption. For example, in a similar study done on the Portuguese Weight Control Registry, the participants were found to also eat a lower-calorie diet, but their diet was higher in fat because the prevalent "diet" in Portugal is the Mediterranean diet, which is rich in higher-fat foods like olive oil, fatty fish, and the like.[65]

Some other behaviors associated with maintenance of weight loss were having healthy foods available in the house, increasing fiber intake, and increasing protein intake (both fiber and protein have been shown to help with satiation).[66] The NWCR in the United States and the Portuguese Weight Control Registry report that the majority of the participants consume breakfast on a regular basis. Furthermore, both report that participants exhibit some sort of cognitive restraint, meaning they do exhibit some restraint in their eating patterns, whether it's counting calories or being mindful of portions, and so on.[67,68]

The Psychology of Keeping It Off

We've talked about the behavioral characteristics of those who have success-fully maintained significant weight loss, but none of it was that surprising. I know what you're thinking: *You're telling me that to successfully maintain a lower weight you have to moderate food intake, exercise on a regular basis, and check your progress every once in a while?* Perhaps more nuanced insights are the psychological patterns of those who successfully maintain weight loss.

These individuals showed a lesser degree of "dichotomous thinking" com-pared to those who did regain weight.[69] Dichotomous thinking is reducing everything to black and white: *I didn't reach my goal weight, so I'm a failure. I ate one cookie, so I blew the diet. I'm not where I want to be, so I suck.* Fortunately, behavior change is generally much more subtle than glowing success versus unmitigated failure. Even walking a few hundred extra steps or getting to bed fifteen minutes earlier can create positive effects.

Those who successfully maintained weight loss also showed a lower amount of comfort or emotional eating, or eating as a way to regulate mood, and "disinhibition," which is uncontrolled eating.[70] The logic be-hind this is pretty straightforward: if you're eating to regulate emotions or cope with stressors, you're going to eat a lot more than you probably need (at least calorically). But this points to an interesting solution: for some, finding a better way to cope with stress—like lifting weights in the gym for Juna or bicycling for me—rather than drastic eating-behavior modi-fication may be the real untapped gold mine when it comes to long-term improvement of health outcomes.

Two factors positively associated with successful weight-loss mainte-nance were perceived benefits outweighing perceived costs and improved body image.[71] These factors speak to two really important things about the psychology of weight loss, or even health-behavior modifications. What-ever you get out of making these changes, it had better be good, and it had better be more than just "I want to look better" (more in chapter 12). If you can really focus on the benefits you might feel when you eat better, move more, hydrate, and so on, it may help you maintain those behaviors. And beating yourself up for how you look won't help you. A poorer body image was associated with weight regain, so don't think you're going to hate your body into submission.

Does This Apply to Me?

Using the NWCR or other similar weight-control registries as the be-all and end-all for weight-loss-maintenance hacks is problematic. For one thing, the NWCR is not a representative sample of the population: about 96 percent of participants are white, 80 percent are women, and 55 percent have a college degree. The founders of the registry themselves have stated, "Because this is not a random sample of those who attempt weight loss, the results have limited generalizability to the entire population of over-weight and obese individuals."[72] Other drawbacks of the NWCR are that all survey data is self-reported, and all the studies conducted are observational, which shows us correlation but not necessarily causation.

Either way, whether you think the NWCR is a valuable database from which to draw research or not, the fact is that none of the findings are that surprising: people who tend to successfully maintain a meaningful amount of weight loss also tend to eat in moderation, exercise regularly, sleep well, eat breakfast, and monitor themselves and their behaviors. Simply put, these are things that we all know to do, and the real question is how to implement them.

The Takeaways

Why All Diets Work

- All diets that result in weight loss are creating a calorie deficit, meaning you are eating fewer calories than you are burning.

- A diet can create a calorie deficit by simply imposing a calorie target, or through other methods such as restricting certain food groups or time windows for eating.

- Foods are made up of macronutrients and micronutrients. Macronutrients (carbohydrates, fat, and protein) contain calories while micronutrients do not.

- Low-fat diets and low-carb diets result in the same amount of weight loss as long as the diets are equated for calories and grams of protein.

Why (Almost) All Diets Fail

- Most people will regain the weight they lose on a diet.

- Dieting, particularly for lean or normal-weight individuals, may predict future weight gain.

- The relationship between dieting and weight gain appears to be bidirectional: those who are predisposed to weight gain are likely to engage in more dieting, but the act of dieting may play a causal role in future weight gain.

- Reasons for weight regain after a diet include the fact that people view diets as temporary, and that after a diet, there is a biological drive to regain weight.

- After a diet, there are many biological mechanisms that prime your body for weight regain, including increased appetite, slowed metabolism, and physiological changes that facilitate fat storage.

- It's likely that your body has a "set range" of weight that it prefers to stay within. Coming out of this range at either end results in significant biological resistance.

- Dietary changes should be viewed as permanent lifestyle changes, not temporary bouts of misery to suffer through until "X" goal is achieved.

4

Weight and Health

The Obesity Epidemic or the Obesity "Epidemic"

Here's a question: Why talk about weight at all? Increasingly, the messaging around healthy eating and exercising is being separated from simply wanting to look a certain way. I think this is freaking awesome, because we all know how frustrating trying to change your body weight can be. Appearances and societal norms aside, is it truly possible to be healthy at any size? Or is there validity to the idea that excess body fat is causing poorer health outcomes? Welcome to the shark-infested waters of the obesity epidemic versus the obesity "epidemic."

Want a surefire way to get a ton of people really angry with you instantly? Make a claim about whether or not obesity is "bad for us." It works like a charm every time. If there's ever a lull in the conversation, or your life is getting too boring, you can just throw it out there: "Yeah, you know the whole obesity epidemic is fake, right?" Or, alternatively, "Yeah, our weight is basically killing us, so . . . yes, I *did* just do my five-hundredth ride at SoulCycle!! Thanks for remembering!" On the one hand, obesity has always been equated to poor health by public-health officials and the media, so *obviously*, it can't be healthy. On the other hand, some will claim that talking about the obesity epidemic in anything but air quotes is blasphemous, a perpetuation of diet culture, and promotes a narrative that fat is bad when there is no scientific evidence to prove it.

Back in 2019, to prepare for an episode of the *Food, We Need to Talk* podcast, I had two interviews scheduled with different experts: one a prominent obesity-medicine doctor at a top hospital in Massachusetts, the other a researcher and associate professor at a top West Coast university. The doctor was adamant that obesity was a disease that needed to be treated as such. Just like heart disease or cancer, it was not the patient's fault, and medications and surgical interventions were vastly underutilized because people saw it as a moral failing, not a true biological impairment.

I finished that call, dialed into the next one (another interview for the same podcast episode), and was promptly told obesity is protective against many diseases and there is no evidence to suggest that it is "bad" for you. If anything, it leads to *better* health outcomes. In the span of one hour, I was being told by two very smart people exactly opposite things. On top of that, I had managed to mildly upset both of them: getting yelled at by one for not using "person-first language"—for example, "person with obesity" (oops!)—and by the other for calling obesity a disease (something I had just been told thirty minutes ago . . . *by a doctor at one of the best hospitals in America*). Needless to say, I was baffled, and also very thankful I had never pursued journalism.

Obesity and Health Outcomes

Obesity is defined as having a body mass index (BMI) of ≥ 30. (BMI is an indicator of relative weight for height; see "Why the BMI Sucks" later in this chapter for more info.) Obesity is a risk factor for type 2 diabetes, lipid disorders, coronary heart disease, hypertension, and even certain types of cancers.[1] Yes, these are "associations," but there is strong evidence to suggest that excess fat tissue, particularly abdominal fat (or visceral fat, which coats our liver and other organs, as opposed to fat on the lower body, which may actually be protective) does play a causal role in our overall health.[2,3]

The implications of getting the causality-versus-association business sorted out are huge. More than two-thirds of the US population is either overweight or obese, so understanding the findings are critical for the majority of us.[4] And for the first time in decades, US life expectancy has been decreasing (since the year 2014, aside from the effects of COVID).[5]

Granted, obesity is only one of the reasons for the decrease in life expectancy (along with increased drug overdoses, deaths from suicide, etc.), but still, understanding obesity and its related diseases is one of the biggest challenges of the twenty-first century.

An early landmark finding in the debate of whether or not it's unhealthy to have obesity came in 2004, when authors from the Centers for Disease Control and Prevention published a study that attributed 400,000 deaths in one year to poor diet and lack of physical activity, second only to deaths from tobacco (some 435,000 deaths).[6] This led to the various warnings along the lines of "Obesity is just as bad as smoking," which you may have encountered.

The only problem: *some* statistical modifications were not copied properly onto some spreadsheets, and so the calculations were actually a pretty big overestimation, leading to the authors having to submit a correction.[7] In the scientific community, this is what we call *the tea*! You do *not* want to issue a correction. (Interestingly, according to Google Scholar, the original, statistically flawed paper has been cited at least ten times as much as the correction. I guess sensationalist headlines are more attractive than "Oopsies, we goofed! Forgot to copy and paste.") Even so, the authors insisted that although the number might have been slightly elevated, it would not change the overall conclusions of the paper: tobacco and obesity were the two leading causes of death in the United States, and obesity, unlike smoking, was increasing.[8]

Of course, the drama of "issuing a correction" was a field day for the obesity "epidemic" skeptics, because it proved what they had been saying all along: the evil health insurance companies and Big Pharma are dying to make obesity seem like a bigger problem than it is so they can continue bringing in the dough at the expense of all the poor souls who are just out here trying to live their best lives without suffering through SlimFast and spin classes forever.[9] The plot only thickened when, the very next year, another CDC researcher came out with a different study, which stated that obesity was only associated with about 112,000 extra deaths in a given year, and being overweight was not associated with *any* excess deaths.[10] A meta-analysis (a.k.a. a study looking at a bunch of studies) in 2013 found a similar result: while *obesity* was associated with earlier death, those who were overweight compared to those who were normal weight appeared to live longer.[11] These findings were slowly building up, corroborating an effect called the "obesity paradox."

How can one study report that being overweight is associated with better health outcomes than being normal weight while another study seems to suggest the opposite?[12]

The "Obesity Paradox"

The obesity paradox has been observed in many contexts: for example, one study found that patients with obesity and coronary heart disease undergoing coronary catheterization had better outcomes than patients with normal weight.[13] Patients with normal weight had higher rates of in-hospital complications, like cardiac death, at one-year follow-ups. In patients with coronary heart disease and hypertension (high blood pressure), the occurrence of death, stroke, and nonfatal myocardial infarctions were lower in people who were overweight or had obesity as compared to normal-weight patients. The paradox continues, though: patients with a higher BMI had a decreased mortality from chronic heart failure than those with a lower BMI. Protective effects of overweight and obesity were also observed in the following diseases: peripheral arterial disease, stroke, thromboembolism, chronic obstructive pulmonary disease, and these are just a few on a much longer list.[14]

The obesity paradox is often cited by proponents as the reason why we shouldn't care about excess weight. If obesity and overweight are, in fact, protective against diseases, then behaviors like dieting are not only a pain in the ass but, in the small percentage of cases in which they do work, they may actually be making us unhealthier. However, several considerations may complicate this black-and-white reading of these associations:

First, let's consider the issue of selection bias. Many of the studies that support the obesity paradox were conducted on study populations of older adults. For example, in a group of nine studies confirming the obesity paradox, eight of them had study populations of an average age greater than sixty-two years. Because there are different risks associated with *where fat is stored*, a plausible explanation of these findings is that those with riskier "abdominal obesity" died at a younger age.[15,16] Thus, the older patients eventually included in the obesity-paradox studies may have been those that simply survived longer with less risky lower-body obesity . . . not a representative sample of people with obesity overall.

Second, the BMI in these studies is not measuring what we think it's measuring. (See the sidebar "Why the BMI Sucks" later in this chapter.) It conflates high body-fat levels with high lean body mass (nonfat tissues such as muscle and bone). In one study, for example, researchers used dual-energy X-ray absorptiometry (DEXA) to measure patients' body composition. I'll spare you the details, but basically, a machine shoots X-rays through your tissues, and in about fifteen minutes, you get a pretty accurate fat-and-muscle map of your entire body. After doing these DEXA scans and having accurate body-composition data, the researchers found that in this group of patients with coronary heart failure (ages sixty-two to sixty-six), BMI was a more accurate predictor of lean body mass (muscle, bone, organs, etc.) than adiposity (fat tissue).[17]

In other words, in this older population with heart disease, BMI acted as a slightly better indicator for muscle mass than fat tissue. In this study, higher lean body mass, and thus lower body fat, was associated with markers of improved mortality in acute and chronic heart disease. Because BMI, in this population, was a slightly better predictor of lean body mass, when you don't look closer, all you see is that higher BMI is correlated with better health outcomes. While this is true, the underlying mechanism appears to be the lean body mass, not the fat tissue.[18]

Furthermore, higher mortality in older patients with low BMI could also be a reflection of the poor health outcomes associated with "sarcopenic" obesity, which is characterized not by high fat mass but by low muscle mass (the scientific rendition of skinny-fat).[19] Basically, the BMI is not a very accurate indicator of what is going on. A higher BMI is indicating a higher weight, but is the higher weight because of higher fat stores or more muscle? If it's more fat, is it riskier abdominal fat or more protective lower body fat? All of these details cause very different effects on disease outcomes. Instead of just using BMI, a proxy measure of both low body fat and high muscle actually appeared to be the best predictor of mortality in men aged sixty to seventy-nine.[20] In this population, low waist circumference (less than forty inches) and above-median muscle mass exhibited the lowest mortality rate.[21]

Another thing to consider is reverse causality (confusing the effect of something with the cause).[22] Think about what happens to a person when he or she gets really sick, often losing a ton of weight. Even if previously obese, patients may be normal or even underweight at the time of death. Therefore, not taking into account history of obesity could have actually misclassified these patients: they may not be having worse health outcomes *because* they're normal weight, they are normal weight *because* they were very sick.

Several studies have also shown an attrition bias: the health effects of obesity take decades to manifest, while the health effects of being underweight play out in a relatively short time; this is because being drastically underweight is often a sign of severe illness and/or malnourishment. Since the average follow-up period of studies is approximately two years, they may be biased toward the negative health outcomes associated with a lower weight.[23]

And finally, we should mention smoking. Smoking, shocking to everyone, I know, is not good for you, like *really* not good. It's associated with many diseases and, more importantly, a very high increase in mortality. Smoking is *also* associated with a lower BMI. (Remember when people used that as a way to lose weight back in the day?) In a meta-analysis of more than 230 studies, looking at thirty million participants, the lowest risk of mortality in *never-smokers* was found at a BMI of 23–24 (well within the "normal weight" category).[24] And when researchers looked only at studies that had a greater than twenty-year follow-up period, again, just looking at never-smokers, a BMI of 20–22 was associated with the lowest mortality. For reference, this is the lower to midrange of "normal weight."

So Should We Be Worried About Our Weight?

What does this mean? Should we all be trying to get down to a BMI of 20–22? Because if so, everyone, say a prayer for me . . . I haven't seen that weight on a scale since age thirteen. But before you order your SlimFast, there are a few things to think about.

Remember that all studies look at these effects "on average." This means that "on average," for nonsmokers, a BMI of 20–22 was associated with the lowest risk of mortality, but that doesn't mean *for you* this is the healthiest weight. Think of someone who had been diagnosed with anorexia nervosa, for example, the most lethal psychiatric disorder, characterized by severe food restriction and being underweight.[25] Does this mean we should stop the person's recovery as he or she barely creeps into the normal-weight category? On the other hand, think of someone who has grown up being active and playing sports, and therefore has an above-average muscle mass. Should we tell the person to starve and stop working out to let his or her body atrophy into the most optimal BMI? Neither of these people are likely see optimal health outcomes at the supposed "optimal BMI." In other words, there is no way to base what your "ideal" weight should be off of population-based studies.

Secondly, as we've seen, the ramifications of losing weight, or should I say "attempting" to lose weight, may be worse than a slightly higher BMI. This is because—breaking news—*it usually doesn't work*.[26] Crash dieting not only fails to produce long-lasting weight loss but, for complex biological reasons, often leads to weight gain, particularly in lean and normal-weight individuals (in other words, it does the opposite of what it's intended to do).[27] Plus, repeated periods of weight cycling (losing weight and gaining weight) are actually associated with a whole host of adverse health outcomes far beyond excess fat accumulation.[28] So if the vast majority of people don't succeed in weight loss, for many reasons far beyond their own "discipline" or capabilities, and if it may worsen health outcomes, it doesn't exactly make sense to chance some supposed improved health markers on an, in all likelihood, failed weight-loss attempt.

Is Fat the Real Problem?

If there actually is some association between a lower BMI and health outcomes, it's important to understand *why*. Why is obesity, or excess body fat, specifically, associated with negative health outcomes? Is it the excess fat? Is it the location of the excess fat? Or is excess fat just a physical indicator of the real cause, namely, eating more than your body needs and the stresses this puts on your metabolic system?

One thing that is pretty clear at this stage is that the location of fat *does* matter. We know, for example, that measures of central fat (fat in the abdominal area) and visceral fat (the fat around your organs) are more associated with chronic health conditions and all-cause mortality than obesity. Put another way: regardless of overall fatness, a larger waist circumference and waist-to-hip ratio predict poorer health outcomes.[29] So it's entirely feasible that you could have a BMI in the "normal" range and still be at higher risk for many chronic diseases because you have a lot of fat around your organs—a reason for even individuals in the "normal" weight category to be careful basing their health status on their weight alone.

Visceral fat is associated with chronic disease perhaps because it produces immune-system chemicals called cytokines (tumor necrosis factor and interleukin-6 are two examples). These chemicals can reduce insulin sensitivity and increase blood pressure and blood clotting, all factors involved in the development of cardiovascular disease and diabetes.[30] Similarly, excess visceral fat can overburden the liver with free fatty acids, thereby leading to insulin resistance.[31]

The problem is, you can't really choose *where* you store fat, and as you gain weight in general, some will get deposited around your organs. Similarly, as you lose weight, you will also lose some visceral fat. Perhaps if we had a magic wand that would only allow our bodies to gain weight in the right *places*, we wouldn't see much of a health impact of obesity at all.

On a positive note, exercise may be the closest thing we have to a magic wand in regard to visceral fat. As we'll discuss in chapters 6 and 7, even with *no changes* in overall body weight, exercise has been shown to lower visceral, abdominal, and subcutaneous fat (the fat you can feel).[32] This is because when you exercise, you can increase your muscle mass while simultaneously losing fat, something not necessarily reflected in your weight. If you start training and the scale doesn't budge, you're probably still reducing the more harmful fat around your organs and abdomen. In fact, there is evidence that exercise, in individuals who are overweight, may cause a relatively greater reduction in visceral fat as compared to subcutaneous fat.[33]

Studies in genetically engineered mice also seem to suggest that it may not be excess fat but rather the thing that leads to excess fat, namely excess calories, that's the issue. We know that when we take in excess calories, some of the fatty acids get stored in our fat cells, and some continue to circulate in the blood. When mice are genetically engineered to be *very good* at fat storage (like they shuttle all the extra calories they eat into fat cells), they don't develop a lot of the negative health markers associated with obesity, such as insulin resistance.[34]

In this way, we can almost see storage of excess calories in fat cells as protective against the burden that excess lipids in the blood places on our bodies. In fact, stopping excess calorie intake (or stopping overeating) will cause immediate improvements in many blood markers, such as triglycerides. This is probably why we see even small amounts of weight loss (5–10 percent) substantially improve markers like blood pressure, glycemia, and HDL cholesterol.[35] It may not be the fact that a person is losing fat but rather that a person is no longer gaining fat, or eating an excess of calories, that seems to immediately improve health markers even with tiny amounts of weight loss.

The One Thing We All Agree On: Weight Stigma

While people may have conflicting views on the dangers of excess fat tissue, something that both the experts I spoke to (in the beginning of the chapter) unequivocally agreed on—and, indeed, almost everyone agrees on—are the dangers of weight stigma. Weight stigma is when people experience verbal or physical abuse due to being overweight or obese. We definitely don't need a study for this, but nevertheless it has been shown that people with overweight or obesity are thought to be lazy, incompetent, unmotivated, noncompliant, sloppy, lacking self-discipline, and lacking in willpower.[36] While other forms of discrimination, such as gender- or race-based stereotyping, are frowned upon in society today, weight-based stereotyping is not.

Here are just a few of the documented manifestations of weight discrimination:[37]

- Compared to similarly qualified colleagues in a thinner body, individuals with overweight or obesity get promoted less, are hired less, and are stigmatized by colleagues and supervisors.

- Hiring managers are more likely to hire a less qualified person in a thinner body than a more qualified person in a larger body.

- People with obesity get paid less than their thinner colleagues; for example, women who have obesity get paid 6 percent less than "normal weight" women.

- In the health-care setting, medical professionals reported having less respect for their patients with obesity, having less desire to help them, and feeling that treating obesity was "more annoying" and "a waste of their time." This may be why people with obesity are less likely to seek medical care and go to doctors' visits, which can severely impact health outcomes because diseases don't get caught as early. In a study of women with obesity, 69 percent reported being stigmatized because of their weight by their doctors. Who wants to go to a doctor's office where the person caring for you is treating you awfully?

- In schools, teachers have been shown to perceive students in bigger bodies as having lower social, physical, reasoning, and cooperation skills. They also have lower expectations of these students.

- In media, people in bigger bodies are more likely to be cast as minor characters, often the object of ridicule, less likely to have romantic partners or friends, and more likely to be depicted engaging in stereotypical behaviors like overeating and binge eating.

Anyone who's lived in America for about two seconds can probably think of examples of all these biases. But there are many who think (though maybe don't explicitly state): *Yeah, you're fat because of your own lack of discipline; you should face the consequences.* Besides just being kind of a shitty way of thinking, I don't think a lot of these people know what the research on weight stigma shows. They think that weight stigma works like a Hollywood movie: Ryan Reynolds, a dorky, fat kid in high school, is in love with his hot cheerleader best friend. He gets bullied for his weight and dorkiness, leaves his hometown, and with a quick fade to black, has turned into a hot, sexy, lean L.A. big shot who gets all the girls he wants (yes, this is the plot of *Just Friends,* and however unreasonable, I watch that movie every Christmas because I am a Ryan Reynolds *stan*). The problem is, this is fantasy that perpetuates weight stigma; making fun of someone's weight doesn't motivate them; it makes them feel like crap, engage in worse health behaviors, and has profound mental and physical consequences.

The psychological consequences of being treated worse because of your weight may be a bit more straightforward. Experiencing weight stigma contributes to poor body image, low self-esteem, social isolation, and risk of depression. In a study of more than nine thousand adults with obesity, researchers found that perceived weight discrimination was associated with current diagnoses of mood disorders and substance abuse.[38]

But what about the idea that you can shame people into exercising or making different food choices? Yeah, it turns out not only is that false, but the *exact opposite* is true. Experiencing weight stigma may actually make people engage in more maladaptive health behaviors, such as binge eating.[39] Eating can be an extremely effective (although short-lived) emotional coping strategy, and being stigmatized for your weight can certainly lead to some emotions that need coping with. In a study of about twenty-five hundred women with obesity, almost 79 percent reported coping with weight stigma by eating more food, and 75 percent reported coping with it by refusing to diet[40] (which, based on our previous chapters is . . . maybe a good thing?). Recent research has also shown that women who were overweight and were exposed to weight-stigmatizing stimuli ate *more than three times* the calories afterward than those exposed to neutral stimuli, and that adults exposed to weight stigma were less likely to engage in exercise, probably because gyms and other exercise settings could be venues for *even further* weight stigma.[41,42]

I don't think I've ever experienced discrimination based on my weight, but I know that even the little comments I would get here and there from my family would trigger an almost spiteful response in me to eat unhealthily. I wanted to start a gym membership in high school, but because my parents were always telling me to exercise, I didn't. The gym has since become one of my greatest loves in life, and I could've experienced it four years earlier if I hadn't been so adamant to not "give in" to what people around me were telling me to do. I'm sorry to break it to everyone who thinks that they can "tough-love" people into submission, but receiving rude comments doesn't make you go, "Wow, that comment made me feel awful; let me make myself feel better by eating some broccoli and hitting the gym." It makes you go, "Screw you; I'm going to eat whatever I want, and I'm not putting myself in a place where I'm going to see more jerks like you."

Adolescents and Weight Stigma

The effect that weight stigma has on adolescents is a relatively new field of research showing some devastating findings. In adolescents, the experience of weight stigma is associated with increased depression, anxiety, low self-esteem, and body dissatisfaction. These associations were found even after controlling for age, gender, body weight, and age of obesity onset, meaning that it was actually the stigma rather than subjects' actual BMI that was contributing to the negative emotional effects.[43] In a study of almost five thousand boys and girls, weight-related victimization was linked to higher risk of depression, while their actual weight status was often not related.[44] Translation: Being made to feel bad about being "fat" instead of actually being fat is what's messing with people's mental health.

Perhaps the most serious and heartbreaking consequences of being bullied for one's weight growing up are its effects on suicides and suicide attempts. Adolescents that experience weight-based teasing are two to three times more likely to report suicidal ideation.[45] One study found that more than 50 percent of girls who experience weight-based teasing from family and peers have considered suicide.[46] Girls with obesity were almost two times as likely to report a suicide attempt in the last year than average-weight peers.[47]

On top of that, weight-based teasing affects children's ability to make meaningful social connections and do well academically. And kids know it: in one study of nine-to-twelve-year-olds, 69 percent report that they thought they would have more friends if they could lose weight.[48] Over-weight adolescents who experience weight-based teasing are more likely to engage in disordered eating behaviors, like binge eating, chronic dieting, vomiting, and laxative use, even after controlling for BMI.[49] Whatever the critics may think about people being "lazy" and "undisciplined," it is hard to ever think that a child deserves to be made to feel so badly about themselves that they would engage in any of these behaviors.

Phew, does it feel refreshing to cover a topic that is not disputed at all in the scientific literature! The evidence is clear: stigmatizing someone because of weight is no way to treat another human. And no matter what someone may think, it's not helping. It causes emotional distress, has psychological and physical consequences, and makes the victim more likely to engage in unhealthy behaviors. I can't believe that I have to write this in a book in the twenty-first century, but, yeah, guys, here's a hot take: treat people the way you want to be treated.

WHY THE BMI SUCKS

The body mass index, or BMI, is calculated by dividing your weight (in kilograms) by your height squared (in meters). As with many annoying things, the idea of using a height-weight ratio was popularized by insurance companies as a way to make money. (Is it just me, or are insurance companies almost always the evil villains in every significant historical debacle?) In the late 1800s, insurance companies started noticing that weight adjusted for height was an independent determinant of life expectancy.[50] In 1959, the Metropolitan Life Insurance

Company published tables of average body weights for heights by gender and by age. The tables were based on data collected from 1935 to 1953 by six different insurance companies on four million people (mostly white men).[51]

These tables were supposed to be a proxy for measuring fat mass, but they didn't do a very good job. The way the tables were set up, for example, assumed that tall people were just scaled-up versions of shorter people. Have y'all seen Simone Biles next to Michael Phelps? Their body proportions are hilariously different. Tall people tend to be narrower and have longer limbs and so have a higher lean-mass-to-fat-mass ratio than shorter people. Because of this, tall people were getting a big advantage in these tables. Even at the same height-to-weight ratios, they routinely had lower death rates than short people just because their weight was not scaling linearly with their height. This especially doesn't make sense because tall people, on average, have worse mortality rates than short people.[52] (Don't worry, tall readers, I said "on average"!) Plus, these tables didn't take into account bone mass, frame size, leg length, and so on—all factors that impact this weight-to-height ratio.

So, in 1972, physiologist Ancel Keys (more on him soon) came out saying these tables were crap, and he instead popularized the use of the Quetelet index, which he called (drum roll please) *body mass index*! This measure (weight/height^2) was created by a Flemish astronomer and statistician in the 1800s, who discovered that squaring the height in the equation reduced the impact of leg length. In other words, it stopped tall people from getting a leg up (hee-hee) just for being taller.

Up until 1995, the National Institutes of Health (NIH) considered the normal BMI cutoff to be 27.8 for men and 27.3 for women. These numbers were based on the National Health and Nutrition Examination Survey. They basically said, "Where do we put the 'normal' BMI cutoff so that 85 percent of people lie below the cutoff?" and got ~27. However, in 1995, the World Health Organization came out with divisions of the BMI into four categories: underweight, normal, overweight, and obese, which were adopted in the United States in 1998. The new cutoff for "normal" was now 25, which overnight converted millions of

Americans from "normal" weight to "overweight." On June 17, 1998, CNN reported "Millions of Americans became 'fat' Wednesday—even if they didn't gain a pound."[53] Indeed, according to the new cutoffs, twenty-five million Americans became "overweight" that day, which should just show you how arbitrary this entire system is.

Putting aside the ridiculousness of how this all was decided, here's a nonexhaustive list of problems with the BMI:

- **BMI was not based on disease outcomes.** If you'll notice in the story of how BMI was created, *none* of it had to do with finding a meaningful predictor of health outcomes. It had to do with finding some sort of cheap, easy way for insurance companies to figure out who was going to die based on the data of mostly white men who lived in the early 1900s. In this data set, BMI was a predictor of mortality, but that doesn't mean it's the best predictor or is universally applicable. It's now being used almost ubiquitously for everything from qualifying for medical treatments to eligibility for medications and procedures.

- **BMI underestimates "normal" weight.** In Western population-based studies, the mean BMI is generally 24–27. Adopting 25 as the cutoff for "normal" therefore automatically puts a large portion of the population in the overweight (later retermed "pre-obese") and obese categories.[54]

- **BMI can't tell us body composition.** While the word "obesity" is supposed to refer to excess body fat, BMI is not a very good measure of body fat. For example, in some populations, BMI has been found to be more highly correlated with lean body mass than with fat mass.[55] For another, women often have lower BMIs than men, even though they carry much more body fat.[56] Athletes, who usually have high amounts of lean body mass, will often qualify as "obese" according to the BMI. One study found that for men with a BMI of 27, their body-fat percentages ranged from 10 percent (hints of a "six-pack at the beach" level body fat) to 32 percent (obesity-level body fat).[57] BMI is not only inaccurate for populations like athletes, it's also dangerous for individuals who have high fat mass but low lean body mass and thus still count as being "normal" weight. This may lead to them getting underdiagnosed and underscreened for medical conditions they may have but aren't "fat" enough to get checked for.[58]

- **BMI doesn't specify location of excess fat.** The fat located in the abdominal area and around the organs has been shown to be much more dangerous than fat in the legs, hips, and butt regions, for example. Abdominal fat is the most highly associated with accumulation of fat in the liver, which may actually lead to insulin resistance and the metabolic issues associated with excess weight.[59] Fat in the lower body (hip and butt region) may actually be protective.[60]

- **BMI was made for white populations.** The BMI was devised by white people for a white population. For example, when researchers tried to match the type 2 diabetes risk faced by white people at the BMI "obesity" cutoff of 30, they found that that cutoff should be 23.9 for South Asian populations, 28.1 for Black populations, 26.9 for Chinese populations, and 26.6 for Arab populations.[61] This means that other ethnic groups may be receiving care later than they should be, which has far-reaching implications for their long-term health outcomes.

What's a Doctor to Say and Do?

Uncertainty and Evolving Science

"How are you at dealing with uncertainty?" the medical school admissions interviewer asked.

"I'm not sure," I answered quickly, which got them to at least crack a smile and gave me a chance to compose a more substantial response.

This is an appropriate question for an aspiring physician because doctors are constantly faced with doubt around a patient's diagnosis and their response to treatment. We also need to adjust our approaches and treatment regimens to match the unpredictability of evolving science. For example, over the course of my career, we have gone from recommending bed rest for heart attacks and corsets for back pain to advocating active rehabilitation for both. We no longer recommend aspirin for the prevention of heart disease because, especially in those over age sixty, the risks outweigh the benefits. Stomach ulcers, previously thought to be stress-related, are now treated with antibiotics to fight the bacteria that actually cause the ulcers. Even if the science were more predictable and straightforward, interpretation of available data can be manipulated by special interests.

Science Corrupted by Special Interests

The work of specialists in my field of physical medicine and rehabilitation focuses on mitigating pain and ameliorating function so that our patients can do the things that they love and need to do. I was initially trained to limit the use of opiates to those with severe pain from, for example, cancer, or immediately after an operation. However, in the early 1990s I went to a presentation by a prominent pain specialist who chastised the audience for not prescribing opiates for pain from common osteoarthritis. We were assured by multiple peer-reviewed studies that the risk of addiction was less than 1 in 200 and could be reduced further if we simply screened our patients by asking about prior problems with addiction. In my effort to remain nimble and provide cutting-edge treatments, I dutifully started prescribing opiates for my patients with everyday knee pain from arthritis. At the height of this craze, I readily provided fentanyl patches with the rationale that their application every seventy-two hours would keep my patients in a continuous state of opiated pain relief. Knowing what I now know about the dangers of long-term opiate use, I cringe when I think about the prescriptions I wrote for dozens of patients, often for many years. It was only years later that I recognized that I and my colleagues were unknowingly complicit in the decades-long opiate scandal that is still ongoing and is still claiming one hundred thousand American lives per year. I am trying to remain only skeptical (but not cynical) as I reasonably challenge whether indeed the classification of BMI is at least in part propelled by pharmaceutical companies promoting anti-obesity medications. (See the sidebar "Why the BMI Sucks.") Will using the BMI be more helpful or more harmful to my patients' health and well-being?

What Do I Say to My Patients?

Although I could dig through the computerized medical records to track my patients' weight charts, I prefer to turn my face away from the screen, toward them, and simply ask, "How are you doing with your weight?" Allowing my patients to answer and share their perceptions of their weight is far more informative and engaging than simply seeing a change in the numbers in the chart. For those who say they are interested and ready to lose weight, I'll ask what health habits they are planning on changing and whether they need assistance, perhaps from a registered dietician, an app, referral to an obesity specialist, or maybe cooking instruction. Occasionally, a patient will report that they have lost a substantial amount of weight, often thirty or forty pounds or more. I then ask about their motivations, strategies, obstacles, and reflections on how they are managing to sustain their weight loss. Their stories often reflect a decision to try to reach a deeply valued goal that was made easier by weight loss, for example, being able to care for children or partners, rather than "so I could look good." Note: You'll be invited in chapter 12 to go through the process of determining what matters most to you.

For those who are overweight or have obesity and say they are not ready or interested in losing weight, I am faced with a quandary. On the one hand, it is my obligation to inform them and offer treatment if I believe that their excess weight is causing medical problems, for example, type 2 diabetes or worsening joint pain in their hips and knees. On the other hand, I try to uphold my oath to "first, do no harm." I do my best to avoid a discussion of a patient's weight that might be perceived as fat shaming or stigmatizing. According to Christy Harrison, author of the book *Anti-Diet,* the negative consequences of weight stigma and fat bias are a much stronger predictor of health than body size.[62] In the midst of the ongoing cultural saga about weight and body image, I seek to remain a support to my patients.

Coming to Peace

Perhaps the best outcome for my patients, and for all of us, is to find a place of peace and balance amid the persistent societal messages to lose weight, the tendency to measure our self-worth by the number on the scale, and the extreme challenge of maintaining weight loss. Although we might be metabolically healthier with even a 5 percent weight loss, the risks to our self-esteem and self-efficacy from not achieving that goal may indeed outweigh the benefits.

In the case of weight, body image, and health, we are in the middle of a fraught conversation charged with a background of sexism, racism, elitism, and the evolving politics of gender identity. To best come to peace with your weight and health, it is vital to acknowledge these forces and then make the best-informed decisions that align with your values, current science, and the best care available to help you reach your goals.

The Takeaways

OK, so I feel like this was a lot of big words and obscure biological mechanisms that sounded confusing. So, *what does it mean*?! Here's the point:

- There's no way to tell from a population-based study what weight is healthiest for you.

- The obesity paradox is likely due to a confluence of biases. Obesity does appear to be linked with worse health outcomes, particularly on longer timescales.

- Excess fat may be a physical manifestation of the real cause of poorer health outcomes: excess calorie intake, which puts a lot of metabolic strain on your body.

- Where fat is located makes a difference. Visceral fat (the fat around your organs) appears to be particularly associated with poor health outcomes and all-cause mortality.

- Weight stigma is associated with a myriad of adverse mental and physical health outcomes.

Because of how incredibly futile it often is to try to "intentionally" lose weight, the best strategy may be this: do healthy stuff (like the nutrition, movement, and lifestyle habits that we outline in the rest of the book) regardless of whether or not you lose weight. Either they will result in some moderate weight loss, which will likely improve health markers, or they won't result in weight loss but almost certainly still improve health markers. It's a win-win. Being healthy—eating better, moving more, sleeping better, reducing stress—will make you better off regardless of whether the scale goes down.

If I could have drilled this into my head at a younger age, I cannot tell you how much suffering I would have saved myself. It's fairly reasonable to conclude that, for a lot of people, not ever engaging in yo-yo dieting would actually have meant a lower long-term body-weight set point. So if you're reading this book early on in your fitness and health journey, and you wanted to buy it to "get your dream body" or impress all your friends at your college reunion, again, I say do what you want, but be aware of the possible and probable consequences.

OK, OK! We hear what you're saying! Enough about weight and diets. Let's shift our focus and start talking about something way more fun: *food*.

5

What to Eat

The First Dietary Recommendations

Before we get into the nitty-gritty of what to eat, we're going to take a slight detour into the ever-so-invigorating history of US dietary guidelines. I know, I know, this topic sounds thrilling to the max, but if you have your doubts, please stick with me, because I promise you, it is quite relevant to understanding a lot of what has gone *wrong* over the past fifty years.

In 1977, the Senate Select Committee on Nutrition and Human Needs released the first ever *Dietary Goals for the United States*.[1] Oh yes! Have no fear! The exact people who are known for being extremely capable and for consistently "getting things right," members of *the US Senate*, are on the job! That year, the committee issued two sets of guidelines. After thoroughly reviewing the available science, they first called for a reduction in overall fat, saturated fat, cholesterol, sugar, and salt and specifically called for decreasing consumption of foods including meat, butter, and eggs.[2]

However, as you can imagine, the meat industry was capital "P" *pissed* about this, and after some pressuring and general sleazy lobbying, they got the committee to change its guidelines in the same year. The new document subsequently stated, "decrease consumption of animal fat, and choose meats, poultry and fish which will reduce saturated fat intake."[3] Not to be dramatic here, but this sentence may be one of the most consequential sentences in the evolution of the American food supply. (Side note: I guess the egg lobby was not too "egg-cellent" at lobbying, because the recommendations on eggs remained unchanged.)

As journalist Michael Pollan points out in his incredible work *In Defense of Food: An Eater's Manifesto,* this directive from the Senate's select committee lumps meat in with poultry and fish, three entirely different food sources, and reduces them to simply a vehicle for the same evil: saturated fat.[4] Secondly, instead of putting the emphasis on the foods themselves, it puts an emphasis on the invisible nutrient properties of the foods: cholesterol, total fat, subcategories of fat, and so on. Rest assured, in order to not step on any toes or piss anyone off, dietary guidelines rarely spoke of reducing a specific *food* ever again and instead opted for the components they contained: carbohydrates, dietary fat, sodium, cholesterol, antioxidants, and so on.[5] Pollan dubs this the beginning of the "age of nutritionism," an ideology that claims that the key to understanding food is its nutrients. Remember this, because we're coming back to it.

Fat Is the Problem

Growing up, there was one thing I knew for sure about health, and that was that fat was bad. I didn't know why, but it didn't really matter. It was undisputed. Magazine covers, infomercials, food packaging, and the behavior of the adults around me were consistent and in agreement. If you cared about your health, you ordered the nonfat latte. You got "dressing on the side." You opted for low-fat muffins and skim milk.

I remember when we first came to the United States, my parents were horrified at the thin, dribbly liquid that passed for "milk." We were one of the only families I knew who stubbornly had gallons of whole milk in our fridge year-round. And when I insisted on getting nonfat yogurt in middle and high school, they would crinkle their noses and say, "How can you eat that?" Clearly, there was no such thing as low-fat in Albania. But surely, the United States is more advanced in their nutritional knowledge than a country that had only recently escaped Soviet rule, right? Well, it turns out . . . maybe not.

Why the demonization of fat? In 1977, when the *Dietary Goals* were first published, it was clear that America's primary "health" problem was no longer nutrient deficiencies and malnourishment, as it had been in the first half of the twentieth century. The problem was basically the opposite: chronic diseases and overconsumption. Heart disease, in particular, was of increasing concern both to everyday Americans and policy makers. And the leading theory for the cause of heart disease at this time was the lipid hypothesis. The logic went as follows: reducing intake of saturated fat reduces serum choles-terol, which in turn lowers incidence of coronary heart disease (CHD).[6]

The Skinny on Fat

First, a little primer on fats will make the rest of this chapter go down a lot smoother, because . . . all this terminology gets annoying *real* fast if you don't know what the heck it means. Dietary fats are in the form of triglycerides— *"tri"* because they have *three* fatty acid chains, and *"glyceride"* because these chains are on a *glycerol* backbone.[7] The thing is: there's a lot of variation in these fatty-acid chains. They can be longer or shorter. They can have zero, one, or multiple double bonds (saturated, monounsaturated, or polyunsaturated). Their double bonds can be in different orientations. And all these variations mean that different fatty acids function differently in the body.[8]

While most foods have combinations of all three types of fatty acids, certain foods are known for having much higher amounts of specific types.[9] For example, saturated fats are most commonly found in animal products: meat and dairy (and are often solid at room temperature, while the other fats are liquid). Monounsaturated fats can be found in olive oil, avocados, and nuts. And finally, polyunsaturated fats can be broken up into omega-3s (most commonly found in fish and certain seeds), and omega-6s (plant oils like corn, soy, or safflower oil). Again, all of these foods have different combinations of all three, but certain foods have much higher amounts of certain fatty acids.

The Lipid Hypothesis

The reason for thinking that saturated fat played a causal role in coronary heart disease is a rabbit hole that not even the most avid of rabbits want to go down. But basically, our homey Ancel Keys (the same guy who ran the Minnesota starvation experiments from chapter 3) noticed back in the 1950s that there was a correlation between countries with high-saturated-fat diets (high in meat and dairy) and deaths from coronary heart disease.[10] This had prompted a few randomized control trials to be run in the 1960s in which saturated fat was replaced by polyunsaturated fats (mostly corn, nut, or seed oils), which showed a substantial effect on cholesterol and a minimal effect on death from CHD.[11] These preliminary findings, although not definitive, were considered adequate to prove that saturated fat increased cholesterol in your blood, which increased death by coronary heart disease.

Meanwhile, the link between *dietary* cholesterol (cholesterol in the food we eat) and heart disease was entirely what in scientific terms we call a hunch. You can see why logically you would think there was something there: dietary cholesterol *probably* has an effect on blood cholesterol . . . because . . . why wouldn't it, I guess? But having a hunch is not exactly a foundation upon which you should be basing dietary recommendations for an *entire population*. But anyway, I digress. Despite the link between cholesterol in food and heart disease being "unproven in clinical trials," as testified to before the Senate committee in 1977 by the director of the National Heart Lung and Blood Institute, the recommendation on decreasing dietary cholesterol (with an emphasis on eggs and butter, in particular) was still put into the report. Like I said: egg lobby, you really need to step up your game.

So with some preliminary science to support the link between saturated fat and CHD, and no science to support the link between dietary cholesterol and CHD, the guidelines were put to the nation: reduce total fat, saturated fat, and cholesterol; they all increase your chances of death by heart disease. As one of the greatest proponents of the lipid hypothesis put it to the Senate committee: "The potential risks are essentially nil, the potential benefits vast."[12] Um . . . yeah. Try making that sentence the exact opposite and you might be closer to the truth.

Shaky Science, Big Effects

The publication of *Dietary Goals* had far-reaching effects, particularly on food engineering and processed-food manufacturing. The processed-food industry is always one of the first to capitalize on changes in dietary guidelines, not because they are particularly interested in improving our health but because they're always looking to get the bag, so to speak. (Note from Juna to Eddie: "get the bag" means "make money.") Considering that ultra-processed foods make up such a large portion of the standard American diet, it's no wonder these changes in packaged-food manufacturing have profound impacts on the overall food supply.[13] The effects were at the same time broad—changing the balance of macronutrients we were consuming (percentage of calories from carbohydrates vs. fat)—and more nuanced, changing things like the sources of these macronutrients (grains vs. refined carbohydrates, saturated fat vs. polyunsaturated and trans fats).[14,15]

The elimination of saturated fat meant it needed to be replaced by *something*, and that something was plant and polyunsaturated-fat-based products, like soybean oil, margarine, shortenings, and so on. Soybean oil, for example, moved from making up 0.006 percent of the average American's calories in 1909 to being the fourth largest contributor to daily calories by 1999 (a greater than one thousandfold increase).[16] The instability of these polyunsaturated oils, however, meant that they had to be partially hydrogenated, a process that causes the formation of trans fats. And so as saturated fat was quietly siphoned out of the food supply, trans fats started to creep their way in.

PS: Here's all you need to know about trans fats: they make processed foods tasty (rich, crispy, crunchy), and they're cheap. Foods containing trans fats have a longer shelf life, so they can live to a ripe old age. Also, did I mention they unequivocally lower good cholesterol, increase bad cholesterol, increase inflammation, and increase blood clotting (among other harmful effects), making them substantially worse for your health than the supposedly nefarious saturated fats they were replacing?[17] In other words, the processed-food industry's dream (a cheap and tasty substitute) is nothing short of a public-health nightmare.

The recommendation for lowering fat also meant that food scientists had to come up with creative new molecules that would mimic fat in mouthfeel, texture, and other properties. After all, who wants low-fat cheese that won't melt, low-fat watery milk, or low-fat icy, noncreamy ice cream? Enter gums, cellulose, dextrin, pectin, and a host of other additives to try to make low-fat food feel as fatty as possible.[18]

The *Dietary Goals*, along with the coinciding shift in processed-food manufacturing to keep up with these goals, also had an impact on the average American's overall diet. Until the 1970s, carbohydrates (most coming from grains), which made up the largest portion of the American diet, had been declining.[19] However, clearly *something* (hm, I wonder what) changed in the 1970s, because all of a sudden, the trend was reversed: overall carbohydrate intake as well as the proportion of calories from carbs started to increase.[20]

The period of 1980 to 1997 also saw an increase in our daily caloric intake of about 500 calories per day, with nearly 80 percent (~430 calories) coming from increases in carbohydrates. But these new carbs were not coming from rice and sweet potatoes. From 1909 to 1997, the per capita use of caloric sweeteners increased by 86 percent, and corn syrup sweeteners specifically saw a greater than twentyfold increase, ballooning to make up 20 percent of the total carbohydrate intake by 1997.[21] Apparently, making things low-fat doesn't make them very tasty. . . but adding a bunch of corn syrup sure does! And a huge surplus of corn crops from American farmers, heavily subsidized by the US government since the 1930s, provided all the high fructose corn syrup one could need.[22]

Interestingly, Americans were never actually able to cut down on their fat consumption. They simply *replaced* the "poisonous" saturated fat with polyunsaturated and trans fats and simultaneously started filling up on a ton more carbs and sugar.[23] Michael Pollan points out that the ideology of nutritionism has as much to do with this as that misguided Senate committee: by reducing foods to their nutrients and nothing more, instead of interpreting the dietary goals as "eat *less* of this food," they were interpreted as "eat *more* low-fat stuff."[24] Here's a piece of human psychology that we don't need to investigate in a study: we almost never want to hear "eat *less*" of anything, but we're all too happy to "eat *more*" of almost anything, especially if it's reduced-fat Oreos.

Low-fat recommendations, put forth by the US Senate committee, sure did change the health of Americans, but it just wasn't the change the committee was aiming to make. It ushered in the era of low-fat muffins, "skinny" omelets, and SnackWell's. It promoted the carbohydrate, demoted the fat, and gave an all-access pass to the *incredibly low-fat* corn syrup. And yet, though there seemed to be less and less fat in food products, America was only getting fatter and fatter. From 1980 to 1997, prevalence of type 2 diabetes increased by 47 percent, while the prevalence of obesity increased by 80 percent.[25]

The Lipid Lie

Not to fast-forward over thirty years of incorrect dietary guidelines, bad science, ingenious food marketing, and uncorroborated hypotheses . . . but we gotta get to what to eat, eventually, so here's the punchline: in 2001, authors from the Harvard School of Public Health, part of the very nutritional establishment that had been touting low-fat diets as the road to optimal health for the past quarter century, stated:

> It is now increasingly recognized that the low-fat campaign has been based on *little scientific evidence* and may have *caused unintended health consequences.*[26]

(PS: I added the italics myself for some extra *pizzazz.*)
Here are some more statements from the same authors:

- The link between dietary cholesterol and coronary heart disease is "weak and nonsignificant."

- There is "little direct evidence linking higher egg consumption and increased risk of CHD."

- Also, BTW, eggs are, apparently, "excellent and relatively inexpensive sources of essential amino acids and certain vitamins."[27] *(Alert the egg lobby!!!! Alert!)*

In fact, while the paper systematically dismantled almost every aspect of the lipid hypothesis, it finds that the *only type* of fat that has been truly linked to poor health outcomes is the exact one that rose to prominence because of their own recommendations against saturated fat: namely, trans fat.[28] It's unclear if the irony of this is apparent to anyone (except maybe Michael Pollan).[29] A perhaps happy end to this part of the story is that the FDA banned artificial trans fats from the US food supply, effective 2018.

Nutrition Research Is Hard

To cut public-health officials a teeny bit of slack, nutrition research is *hard*, like even harder than regular research. We covered this a little bit in our diet chapter, but let's do a deeper dive. While the scientific method relies on isolating variables and measuring the effect they have on a particular outcome, in nutrition research, we can't really do that. We don't eat nutrients in isolation; we eat food. The effects that certain nutrients supposedly have on health outcomes cannot be considered without also considering the vehicle for that nutrient. For example, both dairy and processed meat are high in saturated fat, and yet, in prospective cohort studies, they have completely opposite effects on long-term health outcomes (dairy reduces all-cause mortality; processed meat increases it).[30] By looking at these two foods as simply "containers of saturated fat," you remove all the nuance from the nutritional picture and equate two things that are very different.

Furthermore, not only are nutrients not indicative of food choices, but food choices can't be isolated from overall dietary patterns, and the dietary patterns can't be isolated from lifestyles. Can you attribute the abnormally high life spans in the Seventh-day Adventist community to their diets, their lack of drinking, or their abstinence from tobacco?[31] Is it one of these? All three? Something else entirely? To what degree?

To complicate things further, even if we could isolate specific nutrients, or perhaps isolate food groups, at least, randomized control trials, the gold standard in scientific research, are extremely difficult in nutrition research.[32] We would all love to randomly assign people to diets, have them adhere for a long time, and see who has the best health outcomes, but there are a few logistical issues. Such a study would take decades and tens of millions of dollars. This is not to mention the fact that people are notoriously bad at adhering to dietary interventions and notoriously bad at reporting what and how much they eat. Unless we provide everyone's food or have an invisible person follow them around all day taking notes, self-reported food intake is about as reliable as height on men's dating-app profiles. And of course, the ethics of the whole situation are tricky: Who would ever want to volunteer as tribute for a trial studying trans fats? (Although . . . crunchy cookies and chips are guaranteed!)

Finally, because we *need* a certain number of calories a day, anytime a dietary intervention asks you to take something out, it means you are adding something in to replace it.[33] Therefore, every effect seen in any dietary intervention could be as much about what is being added in as what is being taken out. All of these factors make nutrition science confusing, convoluted, and controversial. However, trials of the past sixty years have allowed us to at least come to some conclusions.

The Dietary-Fat Fallacies

How could we have gotten it so wrong? How could the very guidelines that were supposed to be making us healthier have possibly made things even worse? And why has there been no public reckoning, or, minimally, a public service announcement saying, "Guys, we screwed up! Fat isn't bad! Our mistake!!"

It turns out that while the relationship between saturated fat and serum cholesterol holds true, and the relationship between serum cholesterol and heart disease holds true, this does not mean that saturated fat is, on the whole, *bad* for your health.[34,35]

In the past fifty years, evidence disputing the lipid hypothesis has been slowly piling up (not that anyone would know, because the public-health community hasn't appeared particularly eager to take responsibility or clarify things to the American public).

A lot of nutrition research relies on prospective cohort studies. As a brief reminder, this is where people are enrolled in a study before they exhibit whatever outcome you're trying to measure, and then you follow them for a long time, asking what they are eating and keeping track of their health status. In a systematic review of these studies, there was no association between saturated fat intake and all-cause mortality, cardio-vascular disease, ischemic stroke, or type 2 diabetes.[36] Meanwhile, trans fats were associated with increased risk of all-cause mortality, heart disease, and deaths from heart disease.

As the authors from the Harvard T.H. Chan School of Public Health report, saturated fat intake was associated with heart disease in only two prospective cohort studies, while seven showed no association. Meanwhile, an inverse relationship between polyunsaturated fat intake (the thing we were told to replace saturated fat with) and heart disease was found in *only one study*, and *not found* in six.[37] In other words, the two recommendations that are central to these authors' suggestions, namely that saturated fat increases risk of heart disease and polyunsaturated fat protects against it, are, by their own admission, not corroborated (at least in prospective cohort studies). The authors attribute the confusion in the research to factors like "small study size," "inadequate adjustment for total energy intake," and "lack of control for other types of fat and other components of diet."[38] Translation: Well, the studies just suck, so that's why they don't show evidence for our hypothesis. To which I say: Well, apparently all nutrition research sucks, so why are we ever basing anything off anything?

The overall findings from prospective cohort studies looking at saturated fat and heart disease is a resounding "meh." Some show a tiny increase in CHD from saturated fat intake; others show none. But if only we could run randomized control trials, replacing saturated fat with polyunsaturated fat, and really get to the bottom of this! Oh, wait, we did.

In our latest installment of "Shit That Would Never Fly Today But Did Fifty Years Ago," I bring you: randomized control trials of saturated fat, polyunsaturated fat, and death!!! *Woo!* In the 1960s, when experiments were less regulated than they are now, these trials were conducted largely in institutionalized, hospital, and nursing-home populations. (And we wonder why the public doesn't trust scientists . . .) In fact, it was these very studies that served as some of the first evidence of the benefits of replacing saturated fat with polyunsaturated fats.[39]

One thing is clear in these studies: replacing saturated fat with vegetable oils like corn oil, safflower oil, sunflower oil, and soybean oil, which are high in omega-6 fatty acids (particularly linoleic acid), does, without a doubt, lower serum cholesterol.[40] Perhaps it was this clear effect, and the unwavering confidence that serum cholesterol truly played a causal role in death by CHD, that made these trials foundations upon which scientists based the original diet-heart hypothesis.

However, with reanalysis of these trials, particularly with the inclusion of missing data from two of them (the Sydney Diet Heart Study and Minnesota Coronary Experiment), a very different picture of the health implications of polyunsaturated fats from vegetable oils emerges.[41,42] When saturated fat is replaced by polyunsaturated fat, serum cholesterol goes down, but deaths from all causes and deaths from coronary heart disease *do not*. In fact, some of the data even suggests that death rates went up with such an intervention.[43,44] Ironically, in the Minnesota Coronary Experiment, especially in the subjects over age sixty-five, reduced cholesterol in the blood was actually associated with *higher* risk of death. Researchers have suggested that this may be because while vegetable oils containing linoleic acid do decrease LDL cholesterol, they also increase cells' susceptibility to oxidation, which may increase risk of many diseases, including cancer.[45] Another plausible theory could be that replacing saturated fats with vegetable oils may indeed have a modest effect on reducing death by coronary heart disease, but the increase it causes in other types of death outweighs the modest improvements it creates in CHD.

Perhaps the greatest "experiment" of all was simply what happened in the United States after the 1970s. We've already talked about how diabetes and obesity skyrocketed (in fact, many experts date the beginning of the obesity epidemic to the 1970s), but what about deaths from heart disease?

It's true, deaths from heart disease fell precipitously after the 1980s, prompting public-health officials to call this one of the great achievements in public-health intervention. But was this due to a dramatically lowered incidence or an improvement in medical care? In a paper analyzing the reduced deaths, researchers attribute half of the decrease in deaths to better surgical and pharmacological treatments of heart disease.[46] The authors attribute 24 percent of the decrease in deaths to improved cholesterol . . . and yet also note that two new risk factors were added since 1980: namely obesity and diabetes.[47] So while replacing saturated fat with "other stuff" may have created a modest decrease in deaths from heart disease, its co-inciding and potentially related effects on refined carbohydrate intake and excess calories, and consequently obesity and diabetes, may have simulta-neously increased other risk factors.

If you're just completely lost right now, I don't really blame you. The overall narrative can be summarized as: coronary heart disease was the leading cause of death by the mid-twentieth century. People thought sat-urated fat caused higher blood cholesterol, which in turn caused heart disease. They made recommendations to lower saturated fat and choles-terol. It turns out that this hypothesis is not right. And now we're arguably worse off than we started. The main takeaways I have gotten from this entire mess are:

1. Nutrition research is hard.

2. The government is susceptible to lobbying and flawed science.

3. The egg lobby sucks.

OK, in all seriousness, what can we take away from the disaster of the past fifty years, and how can that inform our future thinking about food?

Nutritionism Is a Problem

Up until this point, you'll notice one trend in all our discussion of nutri-tion: it is based around the benefits of specific nutrients. However, we do not eat *nutrients*, we eat *food*, and it is perhaps this exact focus on nutrients over food that is causing *the real problem*.[48] In their paper dismantling the diet-heart hypothesis, the authors from the Harvard T.H. Chan School of Public Health warn of "the dangers of judging the effects of a food by single nutrients contained in the food."[49]

That is one sentence.

The other ten pages of the paper proceed to go through basically every individual fatty acid found in our food sources and each of their associations with various health outcomes.

(Pause)

Am I the only one about to lose my mind here?

Clearly, approaching dietary guidelines through the lens of nutritionism—the ideology that a food can be reduced to simply its nutrients—has *not worked*. Not only has it *not* improved our health, it has likely made us more sick, more misguided, and more confused than ever. There are *so many* problems with nutritionism, it's hard to know where to begin.

Anyone who has spent five seconds looking through the history of nutrition research can plainly see we just don't know enough about food to be making claims about its nutrient properties and what health outcomes they may or may not be causing. Just look at the evolution of dietary advice. The recommendations go from "Total fat is the problem" to "Saturated fat is the problem" to "Specific fatty acids are the problem" to who knows what? First we think cholesterol is bad, but then we find out there are different types of cholesterol, so we decided LDL cholesterol is bad. And now we've found out there are different subtypes of LDL cholesterol, and so it goes. The recommendations on specific nutrients and health markers change as soon as the next discovery is made.

Second, another problem is the assumption that a complete understanding of a food's "parts" is a complete understanding of it as a whole. Let's say, for the sake of argument, that we *could* actually know every single component of a food. We have a complete list of its vitamins, minerals, and macronutrient properties and there's absolutely nothing more to it. How can this mean that we would understand how this food, as a whole, interacts with the human body? The parts of something often do not equal the whole.

Third, a focus on a certain nutrient allows for equating foods that are simply not equal. The warped lens of nutritionism allows for Cheerios to be marketed as an equivalent "source of whole grains" as brown rice. Omega-3-enriched sparkling water is as good a "source of healthy fats" as salmon. Fortified skim milk is as good a "source of Vitamin D" as the sun. (And you don't even have to go outside or get sweaty!) Indeed, by these standards, many processed foods may in fact be *better* than whole foods. Food scientists can just enrich them with every vitamin known to man and make things like a superfood Oreo.

Nutritionism allows for the puppet masters of the food industry to reengineer whatever "foodlike substance" they are concocting at the time to be remarketed as a "health food," depending on the dietary fad of the week. *This* is the logic that allows the FDA to let Frito-Lay claim that their chips confer cardiovascular benefits, simply because they are fried in vegetable oil (polyunsaturated fats) and may therefore reduce your intake of saturated fats. . . . Really? This is how we get to *chips* reducing risk of *cardiovascular disease*? As Michael Pollan puts it more politely, "So can a notorious junk food pass through the needle eye of nutritionist logic and come out the other side looking like a health food."[50]

Maybe nutritionism was an unavoidable by-product of trying to apply the standard scientific process to food: science is based on isolating variables, manipulating them, and measuring the results. But reducing a dietary pattern to a single food or food group, and reducing a food to nutrients, is never going to give you an accurate picture of what makes for optimal health. Even a cursory glance at the diets of preindustrial societies across the world tells us: there is no evil macronutrient or magic food.

Let's Talk About Food

In the spirit of never having to read the words "fatty acid" for the remainder of this book, let's shift the discussion away from *nutrients* and directly to *food*. What kinds of foods should we be eating? What foods do we know are "good for us"? And what foods do we know aren't? Can science offer any insights into a healthy diet?

When we talk about food in the modern American diet, the thousand-pound elephant in the room is that the majority of our diet is actually not *food*. Around 58 percent of the calories the average American gets everyday comes from ultra-processed foods, "edible foodlike substances," more the products of food science than nature.[51,52] What exactly counts as an ultra-processed food? There's a long answer—largely quibbled over by scholars and getting updated every few years—and a short answer that's fairly useful, though potentially vaguer.

Many foods we eat today require at least some processing. Cooking vegetables is a form of processing, for example. Freezing berries is a form of minimal processing. But, obviously, vegetables and berries are not what we're talking about here. According to the NOVA Food Classification system (not an acronym), which judges diet quality primarily through the degree to which foods are being processed, there are four categories: unprocessed or minimally processed foods (vegetables, fruits, beans, meats, poultry, fish, yogurt), processed culinary ingredients (plant oils, animal fats, table salt, granulated sugar, honey), processed foods (breads, canned vegetables, canned fish, cheese, cured meats, salted nuts), and ultra-processed foods (sodas, cookies, chips, cakes, breakfast cereals, energy drinks, baking mixes, packaged snacks, and so on).

I've included the full definition of "ultra-processed foods" in all its wordy glory in a sidebar, in case you're feeling extra scholarly and want to read it. But this is all a lot of overkill for a pretty simple idea. I think we all, to some degree, implicitly understand what "food" is "junk" (although certain foods may manipulate us by making health claims and using scientific language). I prefer Michael Pollan's decidedly unwordy litmus tests for food: *Real* food is food that your great-grandmother would recognize. *Real* food does not have health claims on its packaging. *Real* food rots. *Real* food is not usually sold where gas is sold. You get the idea.

ULTRA-PROCESSED FOOD DEFINITION
(BASED ON NOVA FOOD CLASSIFICATION SYSTEM)

"Industrial formulations typically with 5 or more and usually many ingredients. Besides salt, sugar, oils, and fats, ingredients of ultra-processed foods include food substances not commonly used in culinary preparations, such as hydrolyzed protein, modified starches, and hydrogenated or interesterified oils, and additives whose purpose is to imitate sensorial qualities of unprocessed or minimally processed foods and their culinary preparations or to disguise undesirable qualities of the final product, such as colorants, flavorings, nonsugar sweeteners, emulsifiers, humectants, sequestrants, and firming, bulking, defoaming, anticaking, and glazing agents."[53]

The Problem with Processed Foods

Here's a moral dilemma: I don't want to be the crazy cuckoo head running around screaming, "Processed foods are evil!" yanking birthday cake out of children's hands as party guests watch in bewildered horror. But at the same time, sometimes I feel that the science behind ultra-processed food may warrant such behavior. Don't get me wrong, I'd die for an Iced Caramel Macchiato on a hot summer day, and Florentine cannolis from Mike's Pastry are the closest thing to my kryptonite. *But* the science around processed food, and more specifically ultra-processed food, unlike some of the science we've discussed thus far, is not convoluted, contentious, ambivalent, debatable, or unclear. Ultra-processed food is not good for us. It's a relatively new influencing factor in our lives, and its introduction to our diets has coincided with proliferation of all manner of health concerns that were effectively nonissues before now.

The associations between ultra-processed foods (UPFs) and health outcomes are robust. In a prospective cohort study of more than forty-four thousand French adults, a 10 percent increase in UPF consumption was associated with a 14 percent increase in all-cause mortality (death by any cause).[54] Another study of more than one hundred thousand French adults found that a 10 percent increase in UPF consumption was associated with >10 percent increase in risk for overall and breast cancers.[55] In a cohort of Spanish university graduates, consumption of UPFs was found to significantly increase risk of becoming overweight or developing obesity.[56] (Wow, a brief tour of Western Europe with those studies—you're welcome.)

In a systematic review of twenty studies, which included 334,114 individuals, consumption of UPFs was found to be positively associated with the following: all-cause mortality, overall cardiovascular diseases, coronary heart diseases, cerebrovascular diseases, hypertension, metabolic syndrome (a cluster of conditions that increase the risk of heart disease, stroke, and type 2 diabetes), being overweight and obesity, depression, irritable bowel syndrome, overall cancer, postmenopausal breast cancer, gestational obesity, adolescent asthma and wheezing, and frailty.[57] Five hundred points to Gryffindor if you could read that sentence in one breath. (PS: A systematic review is a review of the evidence surrounding a specific question.)

By this point in the book, I know what you're thinking: *An association doesn't mean that ultra-processed foods are causing all this stuff!! Maybe there's something else going on!* And to that I say, "Yay; you're paying attention, but also, there actually is evidence to support more than just an association." To summarize why UPFs may be associated with so many poor health outcomes: ultra-processed foods are calorie-rich, nutrient-poor substances that are conducive to overeating and are completely foreign to the human body. Let's dive into some of the crunchy, sweet, salty, greasy details.

Overeating

We know that we eat more than we should.[58] The increase in both diabetes and obesity has happened in parallel with an increase in industrialized food products, particularly from the high-yield and inexpensive crops of soy, corn, and wheat and their various industrialized by-products, which are used as all manner of fillers, additives, and sweeteners.[59] But how do we know that processed food actually is *the cause* of overeating, or at least playing a causal role?

In 2019, Kevin Hall and his colleagues published the first-ever randomized control trial of ultra-processed food consumption.[60] The subjects lived in the Metabolic Clinical Research Unit (MCRU) at the National Institutes of Health for twenty-eight days. While there, they were provided three meals a day plus snacks and water and told to eat as much or as little as they wanted. Each subject had access to around double their caloric needs for weight maintenance. Don't worry y'all, they *definitely* had enough food; apparently, starvation in experiments is more of a 1940s thing (see the Minnesota starvation experiment in chapter 3).

The twist: half the subjects were provided a diet of ultra-processed foods, and the other half were provided a diet of minimally processed or unprocessed foods. The meals between groups were matched for total number of calories available, energy density, macronutrient ratios, fiber, sugar, and sodium content. After two weeks, the two groups switched: those eating the ultra-processed foods got to eat some real food, and those who had been eating real food had to eat ultra-processed food. So what happened when twenty people were locked in a metabolic ward for twenty-eight days with access to twice the amount of food they needed? It depended on which group you were in.

Hall and his colleagues found that participants assigned to the ultra-processed-food diet ate, on average, 500 *more* calories a day than the group on the unprocessed-food diet. This was the case whether the subjects started in the UPF diet group in the first two weeks or in the second two weeks (after eating the unprocessed foods). On the UPF diet, the subjects gained around two pounds over the course of the two weeks, while the group on the unprocessed diet lost about two pounds. And as we would expect, the excess calories observed in the UPF diet came almost entirely from carbohydrates (~280) and fat (~230).

Well, of course people ate more junk food: it's a lot more tasty, isn't it? Interestingly, when subjects were asked to rate the "pleasantness" of the meals, there was no difference between the two groups. The groups also reported similar scores for hunger, satisfaction, fullness, and capacity to eat, suggesting it wasn't an effect of a subjectively higher appetite when fed a junk food diet. Another interesting finding was that the group eating ultra-processed foods consumed their food significantly faster than the group eating unprocessed foods, which we know from previous studies is often associated with increased food intake.

This study shows that ultra-processed food is somehow *causing* overeating, but how? If people don't report liking the ultra-processed food more, or being hungrier, why are they still overeating by 500 calories, the equivalent of about one-quarter of the average person's entire day's worth of calories?

Is Cheesecake Addictive?

You've done it, I've done it: you've got some tasty junk food, let's say Peanut M&M's, at the movies. It's a "Family Size" bag, and you're a non–family-sized person. You decide you'll have like a fourth of the bag. After a while you notice, "Huh, I'm like halfway through this thing." You close it, twist the top, put it in the cup holder.

No more.

Sneakily reach for one, or ten.

No more.

Back in the cup holder.

Sneakily reach for another one, or twenty.

And now . . . the bag's nearly empty . . . so you might as well finish it, right?

Repeating a behavior that causes negative side effects (post-movie-theater sugar crash), even though you cognitively *want* to stop, is a behavior pattern quite consistent with those that characterize substance addiction.[61] But is this just a coincidence, or is the hyper-palatable, a.k.a. extra-delicious, ultra-processed food that has come to characterize the modern-day diet actually having physiological effects in our brains that mimic those seen in addiction?

Ultra-processed food has some interesting similarities to drugs of abuse. For example, addictive substances are usually altered from their natural state—grapes are turned into wine, poppies are turned into opium—and it is only in this altered state that they become problematic.[62] Similarly, lots of natural foods contain sugar (fruits, honey) and fat (nuts, seeds, meat), but in ultra-processed food, these two components are elevated and combined. Sugar and fat almost never appear in nature in the same food, and yet in ultra-processed food (cake, muffins, cookies), they are the dominant components, putting your brain's reward systems on hyperdrive. Another problem is the sheer amount of sugar (or refined carbohydrates) and fat in ultra-processed foods. When looking at drugs of abuse, increased concentration or potency of a substance is associated with higher risk of addiction. Think light seltzers versus hard liquor: Which is more likely to be a drug of abuse? Well, a similar thing may be happening with sugar and fat: they are concentrated in much higher amounts in ultra-processed foods than you would find in nature. Why do we not experience a similar loss of control over a bag of deliciously ripe apples as we do over a bag of multicolored candy-coated peanuts?

Studying food addiction in humans can be quite tricky, so you know what we need to do? Go find some lab rats!!! In one study, researchers separated rats into three groups: one had access to only standard rat chow (from what I hear, pretty bland stuff). Another had access to a "cafeteria diet," a.k.a. some very yummy ultra-processed food for about one hour each day, and standard chow for the rest of the time. And the third group had extended, almost all-day access to the hyper-palatable food.[63]

In the rats with extended, all-day access to the cafeteria-like diet, researchers found that the forty-day junk-food-palooza actually caused changes in the rat brain similar to those seen in drug addiction and, consequently, led to significant overeating and weight gain. The culprit appears to be the brain's dopamine reward system. Basically, eating junk food is *so pleasurable* that your brain starts to become less sensitive to the large floods of dopamine experienced when eating it. This *hyposensitivity* to the reward stimulus, a.k.a. the junk food, means that you need to eat more and more to cause the same reward response in your brain.[64] Just as we see in drug addiction, consistent consumption of junk food may mean that you need to eat more and more to get the same pleasure you originally got from smaller quantities.

Interestingly, the rats with only one-hour access to the hyper-palatable-food diet started exhibiting binge-like behaviors, eating two-thirds of their daily calories in that one hour and allocating the other third to the standard rat chow throughout the rest of the day. I have to say, these rats are giving me some pretty strong déjà vu to long days of trying to "eat clean" and then going to town the second I had access to treats.

The reward deficit (diminished response to food in the brain) seen in the rats persisted for two weeks after their access to hyper-palatable foods was taken away. (Interestingly, similar reward deficits after rats self-administer cocaine goes away after forty-eight hours.) When the rats went back to eating their standard laboratory chow, they ate substantially less, almost as if they would prefer to starve than eat regular food. Just some hyper-palatable food for thought.

It should be said, there are many differences between the concepts of food addiction and drug addiction.[65] For one, unlike with drugs of abuse, we need food to survive. Thus, there is no such thing as abstinence from food. For another, the overlap between food addiction and binge eating disorder also muddies the waters: Is it addiction or is it an eating disorder? Or is food addiction the underlying mechanism that explains binge eating disorder?[66] Finally, the food environment of rats is very different from the food environment of humans, so the extrapolation of rat data into human data still needs further research.

The Gut and the Brain

Whether or not you are swayed by the literature on food addiction, there is a whole host of other mechanisms, physiological and otherwise, that may explain how ultra-processed foods influence eating behaviors. The higher fat and refined-carbohydrate content of these foods not only makes them extremely tasty and craveable, it also makes them extremely calorie dense.[67] This means for the same amount of volume, ultra-processed foods contain way more calories. Think of a bunch of broccoli, which might be 200 calories, versus three Double Stuf Oreos, also around 200 calories. Ultra-processed foods take up less room in your stomach, which means it takes more of the food to make you feel "full." UPFs are also extremely low in fiber and protein, both nutrients that are known to increase fullness, or satiation.[68]

Furthermore, there is emerging evidence that ultra-processed food alters the way your gut communicates with your brain, which may also play a role in overconsumption and impaired reward signaling.[69] For example, in unprocessed food, how sweet a food tastes is directly proportional to how much sugar that food contains. Grapes taste sweeter than something like celery, and obviously that is because they contain much more sugar than celery does.

Many ultra-processed foods, however, use a combination of caloric sweeteners and noncaloric sweeteners, such as Splenda or stevia leaf extract. This means that how *sweet* the food tastes is actually disproportionate to the amount of sugar in the actual thing you're eating. New evidence seems to suggest that this mismatch between taste and the actual caloric properties of the food disrupts how your gut communicates to your brain.[70] It's confusing because your body evolved with sweetness being a signal of calories, but in today's food environment, that's not always the case. Researchers believe that mixing artificial and caloric sweeteners means the energetic value is not being accurately communicated to the brain. This, in turn, may also dysregulate food reward systems (making you eat more) as well as nutrient storage. Yet, again, a piece of food engineering meant to sell us on the "health" of ultra-processed foods, namely zero-calorie sweeteners, may actually be doing the opposite.

Portions and Packaging

Other aspects of ultra-processed foods, beyond their nutrient properties, may cause overeating. Ultra-processed food is not only hyper-palatable, it also usually comes in larger portions. We've all experienced the "portion-size effect," a.k.a. the tendency to eat more when you are served larger portions.[71]

Even the marketing around processed foods has a dramatic effect on how much of them we eat. Getting back to the processed-food-companies-capitalizing-on-dietary-fads debacle, a series of studies published by the Cornell Food and Brand Lab found that when M&M's were labeled "low-fat," participants were likely to consume 28 percent more of the candy.[72] Even though low-fat products, on average, had 59 percent less fat than their full-fat counterparts, they actually only had about 15 percent fewer calories (remember, when you take out fat, you have to add something else to make the food taste remotely good). Combined with the fact that people underestimated calories *the most* when foods were labeled as "low-fat," it seems that low-fat labeling actually makes you eat *more* than you would of the full-fat product.[73]

This perfectly aligns with the fact that Americans, after the dietary-fat guidelines were released, did not really reduce overall fat (although they did reduce saturated fat), and also started to eat way more total calories.[74] Researchers found that just labeling something as "low-fat" decreases perception of calorie density, increases what you think the "appropriate" serving size is, and reduces subjective feelings of "guilt," which may also contribute to people eating more.[75] This is just one example of how a supposed health claim on a food can have a dramatic effect on perception of the food and portion size. Now think about how many health claims you see in the supermarket every single day.

The amount of money spent by processed-food companies is astounding: in one year, $11.26 billion was spent on food-related advertising. Does anyone want to guess how much was spent on the glamorous task of glorifying plants and whole foods? Well, the US Department of Agriculture, in that same year, spent a whopping $268 million dollars on nutrition education.[76] To save you some quick math, that's just about 2 percent of the money spent by "food" advertisers.

How many commercials have you seen for kale? Mushrooms? Salmon? Black beans? I would guess a big, gaping zero. Now think back to your childhood Saturday mornings: between episodes of your favorite cartoons, Do you remember commercial after commercial of happy children with young, smiling moms getting the newest flavor of Lunchables, Toaster Strudels, and Pop-Tarts? Every other ad was for some version of sugar-flour clumps, sold to you by a leprechaun, toucan, or sea captain, complete with a "heart healthy" badge because they were now "made with whole grain." And these ads have effects. One 2014 study found that those exposed to food advertising ate 28 percent more of the unhealthy foods than those exposed to nonfood advertising.[77] In children, the effects are even more dire. In one study, children consumed 45 percent more after being exposed to food advertising.[78] The bottom line: a lot of money is spent on marketing these substances as "food," and all that money really pays off.

Finally, let's briefly consider the way in which ultra-processed food is consumed. These food products are convenient, cheap, ubiquitous, and either ready-to-eat or ready-to-heat. Thus, they can shift our eating patterns, promoting snacking, eating while doing other tasks, and mindless eating.[79] How easily can you mindlessly eat an avocado versus something like a sleeve of Oreos? If you've spent an hour preparing a dish versus two seconds opening a package, how attentive are you likely to be when eating that food? Ultra-processed food often turns our mouths into autonomic human vacuums, with the sounds of crunching or crinkling merely serving as a backdrop to the newest episode of *Euphoria* we may be watching that night. Research shows that the rapid eating rate and inattention often associated with UPF actually interrupts digestive and neural mechanisms that usually tell your brain "Hey! We can stop eating now! We're good!"[80] Anyone who has sat on their couch elbow-deep in a bag of salt-and-vinegar chips with *Grey's Anatomy* on blast knows: it's almost impossible to stop.

Overfed and Undernourished

In reading about nutrition and food, so much of the discussion is focused on what to *avoid*: dietary fat, cholesterol, refined carbohydrates—the list goes on and on. Besides the general advice to "eat more fruits and vegetables," very little is actually said about *why* this almost universal advice is given. I say "almost" because in this week's episode of "New Controversial Hot Take and Diet to Sell Your Instagram Plan," there are actually people on social media and beyond giving "advice" to avoid certain fruits and vegetables. Oh yes, the carnival continues!

Back to the matter at hand: one reason (almost) everyone advises us to increase fruit and vegetable intake is because they are remarkably high in fiber and micronutrients, a.k.a. vitamins and minerals. Although the focus is generally on plants, they're not the only stars of the micronutrient show; other food groups, including meat, fish, eggs (thank you, Harvard T.H. Chan School of Public Health, for the update), mushrooms, legumes, and nuts, are vitamin and mineral *packed*. What do all these groups have in common? Well, they're *real* food, mainly minimally or unprocessed. Cookies, cakes, cereals, TV dinners, and chips? Not so much.

Ultra-processed foods make up a majority of the average American's diet, and they're overwhelmingly made up of fat and refined carbohydrates (usually in the form of sugar). Thus, a big focus is put on how eating a ton of processed foods means that the average person's diet is also extremely high in fat and refined carbohydrates. But what about all the things we're lacking by eating so many processed foods?

Because a lot of the diseases that we deal with today are diseases of overconsumption, we don't often think of ourselves as "malnourished." We don't think about the fact that having excess calories can simultaneously exist with poor nutrition. Therefore, we don't ever pay attention to micros. When was the last time someone told you, "Yeah dude, I'm really trying to up my micros." Or, "I'm tracking my micros." But micronutrients are just as important as, and maybe even more important than, overall calorie and macronutrient intake.

Micronutrient deficiencies are among the twenty most important risk factors for diseases, and at least half the world's children (most of whom are growing up in developing countries) are deficient in at least one micronutrient.[81] And although there can be other reasons for micronutrient deficiencies, like certain diseases, the most common cause is, you guessed it, insufficient micros in the diet.[82] But how big is the difference in micronutrients between ultra-processed food and minimally processed food? I mean, ketchup has tomatoes in it, right? There's some dried fruit in that cereal somewhere, I think.

In a study looking at UPF intake in the Brazilian population, the ultra-processed foods most common in the Brazilian diet were found to have lower levels of sixteen out of the seventeen micronutrients measured.[83] And for ten of them—vitamins B12, C, D, and E, and niacin, pyridoxine, copper, magnesium, manganese, and zinc—the amounts found in the ultra-processed foods consumed by the subjects was less than half of that found in minimally processed foods. That's not to mention the fact that many ultra-processed foods are fortified with micronutrients, which also inflates their perceived health "benefits." By the way, researchers also found that diets high in UPF, compared to those high in minimally processed food, provided 2.5 times the energy per gram (calorie density), 2 times more free sugar, 1.5 times more overall and saturated fat, 8 times more trans fats, 3 times less fiber, and 2 times less protein.[84]

When I was first getting into health and fitness, micronutrients seemed completely irrelevant to me. If they're not contributing to my plan to "look hot for summer," what was the point of caring? But you can only go so far with an attitude like that before you face the health consequences of eating a diet entirely of protein bars, protein powders, and low-calorie "healthy" food items.

Vitamins and minerals are crucial for cell signaling, hormone production, immune responses, and overall maintenance of pretty much every vital function. Unfortunately, micronutrient deficiencies aren't something you'll notice overnight: it's not like your hair will start falling out the second you stop eating enough vitamin E. But subclinical deficiencies are pretty common. I don't know what I could've said to my younger self to take micronutrients seriously, but here is a brief and abridged list of just a few things micronutrients are needed for.[85]

- Lack of sufficient iron, zinc, and vitamin A are among the biggest problems in the world (affecting mainly pregnant women, children, and populations in developing countries). These deficiencies can cause stunted growth and increased fetal and maternal mortality.

- Iron, zinc, vitamins A, C, D, and selenium and riboflavin act as immunomodulators, which impact your susceptibility to infectious diseases as well as how sick you get if infected. Given the context of the COVID pandemic, this seems particularly relevant.

- Having enough vitamin D, calcium, magnesium, and phosphorus is crucial for growing strong healthy bones and maintaining them as we age.

- The B-complex vitamins, including thiamine, riboflavin, pyridoxine, and niacin, are crucial for cognitive functioning.

- And, of course, micronutrients that act as antioxidants have crucial functions in the etiology and development of chronic diseases.

The share of ultra-processed foods in our diets is only increasing, which means that the amount of these micronutrients in our diet is rapidly dwindling. Who would have guessed that we are at the same time overfed and undernourished? This trend is particularly of concern in children. Several studies have shown that children's diets have the highest proportion of ultra-processed food: in countries like the United Kingdom, the United States, and Canada, well over half of the average child's calories come from UPF.[86] Obviously, childhood and adolescence are crucial times in our development, physically and cognitively. And malnourishment at these stages may have life-long consequences.

Beyond the Nutrients

Here's a question for you: If we know that we need all these micronutrients, and we know we need to not overeat certain macronutrients, couldn't we just engineer some perfect food that meets all these criteria? Is it *just* the nutritional profile of ultra-processed foods that makes them so bad for our health? Or is there something about the actual "processing" part, something separate from the fat, sugar, and vitamin content? After all, we've spent pages and pages in this book discussing specific nutrients, what they're for, why they're helpful or unhelpful. Isn't this upholding the very nutrition-ism we previously slandered? And if we're buying into it, shouldn't we use this knowledge for good, rather than evil, and create an ultra-healthy food (UHF)? (Sidenote: Must trademark this new acronym ASAP.)

Well, here's the problem: nutritionism falls short. Research suggests there's something beyond the nutrients here. Yes, UPFs make us overeat. Yes, they are high in sugar, fat, and salt. Yes, they are devoid of any mean-ingful vitamins and minerals. But also, there's something else going on.

For example, there was still an association between ultra-processed food and obesity, even after researchers adjusted for saturated fat, trans fats, sugar, and fiber intake, suggesting it's not just the nutrients impacting risk of obe-sity. In a study in the *American Journal of Hypertension*, researchers found an association between ultra-processed food and hypertension, even after adjust-ing for sodium, fruit and vegetable intake, and Mediterranean dietary pattern score. In yet another study, while consumption of processed or ultra-processed food was associated with metabolic syndrome, carbohydrate, fat, protein, or fiber intakes were not.[87] All of this suggests there's something beyond the nu-trients about processed foods that is adversely affecting our health outcomes.

We can also see this effect more acutely. For example, one study tested the effect that cream versus butter had on acute blood cholesterol.[88] In case your parents didn't grow up in rural Albania, like mine did, butter is just churned cream, that is, a more processed version of cream. Despite supposedly being the same thing, cream was found *not* to increase blood cholesterol, while butter did. The authors suggest that the reason for this difference is that cream has almost double the milk-fat globule membrane (MFGM) on a per-gram-of-fat basis as butter, which may lower serum cholesterol. Apparently, the MFGM gets greatly reduced in the churning process, where it mostly transfers to the buttermilk portion. To be honest, knowing about MFGM and the process of making butter is about number 1,032 on my list of things to care about, but the fact that something *just being churned* changes the way we respond to it is reason enough to think more carefully about what we're eating and what state it's in.

Similar effects have been found with sugar versus honey, or even artificial honey versus real honey: despite the sugar content, calories, and even molecules matching, the sugar *and* imitation honey both have worse health effects on people's blood-sugar levels than the real honey.[89] In another study, researchers tested full-fat cheese versus low-fat cheese plus butter.[90] The researchers matched the macronutrient profiles of the groups (meaning they were eating the same amounts of fat and protein) as well as the casein and calcium content. A strictly nutritionist reading of this experiment would make you think that there shouldn't be a differing effect on serum cholesterol or LDL cholesterol. And yet the study found that the low-fat-cheese-plus-butter group saw significantly increased serum cholesterol, while the full-fat cheese group did not. Again, the nutrients were the same, but the effects were different. Fun fact: the reason researchers wanted to run this experiment was to partially explain why cheese seems to have a positive effect on health outcomes, despite cheese being supposedly "bad for you."

What to Eat

After a harrowing journey through egg lobbies, Senate committees, low-fat M&M's, and more, I am delighted that we have made it to this section of the book: what to eat. On the next page, you will find all micro- and macronutrients, in alphabetical order, with their recommended dosages, timings, and suggested sources. Alternatively, on the website for this book you can purchase a cocktail of these nutrients, attractively packaged, and sweetened with zero-calorie sweeteners, complete with free shipping for your first thirty orders! Enjoy!

OK, sorry, I am being annoying here, but seriously, if you believed that I would just give you a list of nutrients and amounts . . . please reread the chapter! If I've learned anything, it's that much smarter people than I have not been able to piece together exactly what to eat, so the idea that I will come up with a new formula never thought of before is hilarious.

There's actually a lot of nutrition research that people agree on, and have in fact agreed on for the past fifty years. For example, those same *Dietary Goals* from the 1970s also advised the following:[91]

- "Consume only as much energy (calories) as is expended."

- "Increase the consumption of complex carbohydrates and 'naturally occurring' sugars."

- "Reduce the consumption of refined and processed sugars."

- "Increase consumption of fruits and vegetables and whole grains."[92]

Sure, you can find some fringe Instagram "nutrition experts" who disagree, but the vast majority are going to say, "Yeah, this all sounds good." These recommendations have been consistent for the past several decades and have stood the test of time scientifically. We'll go through some more general tenets to guide your food decisions in the sections below.

From the Doc: What to Eat

When I speak to my patients about their eating, I try to address their overall diets rather than putting them *on* a diet. All of us can make some tweaks toward higher-quality food and healthier choices for our meals and snacks. The results are dramatic. Transitioning from the standard American diet to a more optimized diet by eating more vegetables, legumes, whole grains, and nuts and less red and processed meat could translate into a decade of increased life expectancy for young adults and a 7 percent or more increase across all age groups and sexes.[93] You can instantly estimate the impact of changes in your diet on your life expectancy at www.food4healthylife.org.

The recommendations I make are evidence-based and give concrete, measurable changes that are realistic, small substitutions.[94] These incremental tweaks can have measurable changes on your health metrics and improve your sense of self-efficacy and confidence to move on to larger changes in your diet and other health behaviors. These changes will not necessarily tip the (bathroom) scale, but they are a reasonable, usually acceptable, and achievable place to start a conversation. You need not make all these changes: even choosing one can get the process started toward an improved diet.

Drinks

Decreasing consumption of regular sodas, juices, and other sugar-sweetened beverages by one serving per day and replacing it with water, flavored water, coffee (without lots of added sugar and milk), or tea is often one of the easiest tweaks to improve diet quality. You don't need additional planning or a special trip to the supermarket to choose a different drink from the store or vending machine. The ease of this transition may be part of the reason why consumption of sugar-sweetened beverages showed a marked drop from 1999 to 2012.[95]

Vegetables

Increased vegetable consumption, whether fresh, frozen, or canned, provides myriad benefits, especially from the high fiber content and low caloric density of vegetables. Even for the small minority of us who do consume the recommended five daily servings of fruits and vegetables, the extra vegetables are a very healthy addition. Start simply by having carrots in your fridge, perhaps washed and cut and ready to grab at any time.

Fast Food

Plan to decrease one fast food meal per week and replace it with prepared food from the supermarket or a meal made at home. Almost any food you make at home will have fewer calories and healthier ingredients than what you will find in prepared food.[96,97]

Ultra-Processed Food (UPF)

Cut back or avoid ultra-processed food products to improve health and to limit excess calorie intake. These products feature added salt, sugar, and fat and are engineered to be highly palatable. This was summarized in the iconic potato-chip ad slogan "Betcha can't eat just one."[98]

Snacks, Chips, or Crackers

Aim to eliminate one serving each week of chips or crackers by swapping it for a handful of nuts. This healthy diet hack may involve simply choosing peanuts instead of chips at the store or market. The health benefits of most nuts are considerable despite the high levels of fats and their energy density.[99]

Whole Grains

Whether in the grocery aisle, at a restaurant, or ordering a pizza, opt for the whole grain option to increase your intake of fiber, vitamins, and minerals.

Desserts

Try to decrease your desserts by one serving each week and replace one sugary sweet or dessert with fruit or a handful of nuts. You need not even give up dessert completely. A healthy "dessert flip" might be trading a piece of chocolate cake topped with strawberries for a serving of strawberries dipped in chocolate. Or rather than giving up a dessert, try making one at home. Almost anything you bake at home will include healthier fat, fewer calories, and less sweetener than something you buy at a store or restaurant.

Fruit

Increasing fruit consumption by one serving per day (whether the fruit is fresh, frozen, or canned) may reduce cardiovascular deaths by 8 percent, saving sixty thousand lives in the United States each year and preventing 1.6 million deaths across the world.[100] As the new saying might go, "An apple a day keeps the grim reaper away."

Processed Meats and Red Meats

Consider trading one meal of ham or other processed meat for a serving of beans, nuts, chicken, or fish each week. Making this switch can be as complex as planning a different dinner entrée or as simple as choosing tuna fish instead of roast beef for tomorrow's lunch. Another option is to substitute processed meat with any kind of meat cooked at home.

As small as some of these changes might seem, it takes planning to accomplish them. For example, try buying fruits and vegetables to have ready to eat at home or to take with you. Meal planning is not a trivial task. For many of us, thoughts about dinner don't arise until we start to get hungry. Interestingly, it is becoming increasingly popular for physicians to advise patients on food planning and preparation as part of culinary medicine and a program called CHEF Coaching (Culinary Healthcare Education Fundamentals).[101,102] The Health meets Food™ culinary medicine curriculum launched at Tulane University School of Medicine in 2012 has spread to more than fifty-five medical schools, residency programs, and nursing schools. The curriculum encourages students to trade in their white lab coats for a white chef's apron as they learn to cook as part of their education.[103]

EATING FOR THE PLANET

No discussion of "what to eat" in the 2020s would be complete without considering the impact of our food choices on the planet's health as well as our own. We really can't go much further down our self-centered path without acknowledging the herd of elephants in the room.

How do our individual food choices affect the health of the planet? What on earth can we do to help the earth while feeding ourselves beneficially?

At the risk of inducing stress eating by focusing only on the dire predictions for our climate emergency, let's state the facts and find a path forward. According to the EAT-*Lancet* Commission 2019 report:[104]

- 2 billion people are overweight or have obesity.

- 820 million people lack sufficient food, and many more have low-quality diets.

- Unhealthy diets now pose a greater risk for death and disease than unsafe sex and alcohol, drug, and tobacco use combined.

- Global food production threatens climate stability and ecosystem resilience and is the largest single driver of environmental degradation.

The transformation to healthy diets will include doubling the consumption of fruits, vegetables, and legumes, and a more than 50 percent reduction in consumption of less healthy foods, such as added sugars and red meat. The solution may be simple but not necessarily easy to achieve.

"A diet rich in plant-based foods and with fewer animal source foods confers both improved health and environmental benefits."[105] This is basically a "flexitarian" diet, largely plant-based but accommodating modest amounts of fish, meat, and dairy foods. Adopting these dietary changes from our current eating patterns could prevent an estimated eleven million deaths per year and dramatically decrease stress on the environment.

"Food is the single strongest lever to optimize human health and environmental sustainability on Earth."[106]

Eat well for yourself and for the planet.

The Takeaways

Here are some practical tenets to guide your food choices, minus lobbying and food-industry influence:

1. **Eat real food.** It's not that complicated: we need to eat real food, not creations of food science. Real foods are usually on the perimeters on the grocery store. They go bad; they are minimally processed or unprocessed; they don't have health claims on the packaging; they would have been recognized a hundred years ago. Focus less on nutrients and more on where those nutrients come from.[107]

2. **Diversify your food.** No one food can give you all the nutrients you need. Therefore, eating as wide a variety of foods as possible ensures you are getting as wide a variety of nutrients as possible. This includes *a lot* of plant foods (fruits, vegetables,

legumes, nuts), some animal foods (meat, seafood, eggs, fermented dairy), and fungi (mushrooms). One thing that almost all dietary guidelines agree on: increased food diversity = increased diet quality and better health outcomes.[108]

3. **Prepare your own food.** Maybe it's because it takes more time and work, forcing you to slow down; maybe it's because it makes you look up new recipes, try new vegetables, and eat more real foods, but whatever the reason, cooking your own food seems to improve diet quality.[109] Meal planning is also associated with a better diet.[110] So let's bust out the pots and pans, folks.

4. **Eat the right amount of food.** No matter how "healthy" you eat, overeating is not good. If you focus on the rest of the advice, though: enjoying a diet primarily based on whole foods, you'll likely find it relatively easy to stick to the right amount. PS: We all overeat sometimes, and that's OK! We're talking here about eating the right amount on average.

5. **Enjoy your food.** So much focus is placed on overeating and what foods are "bad" for us that we often forget the following: food keeps us alive. It nourishes our bodies. Eating food should be a pleasurable experience.[111] Slower and more mindful eating helps reduce binge eating, emotional eating, potential overconsumption, *and* makes us *enjoy* food, as we're supposed to.[112]

And now, we move to the other side of the equation, and Eddie's and my favorite topic, the "energy out." Since this is Eddie's whole specialty as a physician, I'm going to let him take the lead.

6

Exercise: The Magic Pill

How the Doc Discovered Exercise

One of my earliest memories is of watching my father do his daily push-ups. Unable to copy his movement, I was thrilled to participate in the routine by climbing on his back and hanging on for the ride. He would flex his biceps like Popeye and regale my sisters and me with stories of his glory days as a high school football player. These were the days when players played both offense and defense, helmets were crafted from soft leather, and the hard, plastic, modern face guards and protective gear were nowhere in sight. I was enraptured, listening to him recount the tale of how he once played football at Ebbets Field, the home of his beloved Brooklyn Dodgers. My father also had a short boxing career. "I could have been a contender," he insisted in his gruff New York accent, "if my father hadn't shown up and pulled me outta the ring." I was never a football player. I never tried my hand at boxing. Nevertheless, I was imprinted with my father's athletic predilections, with the glimmering prospect of making my body strong enough "to be a contender."

As a teenager, I stumbled upon a book detailing the complex kinematic interplay between the human body and the bicycle. I understood precious little of the book's dense mathematics, but I was fascinated by the perspective of our bodies as mechanical masterpieces. These experiences literary propelled me into a multidecade career of intensive martial arts training. I yearned to be an expert in the mechanics of human movement, to understand every gear, lever, and system animating our beings.

At first, memorizing the myriad movements felt like an insurmountable task. However, what I eventually came to learn was the almost poetic commonality underscoring all human movements: you can only punch or kick or walk in so many ways.

Out of the thousands of students in training at the dojo I attended, only two or three were awarded black belts per year. Achieving this rare distinction required endless hours of training and dedication. To earn the belt, it was not enough to simply demonstrate one's strengths. The true mark of an advanced martial artist was the capacity to overcome one's weaknesses. For me, physical strength was my greatest asset, but exhibiting gracefulness and precision with several weapons proved to be the biggest challenge. At the height of my training, I planned to devote a year of full-time training to achieving my black belt between college and medical school. When I realized that I would not earn my black belt within that year, I wrote *the letter of my life* to convince the medical school to delay my entrance for another year so that I could fulfill my dream of becoming a black belt. I knew that accomplishing this goal would eventually enable me to become a better doctor. The school granted me the deferment, and I earned my black belt just a few months before medical school started.

Now, decades later, I no longer practice the punching, kicking, and sparring that defined my adolescence and early adulthood. What I have carried with me from my prior intensive physical and mental training is the continued practice of the movement of my *energy* (variously described as chi, prana, life force) through tai chi, yoga, and meditation.

Specializing in Exercise

Students entering medical school are like pluripotent stem cells, confronted with a plethora of different paths toward becoming a specialized physician. There is a critical stage in the final years of medical school in which future doctors begin to differentiate. Absent purely financial considerations—choosing a higher-paying specialty to pay off egregious debts incurred by becoming a doctor—students get to dedicate their careers to whatever field of medicine fascinates them the most. If the heart is your beat: cardiology; if skin covers it: dermatology; if lungs inspire you: pulmonology; or if the brain gets you thinking: neurology. Absent a cringeworthy pun, I chose to specialize in physical medicine and rehabilitation (PM&R). Rehab specialists, more correctly called *physiatrists,* are the healers, *iatrists,* of the body, *physia* (not to be confused with *psych*iatrists who heal the *psyche,* or mind). While other physicians care for your skin, brain, heart, or kidneys, we care for your muscles and, by extension, your ability to move and function. Our brains issue instructions, transmitted through our nerves, which fire the muscles that pull on our bones to make the joints move in whatever manner we like. And all of this, remarkably, while balancing on two legs.

Imagine my thrill when I discovered a specialty that would allow me to study gait, treat joints and muscles, and devote my working life to what has always fascinated me most: our innate physicality. I found that practicing as a physiatrist paralleled my transformational experience in the karate dojo. As a young martial artist, I focused on the internal exploration of my own movement, but as a physician, I get to orient that focus externally, toward my patients, toward each person's specific pain and physical dysfunction, and guide them toward improved strength, balance, and agility so that they may rely on their bodies to move with less pain and more confidence.

There is an adage that "physicians treat their own disease." It's true that medical professionals are often motivated to select specialties based on personal or familial medical concerns and challenges. Early loss of a parent to cancer (and increased personal risk) is a common inception for a future oncologist. My early experience showed me the dramatic therapeutic capacities of exercise. At age five, I had both a "lazy eye" and a lisp. Eye exercises and speech therapy—which retrained the movements of my eye and the positioning of my tongue—enabled me to evade both corrective eye surgery and the orthodontics that plagued my two sisters. If exercise could be used to strengthen tiny eye muscles, imagine its capacities when therapeutically applied to larger muscles of the body.

In my more than thirty-year-long career in physical medicine and rehabilitation, I have devoted myself to using exercise to help patients who have lost limbs, suffered strokes, undergone joint replacements, sprained ankles, and more to regain a functioning body. Time and again I have witnessed how allowing these patients to restore their movements enables them to regain their lives, to do what they need and love to do. This transformation is primarily accomplished through therapeutic exercise steered by physical and occupational therapists. If exercise is such a powerful tool for those with disabilities and injuries, the logical extension seemed obvious. Why not apply exercise to the broader population?

Lifestyle Medicine

More than twenty years ago I coauthored a textbook chapter exploring the science of motivation for patients entering rehabilitation. I soon broadened that investigation to explore how physicians (and indeed all clinicians) might help motivate patients to become and stay more physically active. For decades the central scholarly question propelling my work has been, "If exercise is so damn good for us, then why don't more people do it?"

My fascination with exercise led to my role as a pioneer and thought leader in the rapidly evolving field of lifestyle medicine. However, I soon came to understand that not all my patients (nor my colleagues in lifestyle medicine) shared my passion for exercise. In some cases my patients were already getting an adequate amount of exercise, and they wanted to focus more on other areas, such as stress management, getting enough sleep, or deepening their relationships. With other patients, bringing up exercise immediately induced disinterest or an aversive reaction. This diverse set of patient needs and experiences led me to conclude that clinicians need to promote exercise, but only as one of several tools.

In scenarios wherein it is appropriate to discuss exercise with my patients, I aim to demonstrate how certain types of physical activity can directly aid each individual's ailment or illness. For example: "You should know that getting in more steps per day will help you manage your diabetes and possibly cut down on your need for insulin." If your goal is to improve your mental health, improve sleep, or maintain or lose weight, then you should know how exercise might be helpful. But first, let's define physical activity and the different types of exercise that you might consider.

Exercise Defined

Physical activity is defined as any bodily movement produced by skeletal muscles that results in energy expenditure.[1] In other words, if you are not sedentary and your body is in motion, you are being *physically active*. Physical activity is, for some of the population, naturally embedded in our daily lives as part of our occupations, household tasks, or hobbies. As a result, physical activity is more approachable and perhaps more enticing than *exercise*. Exercise is formally defined as "a subset of physical activity that is planned, structured, and repetitive and has as a final or an intermediate objective the improvement or maintenance of physical fitness."[2]

In a clinical setting, I rarely ask my patients about "exercise." For so many of us, the term "exercise" is laden with negative associations like guilt and discomfort. If the topic does come up with my patients, they will often respond with statements such as the following:

- "I don't like exercise; that's what they made me do in the Army."

- "I don't like to sweat and be out of breath."

- "I would do it if only I could find an exercise that doesn't mess up my hair."

- "The gym is too expensive, too far away, and I don't feel comfortable there."

- "I guess I would exercise, but I can never find the time."

Early in my career, I felt it was my duty to advocate for exercise regardless of these aversive responses, but I have come to realize that emphasizing "physical activity" is oftentimes a more effective approach. Either way, *physical fitness* is the outcome of your exercise *or* physical activity, and it is defined by the enhancement of endurance, strength, flexibility, balance, and so on.

Next, let's consider the quantity and intensity of physical activity one should ideally do each week to benefit health. Physical activity is a very potent intervention that improves almost every function of your body, and one need not ever sweat or get out of breath to successfully complete one's weekly minutes of recommended activity. It is important to note that the guidelines for physical activity are generalized recommendations and do not account for the nuances of every individual's needs and capacities.

According to the "Talk Test," while performing *light*-intensity physical activity, you would be able to talk in full sentences and sing. At *moderate* intensity, you could talk but not sing, while at a *vigorous* intensity you would no longer be able to talk in full sentences without stopping to take a breath.[3] Remember that these measures of intensity are relative to you and your level of fitness. For example, when I run with my wife—who has a much higher cardiovascular endurance than me—I work *vigorously* to keep up while she is capable of cruising along at a *moderate* intensity. This gives me the opportunity to become an excellent listener, as she can easily talk about her day, while I can only grunt short phrases of encouragement: "Then what happened?" "Wow," or "No way!"

The application of this three-tiered approach to physical activity means that you have the power to choose what degree of intensity is right for you on any given day without sacrificing the benefits of regular physical activity.

Unlike the drama and controversy of the government's dietary guidelines (see chapter 5), the *Physical Activity Guidelines for Americans* are consistent with those of the World Health Organization and are followed in multiple countries.[4] They state that we should get the following:

- 150 minutes of moderate-intensity physical activity per week, *or*

- 75 minutes of vigorous physical activity in bouts of any length, *or* an equivalent combination.

- For sedentary individuals (performing neither moderate nor vigorous physical activity), adoption of light-intensity activity is beneficial.

For more extensive health benefits:

- 300 minutes of moderate-intensity physical activity, *or* 150 minutes of vigorous physical activity, *or* an equivalent combination.

- Resistance training (muscle strengthening) at least twice per week.

If you do vigorous-intensity physical activity, you can cut your workout time in half. However, the same benefits can be achieved from briskly walking 30 minutes a day with your dog. A swim at a local pool or a class at your community center can get you on the right track as well. Even if you are not getting a full 150 minutes per week of moderate-intensity physical activity, you still benefit from the minutes that you are active.

Surveys report that many Americans struggle to reach these guidelines. Just more than half of the population meets these recommendations for weekly cardiovascular activity, and if you include the recommendation for twice-weekly resistance exercise, that number falls to about one in five Americans.[5]

Cardiovascular Activity and Weight

If you have a specific goal in mind, such as training for an athletic event or maintaining weight loss, you will likely need to do more than three hundred minutes of moderate-intensity activity per week.[6] Even then, the number of calories burned doing this higher level of activity is usually not sufficient on its own to lose weight.

Why is it so hard to lose weight just from exercising? As we discussed in chapter 3, exclusively measuring *calories in* and *calories out* is not the only or necessarily the best way to estimate weight loss. Even so, the numbers are instructive. A pound of fat contains around 3,500 calories of energy. Humans tend to be very energy efficient when it comes to walking; the average adult male burns about 100 calories per mile. If you were to walk briskly for three hundred minutes, or five hours, per week at 4 miles per hour, you would cover twenty miles. This activity regimen would burn about 2,000 calories, and you would theoretically lose just over half a pound of fat per week. However, this regimen is not necessarily the recipe for weight loss, because increased physical activity is often accompanied by increased hunger and increased food consumption, as well as potential downregulation of other metabolic functions (thereby decreasing your caloric expenditure), depending on the intensity of the activity (see chapter 2). That being said, regular physical activity is one of the best tactics to *maintain* weight loss. The National Weight Control Registry, which tracks individuals who have lost at least thirty pounds and kept it off for at least a year, reports that females expend >2,500 calories and males >3,330 calories in weekly physical activity to maintain weight loss.[7]

The efficacy of exercise as a tactic for maintaining weight loss may be better explained by the role that physical activity plays in enabling the termination of restricted food intake and in helping the body maintain lean muscle mass. As revealed in chapter 3, once you have lost weight, you have effectively lowered your basal metabolic rate by becoming a smaller person: you have reduced your body mass, and thus your body takes less energy to maintain itself. If you "end your diet" and resume eating at your prior, habitual amount, over time you will regain your prior weight. This formula outlines the experience of the vast majority of dieters who regain weight in the months and years after their periods of restriction end. As an antidote, burning off additional calories from resistance training or cardio may slow the weight regain or help keep you at your new weight.

If cardiovascular exercise is not the magic pill for weight loss, then why do it? The *Physical Activity Guidelines for Americans* concludes that greater volumes—that is, more than 150 minutes per week—of moderate to vigorous physical activity are associated with:[8]

- preventing or minimizing excessive weight gain in adults;

- maintaining weight within a healthy range and preventing obesity;

- relative reduction in risk of all-cause mortality;

- reduced incidence and mortality of cardiovascular disease; and

- reduced incidence of type 2 diabetes.

Also, even if you were never to lose weight, becoming more physically active confers similar benefits on those who are overweight or have obesity as on normal-weight individuals. As a bonus, physically active women are less likely to gain excessive weight during pregnancy, develop gestational diabetes, or develop postpartum depression.

BENEFITS OF CARDIOVASCULAR EXERCISE

- prevents obesity and mitigates its risks

- reduces development and improves management of diabetes

- prevents and treats heart disease

- lowers risk of some cancers

- treats hypertension

- prevents osteoporosis and fractures

- manages depression and anxiety

- reduces risk of dementia

- decreases risk of premature death[9]

Lifting Weight to Lose Weight

Getting enough cardiovascular exercise will help you maintain a healthy body, but the final recommendation in the guidelines for *resistance training* (muscle strengthening) *at least twice per week* provides numerous additional metabolic, functional, and aesthetic benefits. (See sidebar "Benefits of Resistance Training" later in this chapter.) Resistance training may also become an important element in losing weight. My introduction to resistance training (a.k.a. weightlifting) was not in medical school but instead was the result of a revelation that emerged from a course that I ran.

One of my favorite professional activities is organizing and directing large training courses for colleagues to learn how to keep both themselves and their patients healthier. Before the COVID-19 pandemic, medical professionals from around the world would travel to Boston for these lifestyle-medicine events, but during the pandemic, this course—and the community accompanying it—had to transition to online.

About seven years ago, in his presentation at "Active Lives," a continuing medical-education course in Boston, Dr. Wayne Westcott spoke about the significance of resistance training for general health. He presented himself as a case study and noted that through the aging process we lose, on average, about 3–5 percent of our lean muscle mass each decade. This means that even in maintaining his college weight of 160 pounds for the ensuing four decades, he would have lost about 24 pounds of muscle mass. The same weight would have been replaced by 24 pounds of fat in Dr. Westcott's body. This poignant message, that our advancing age turns us into bowls of Jell-O, was punctuated by one word that changed my life: "unless."

The entropic inclination of our bodies destines us toward gelatinous decay *unless* you maintain your muscle mass by training it and providing modest but regular stress to it, that is, resistance training. Put simply, humans are adaptation machines. If you stress your muscles, they will stay strong and even improve. This improvement could manifest as the power to lift more weight, the ability to take longer walks, or a sustained capacity to carry your grandchildren. However, in the absence of stress, muscles will adapt in the opposite direction and begin to atrophy. "If you don't use it, you lose it."

Westcott's studies found that subjects placed on caloric restriction (a.k.a. a diet) along with a resistance-training regimen of two to three sessions per week for ten weeks experienced, on average, the loss of four pounds of fat and the acquisition of more than three pounds of muscle.[10] These research results mirror the experience of my patients who take on a regimen of resistance training alongside a reasonably reduced caloric intake. Demonstrating a tightened belt, patients say, "I haven't lost much weight, but I am losing my pants." Maintaining or increasing your muscle mass can have profound effects on your overall health (see sidebar "Benefits of Resistance Training") and on your weight.

Body fat has very limited metabolic expenditure, meaning that it does not burn up many calories. On the other hand, the process of repairing muscle-protein breakdown after resistance training and building new muscle results in a higher rate of resting energy expenditure (see "Metabolism and the Physiology of Weight Loss," chapter 2).

Untrained muscle mass burns about 5–6 calories per pound per day.[11] If that muscle is *trained* it burns 50 percent more calories, more than 9 calories per pound per day.[12] The logical extension of this science means that maintaining more muscle mass enables you to eat a bit more and stay the same weight. There are increased energy requirements (i.e., burning extra calories) for seventy-two hours after a standard session of resistance exercise to repair the microtrauma and remodel the newly trained muscles. This additional energy expenditure, which equals around 100 calories per day, adds up to the energy stored in almost a pound of fat, that is, more than 3,000 calories each month that you perform twice-weekly resistance training. This science is the foundation of the recommendation that you can "lift weights to lose weight."[13]

The incorporation of resistance training into your weekly routine does not need to take up a lot of time, nor does it demand a gym full of fancy equipment. With a bit of research and creativity, resistance training can be one of the most accessible forms of exercise, due to the vast array of bodyweight resistance exercises. From your muscle's point of view, it doesn't know or care whether the stress on it is from using a machine in the gym or lifting weights at home or using a resistance band in your office. You don't have to actually lift any weights. For example, you could try taking your next phone call while standing and performing heel rises (going up on the balls of your feet) or while doing repeated partial squats (feet out at 45 degrees and gently lowering your buttocks to a chair or the arm of a couch). The same recommendations apply to those with disabilities. My patients with paralysis of their legs are encouraged to perform strengthening exercises to improve the function of their core and upper body. This enhances their ability to transfer independently and push a wheelchair safely.

You can perform a spontaneous body-weight-resistance exercise session almost anywhere, with essentially no equipment and minimal training. A few years ago, my wife and I were traveling to visit our son in college and inadvertently chose a place to stay featuring "the worst hotel gym in America." The large exercise room had eight treadmills, bikes, and ellipticals, four of which were plastered with OUT OF ORDER signs. I can only assume that the hotel's copy machine was also out of order because there were another couple of machines, without signs, which were also not working. There were several hotel guests waiting impatiently to use the last two working treadmills. Having lost our opportunity for our planned cardiovascular session on the machines, my wife pivoted quickly by writing down eight different body-weight exercises (see sidebar "Common Body-Weight Exercises") that we would commonly do as part of our boot-camp workouts at home. She then set her phone timer to thirty seconds of movement followed by fifteen seconds of rest. This routine, commonly known as Tabata, is a style of high-intensity interval training (HIIT), which allows for a short bout of maximal effort, in this case for thirty seconds, followed by a short recovery (of fifteen seconds). We started our session, doing squats, lunges, push-ups, and crunches. After a short while, one of the hotel guests waiting for the treadmill said, "That looks great. What app are you using?" I responded, "It's nothing fancy, just the timer on the phone," and she then joined our spontaneous boot camp. (There are multiple free downloads available for HIIT to mimic our workout with your choice of exercises.)

BENEFITS OF RESISTANCE TRAINING

- decreases risk of injury

- decreases risk of osteoporosis

- increases basal metabolic rate

- decreases fatigue

- increases performance

- increases muscle mass

- promotes aesthetic changes (you look better)

- increases quality of life, strength, endurance, and bone mineral density in early postmenopausal years

- decreases body fat

- improves lipid profiles

- improves glucose tolerance

(Note: These benefits are in addition to benefits from cardiovascular exercise.)[14,15]

STRENGTH-TRAINING GUIDELINES

- **exercises:** all major muscles (8–10 exercises)

- **frequency:** 2–3 days per week

- **sets:** 2–4 sets per muscle group

- **repetitions:** 8–12 repetitions per set

- **resistance:** 60–80 percent of maximum resistance

- **speed:** controlled concentric (shortening the muscle, e.g., a biceps curl); and eccentric (lengthening the muscle, e.g., straightening the elbow slowly with a weight in hand)

- **range:** full range of joint motion

- **breathing:** exhale on the concentric, inhale on the eccentric[16]

My Exercise Routine

Dr. Westcott's presentation at the "Active Lives" course profoundly influenced me. For the first time in my life, I was inspired to intentionally incorporate resistance training into my weekly routine with the hopes of maintaining my body's function as I age. In addition to my regular boot-camp resistance training, along the way, I have also dutifully dallied with nearly every exercise fad of the last few decades. I have tripped my way through Zumba, felt "the burn" in Pilates, pedaled on a Peloton, competed at the World Rowing Indoor Championship competition (don't be impressed; anyone can join for thirty dollars), strained unidentified muscles in barre and Gyrotonic Method, and sweated to the oldies under the guise that it is my professional responsibility to try every new exercise class and machine so that I can better understand how to best advise my patients. I can now knowingly suggest, "You might consider Pilates to strengthen your core," but also to understand the mechanism of injury. That's the medical term for understanding exactly how twisting your knee the wrong way can rupture your ACL, or, on a more personal level, how far I can extend my back in a yoga class before I feel back pain, because, yes, you can get injured in yoga. But there is something more that beckons me to these activities beyond my field of medicine. I remain enduringly and radically amazed by the physicality of our bodies, by all the ways that we can move with grace, creativity, and strength.

The exercise routine I follow with my wife has a loose rhythm to it, based on the cycle of the seasons and the balance of the days of the week. During the summertime, when we commit ourselves to train for triathlons, this routine includes a rotation of swimming, biking, running, strengthening, stretching, and resting. Flexibility—both literally and figuratively—is key. We do yoga stretches to protect our joints and muscles, but we also exercise the principle of flexibility when it comes to switching up and reordering exercises based on the weather, soreness, and injuries. For example, one of us might say, "I don't feel like I could run today, so let's go for a swim," or, "The weather is great for biking tomorrow." Rotating our exercises seasonally helps us reduce the risk of boredom, appreciate the environment, and avoid overuse injuries. In warmer months, we cherish the opportunity for open-water swimming in local ponds. When the snow falls and the lakes freeze over, we embrace the winter and the opportunity to strap on cross-country skis for a jaunt in the forest. My embrace of exercise engages me mentally, physically, and creatively. By doing my best to stay strong and in shape, I have the confidence to try new sports or activities and, when appropriate, to share my passion for exercise with my patients.

WAYS TO DO RESISTANCE TRAINING

- traditional free weights

- dumbbells

- weight machines

- body weight

- elastic bands or tubing (a.k.a. resistance bands)

- medicine balls

- common household products, like milk jugs filled with sand, or soup cans[17]

Counseling My Patients

When my patients present with concerns and frustration about their weight, our discussions can be loaded with emotional baggage and confused by the latest fad diet to hit their social media and seemingly conflicting scientific studies. Fortunately, there is much less emotion and controversy about exercise. Also, I can more easily inspire fascination, joy, and passion for physical activity because it enables my patients to add something positive to their lives without a perception of having to give up something.

In my exam room, I will simply ask, "How's your weight? Is it going up or down, or is it about the same?" I may have that data in front of me in the medical record, but I would rather engage with my patients than scan the computer screen. A patient's personal perspective concerning his or her weight is, in most cases, far more instructive than any number. Similarly, I'll ask, "How's your physical activity?" "What are you doing now?" "What sport or activity would you like to be doing?" These questions may be the most important ones I ask. Receiving the aspirational response, "Well, if I were in better shape, I might be able to get back to tennis," orients the conversation toward what matters most to the patient. Positive, effective behavior change is only sustainable if it propels someone toward what they deem to be most important. Being told to exercise because it will reduce your risk of future heart disease, cancer, or diabetes is usually not enough motivation to inspire changing existing habits. But if your exercise routine allows you to feel better right away and noticeably improve your function— for example, "I can now walk with my partner"—you are more likely to stick with it.

Focusing on the physical, mental, and emotional effects of exercise in the present moment usually offers a more compelling source of motivation than a distant health goal. Studies show that emphasis on the health benefits of exercise can backfire, making the activity less fun and consequently less enjoyable to continue to do. In one study, subjects who were instructed to walk one mile "because it was fun" were compared to subjects doing the same walk "for exercise." When they were then offered the same "all-you-can-eat" buffet, the "exercise is fun" group served themselves and consumed less "reward" foods (M&M's, soda, and chocolate pudding). To avoid the perceived work of exercise and the temptation to then reward yourself with food, go for a walk because it is fun and makes you feel better.[18]

COMMON BODY-WEIGHT EXERCISES

- heel rises (Hold on to the wall or an immovable object for balance. For an extra challenge, try it on one foot at a time.)

- partial squats

- lunges: forward, side, reverse

- push-ups (modifications on knees or against a counter or the wall)

- bridging (Lying faceup, heels to buttocks, raise the pelvis to create a "bridge.")

- crunches

- planks

- tricep dips (With your hands on the arms of a chair, raise and lower your butt without using your legs.)

Motivation to Get Moving

If you are largely sedentary, mostly sitting behind a desk and not accumulating enough moderate-intensity physical activity, replacing some of that sedentary behavior with light-intensity exercise is a great place to start. Your chance of developing diabetes, dying from cardiovascular disease, and generally dying from any cause is minimized by the regular incorporation of movement into your routine.[19]

If you feel intimidated by having to carve out time for a forty-five-minute cycling class, or by paying a hefty sum for a gym membership, rest assured that *any type* of physical activity of *any length* contributes to the health benefits associated with accumulating enough physical activity each week.[20] Exercise goals are more easily and enjoyably attained once an all-or-nothing mentality is abandoned. Every step and every minute of exercise counts. So make sure to get in the minutes you can, even if you don't reach your goal: zero minutes equals zero benefits.

When you write yourself an exercise prescription, choose activities that bring you joy. No type of movement is discredited. You are more likely to maintain your exercise routine if you choose enjoyable activities that will sustain your interest. Maybe you feel moved to dance one day, to garden the next, to hike the weekend after that. Flexibility and creativity when it comes to experimenting with a variety of different exercises will reduce boredom and your risk of injuries from repeating the same movement. You will keep up with your activity if you feel in charge of your choice.

Instead of framing your exercise session as an unpleasant chore, I encourage you to think of it as a gift that you give yourself at the beginning, end, or any time throughout the day. Your day can be a treasure hunt filled with hidden opportunities to get your body moving.[21] The more you see and experience the wonder of our physicality and myriad ways to move our bodies as a privilege and not a punishment, the more you will experience being active as a gift that you give to yourself rather than an unpleasant event to endure. One of the most compelling aspects of achieving physical fitness is the freedom, confidence, and fun of going on a hike to a spectacular vista, jumping in a kayak for a paddle across a quiet lake, or even spontaneously joining an Ultimate Frisbee game.

We're human. Sometimes injury, exhaustion, or stress can inhibit us from completing our regular exercise routines, and this is OK. There are some situations in which exercise can help rectify ailments, but there are others—perhaps in the case of an eating disorder, surgical recovery, or an exercise addiction—where physical activity is not advised. So long as we continue to strive for movement in whatever ways our bodies are able, when we are able, physical activity can be a powerful, joyful, and healthy addition to our lives.

While the health benefits of staying active are important, for many, those outcomes may be too far in the future. Be active for enjoyment, fun, and pleasure. Be in touch with the power of immediately feeling better, functioning better, and sleeping better.[22] Be clear about your *why*. Determine what matters most to you and the power of exercise will help you fulfill those goals. Connect exercise to its power to help you do what you find is most vital.

You've Got Q's; We've Got A's

Q: Is my walking enough?

A: Yes, walking briskly, which is slightly quicker than a pedestrian pace—that is, faster than 3 miles per hour—for 150 minutes per week will provide the majority of health benefits from physical activity. However, adding resistance exercise provides many additional benefits (see sidebar "Benefits of Resistance Training").

Q: Do I have to sweat and be out of breath?

A: No. You may choose to exercise at a vigorous intensity, indicated by not being able to talk in full sentences, but you can gain the same benefits from moderate-intensity physical activity without getting out of breath or necessarily sweating.

Q: I've never lifted weights before. How do I get started?

A: While getting started with a walking program should not take much coaching or instruction, learning to do resistance training is best supported by a qualified physical therapist, exercise physiologist, or personal trainer with credentials from well-recognized accrediting agencies.

Q: Won't lifting weights make me bulk up?

A: No! It takes *a long time* to build muscle and, especially for women, who have lower levels of testosterone, getting a "bulky look" is almost impossible without exogenous hormones (e.g., hormones taken as a supplement). Plus, if you ever feel like you've gotten too bulky, you can stop doing whatever you're doing, and it will atrophy in a matter of weeks. So just try it!

Q: What did we do to stay strong before weight machines were invented?

A: Our lives used to intrinsically incorporate physical activity. At certain periods in history, it was hunting and gathering, at other times, it was agricultural work. We didn't need to set aside time to "work out," because it was naturally incorporated into our daily lives.

Q: Does it matter whether or I lift weights or use a machine, resistance bands, or the like?

A: No, your muscles do not know (or care) what is causing the stress. Your muscles will strengthen if they are given unaccustomed stress.

Q: Does yoga count as resistance training?

A: Parts of your yoga routine, especially holding a plank position or the warrior poses, will strengthen those muscles stressed by the pose.

Q: What if I start exercising and I do not see the results that I want?

A: First, exercising just for aesthetics is a dangerous road to go down, because you will be quickly frustrated. Instead, focusing on how exercise makes you feel is a recipe for having fun and sticking to it. Second, if you regularly exercise for a period of a few months, you will see changes, whether they are physical, in your strength, or in your abilities. Your body is built to adapt, and if you are consistent and patient, it will do its job.

Q: What are my options if I cannot afford a gym membership or workout equipment?

A: You don't need to go to a gym to get a good workout. First, we have the great outdoors, which is free to everyone. Second, there are countless free resources online to help you learn and perform at-home workouts.

Q: What happens if I stop exercising for a few weeks? Will I lose my progress?

A: Remember that we are exercising to improve our health and to have fun . . . hopefully for the rest of our lives. In the grand scheme of things, a few weeks is nothing. Will you potentially take some time to rebuild your endurance or strength when you get back? Yes. But you never lose your capacity to improve your cardiovascular fitness or get stronger, no matter your age.

7

A Love Letter to the Gym

Me and Exercise—It's Complicated

I would like to preface this chapter with a disclaimer. Just so we all understand where I'm coming from here . . . I am *not* by any means an athletic person. I never played any sports growing up. I was never fast or strong. Not only did it not particularly appeal to me, but it didn't even really bother me that it didn't appeal to me.

Part of it was that I'm legally blind. This meant that no one made a particular effort to get me playing sports. When I was in elementary school, I played at recess with everybody else, and it had never occurred to me that maybe the reason I was always "it" in tag was because . . . I couldn't see the other kids once they were any farther than six feet from me. A monstrous, epic collision with Danny O'Malley during fourth-grade kickball was probably the most significant moment of my short and illustrious career in any sort of sporting event. And then it was middle and high school where gym teachers never really bothered putting the blind girl into the dodgeball game. Most made no effort and just let me have a study period. Those that tried would have me do twenty crunches and *then* do the study period. Either way, this was fine by me, because who the hell wants to actually go to gym class?

Other than that, I had a brief stint in swimming lessons, which, as you can imagine, is every large-chested, insecure teenage girl's dream. I would get a two-dollar summer student membership to the Y and pretend to "use the bike" for a few days each summer. And I did abs: my own personal specialty. My stomach is and has always been my insecurity. It was the thing that my family members would always comment on: "Juna, you would have such a nice body . . . but you really need to work on that stomach," and so on, and so forth. (PS: I swear, my family is made up of kind and loving people, but commenting on people's bodies, good or bad, is common practice in Albania. To this day, they don't get why it upsets me, but they're getting better!) I would obsessively get into ab routines. This could be doing leg raises during commercial breaks or crunches in my room after dinner. After a week or two of no results, I would quit.

In college, exercise became something very different. My tuition included a gym membership that was now year-round, not only in the summers. And more importantly, my parents were not there to watch me. You see, my parents were always encouraging me to "be more active," usually on the tail end of some comment about my weight. Therefore, the *last thing* I could possibly ever do was to be seen following their recommendations. If they wanted me to be active, I could, under no circumstances, let them see me being active. So for most of high school, my ab routines and gym sessions were as secret as I could keep them. But in college, no one could watch me, so I was finally free.

Back then, my very complex and nuanced understanding of human metabolism went as follows: I hate my body. This is because I weigh too much. This means I eat too many calories. Therefore, I need to exercise. With logic this solid and a body image this immaculate, how could anything possibly go wrong?! I jumped in headfirst.

Every year, when I inevitably got on a weight-loss kick, I would start eating plain Greek yogurt and salads for all meals. And I would go to one of the gyms on campus called "the MAC." The effort it took me to get to the MAC was monumental: it was basically like, could I muster up enough self-loathing to force myself to do this horrible activity I hated? If so, I would put on my one pair of *cropped* Lululemon leggings (yes, they looked just as bad as you are picturing; my petition to ban all cropped leggings can be found in the appendix to this book), and I would drag my ass to the gym. I would head straight upstairs to the chaotic cardio area, and then I would run at around a ten-minute-mile pace for thirty to forty minutes, depending on how much life energy my Fall Out Boy playlist could breathe into me. I did anything to pass the time: count steps forward, count steps backward, count every other step, watch the time tick by, and the second, and I mean *the second*, the calorie counter on the treadmill hit 300, 350, 400—whatever my goal was for the day—*slap*, I would hit that red button with the force of a thousand suns, and I would scurry my ass outta there faster than I had ever moved on the dang treadmill.

In the back of my mind was the constant thought: *I have to do this to burn calories to lose weight.* I never questioned *why* I wanted to lose weight. I never questioned *why* I hated my body so much. I just knew: to be happy, I needed to be thin. When I was feeling especially self-loathing-y, or "motivated," depending on which way you twist it, I would head over to a squishy mat in the corner to do some of my old go-to moves: leg raises, reverse crunches, planks, and butterfly kicks. If someone started to approach the mat, or God forbid, lie on the gigantic Harvard shield next to me, it was "game over." Abort mission. I cannot be seen doing abs, because people will think (a) why is this clearly unfit girl doing abs, and (b) they will see my stomach bulging over my cropped Lululemon legging waistband as I do my crunches. *Nope,* not today people. I'm out.

It never occurred to me to *like* exercise. I never saw any results in my abs, and every year, my weight would follow its annual "U" pattern. New high weight at New Year's, bust my ass, low weight in June, run out of steam, increase again just in time for an existential crisis by the next New Year's.

This cycle was set on its usual trajectory until New Year's in 2017, when one thing happened, one thing, that literally changed my entire life. (PS: I know my therapist Brian says I have a "flair for drama," but this time it's actually not an exaggeration).

I had gone to celebrate New Year's with the family and had gotten the typical weight comment from an uncle. This had sent me into a spiral of shame, and my usual frenzy of "I need to fix myself" had begun. I started doing my usual internet searching, desperately looking for people who had lost significant amounts of weight and how they had done it, when I came across a YouTube video of a girl, and my jaw dropped. She looked like a Barbie, I thought. An actual human Barbie.

This girl was lean, but she was curvy. She didn't look like the stick-skinny models I had grown up seeing in magazines and on TV shows. She didn't have much fat on her body, but she looked fuller, not unhealthy. This is the look that today we call slim-thick. And the weirdest part of all: she was lifting weights. In every single video she had posted on YouTube, she was in the gym, squatting, lunging, bench pressing, doing lat pull-downs. She was preparing for a "bikini competition"—whatever that was—but I was astonished. I had never in my life seen someone who looked as beautiful as she did.

I ordered a scale that would sync with my phone, some protein powder, protein bars, branched-chain amino acids, as well as new pre-workout and gym clothes. I got back to campus, and in a cloud of chemical-fruit-smelling dust, opened three Amazon packages filled with different colored powders. I wanted to be just like the gym girls I saw posting their weightlifting workouts on YouTube, and I became obsessed.

My first forays into the gym to lift weights were embarrassing on a level that is alarming even for me. I wore dark colors, long sleeves, and loose fits because I was so insecure about the way I looked. If you think going to the gym for the first time is awkward, try doing it while being legally blind. How the hell was I supposed to figure out where everything was, how much the plates weighed, what each dumbbell was labeled? I took a "before" photo in my tiny dorm-room mirror, took a scoop of pre-workout powder, put on my giant silver Bose headphones, and made my way over to the MAC, looking like a silver alien (my Bose) that had discovered the T.J. Maxx clearance athleisure (my outfits). This time, instead of going upstairs, I went down to the weight room.

In retrospect, my closest school gym (shout-out to the MAC) has a tiny weight room that is almost hilarious to think back on. There were only two squat racks, two bench presses, and a bunch of machines, but at that time it seemed huge, scary, and, most uncomfortable for me, filled with men. My strategy was simple:

1. Watch YouTube videos obsessively and try to memorize all the new words: dumbbell, barbell, row, press, and so on.

2. Gather equipment I needed into the little dark corner outside the weight room, partially under the staircase, where I could hide.

3. Perform exercises as similar to YouTube videos as possible while listening to old motivational self-help videos of Tony Robbins and picturing how awesome it would be to look like Barbie upon graduation (five months away).

4. Pray to the dear lord, baby Jesus, Allah, Yahweh, and/or the alien simulation that controls our universe, that no one ever found out about step number 3, especially the part about Tony Robbins.

I did this every day, religiously. Three months was going to be my marker. When I reached three months, I would evaluate whether or not I saw any changes. This was a suggestion I had gotten from a YouTube video. Progress pic, pre-workout, gym. Repeat. Progress pic, pre-workout, gym. Repeat.

Did my undying devotion to the gym start off for the wrong reasons? Yes. I spent all the time in those first few months just picturing my body turning into what I wanted it to. It was all driven by aesthetics and fulfilling some arbitrary thin ideal that I felt like I needed to fit in order to be happy. But something started to slowly happen to me as I started to work out.

When I had lunch with my dorm mates, all I could talk about was how I had added *another fifty* pounds to my leg press. *"Can you believe it?!"* I would exclaim, getting mostly blank stares. *"I had six plates! Six!"* I became obsessed with pull-ups, researching endlessly about how to get strong enough to be able to do one. I started writing down my workouts, weight, sets, reps. I had a proper "workout split" (this is what us gym rats call our workout schedule). Every day I would wake up and flex different parts of my body to check if they were sore from the day before. If they weren't, I had failed; if they were, I'd done something right. On Sunday mornings, my "mandatory rest day" (according to YouTube videos), I would wake up in my twin dorm-room bed and go through every part of my body: Flex quads. Sore? Check. Flex my hammies. Sore? Check. Raise my arm. Sore shoulder? Check. If everything was sore on Sunday, I had won.

The change was so gradual that I didn't even realize it was happening. I started off not wanting to be "bulky" or "muscular." I just wanted to get toned. I started off mostly caring about the fat loss, and if the strength gains came along with it, who cares? I found it strange when girls I watched online used words like "jacked" or "built" as things they were aspiring to be. But the fitness bug had bit, and I was hooked.

How can I describe how much the gym means to me, especially to people who don't go to the gym? I think we can start here: for my entire life, I had wanted to be smaller, take up less space, be thin, be pretty, and be elegant. And that's how I started off at the gym, too. But there was something about lifting weights, seeing my numbers increase week to week, seeing myself progress, feeling my body get hard and strong—it was indescribable. At first, I wanted to just tone my muscles, then I wanted to build a few certain parts: my butt, my abs. Then it morphed into wanting to be able to *do* stuff. I wanted to do a pull-up, I wanted to learn a back-flip, I wanted to get good at handstands, splits, deadlifting three hundred pounds, benching my body weight. It was like all the fixation with my body not being good enough, not looking the way I wanted it to—all that didn't matter when I felt like I was progressing in the gym.

It may not come as a surprise that my family was not on board with my newfound obsession. After losing fifteen pounds over the course of spring semester, I started to get compliments from my parents, saying I looked "really good." And that lasted all of two weeks, before I got comments like, "Don't you think your shoulders are getting a little manly?" or "Don't you think you shouldn't be going to the gym as much?"

I was furious. Here I was, busting my butt every day, eating healthy, lifting weights, and I had finally found a form of exercise that I not only didn't hate but felt excited about, and even that was not what people wanted me to do. I felt self-conscious about my body getting more athletic and thought to myself, *Should I skip upper-body days altogether?* Maybe they were right. Who wanted strong shoulders when you were wearing spaghetti-strap dresses? But for some reason, I couldn't stop. Why would I ever choose to get weaker when all I wanted to do was get stronger?

The appeal of fitness and the gym to me was not about my body. It was about how everything in the gym applied to my life outside the gym: Every workout I showed up and busted my ass, sweating, grinding, putting in the work. And when I came in the week after, I could add ten pounds to the bar, I could squeeze out one more rep, I could get an inch lower on my squat. While progress in the rest of life was abstract, progress in the gym was tangible, numerical, clear, and easy to track. When I had an off day, it didn't matter, because, as I learned, progress was not linear. It went up and down: some days I felt like it, other days I didn't. But the point was, I was always striving to get better, and as long as I did that, I did get better.

It taught me discipline, confidence, work ethic, and the ability to continue doing something I loved no matter what the people around me were saying about it. I never associated being strong with being a woman. I never felt like athleticism was "hot." I never thought I would want to "get swole," but experiencing the profound impacts lifting had on my mental health, it literally saved me.

In the depths of my eating disorder, I would lift. In the highest points of my success, I would lift. When I was lost with no career prospects, having decided not to pursue piano any further and having no future direction after college, I would lift. On Friday nights, when I was alone and all my friends had moved away, I would lift. Horrendous binge-eating episode? Glutes and hamstrings. Told that my podcast would be canceled? A push workout. Sexually assaulted on a date and not sleeping for more than twenty-four hours? I deadlifted 225 for four sets of five like it was nothing.

Never in my entire lifting career have I felt like I "looked the part." I never got my body to be like a Barbie. I never felt like I was a credible source of information, because I was never thin enough. But sharing my insecurities, my victories, my failures, and my progress on social media became one of the most rewarding parts of going to the gym. If the gym had so completely turned around my attitude toward my body and myself, I was convinced it could for other people, too. It's one of the things I'm most passionate about on this planet.

How It Works

As Eddie mentioned in chapter 6, your body is an adaptation *machine*. When you apply stressors to the body, it adapts in order to better cope with similar stressors in the future. A very concrete example of this is sun exposure: when you lounge by the pool, the sun is a stressor to your skin. In response, your skin produces melanin, the pigment that makes skin tan and also protects skin from future sun exposure. We've also seen this phenomenon in our discussion of metabolism in response to crash dieting or sustaining high amounts of physical activity, but it's a pretty universal concept that applies to all stressors that our bodies encounter—and exercise is no different.

Exercise can be broken down into two categories: aerobic, or endurance exercise (often called cardio by gym rats and fitness enthusiasts), and anaerobic exercise, or strength/power training (lifting).[1] Endurance exercise is generally performed against a relatively low load for a long period of time—think jogging, cycling, swimming and so on. Strength training is generally performed against relatively higher loads for shorter durations of time—think squats, push-ups, pull-ups, and so on.[2] Of course, in reality, it's much more complicated than this, because a lot of forms of exercise are some combination of the two, also called concurrent training, but when we talk about the effects of each, it's useful to maintain this dichotomy.

When we engage in endurance exercise, our body responds in a way that makes it better able to perform future endurance exercise. Technically, doing cardio results in "enhanced cardiac output, maximal oxygen consumption, and mitochondrial biogenesis."[3] Translation: It increases your ability to perform a repetitive movement such as running for longer distances and longer times. Resistance training (RT), on the other hand, increases muscle cross-sectional area, neural adaptations, and maximal force output.[4] Translation: It makes your muscles bigger and stronger. Again, in reality, things are often more nuanced: recent research has shown that short bouts of high-intensity exercise can lead to endurance adaptations, and long bouts of low-intensity exercise, if taken near failure (the point at which you can no longer perform the exercise without breaking proper form), can lead to strength adaptations.[5] But you get the idea. Your body will get better and prioritize the adaptation to whichever stimuli you throw at it.

Up until fairly recently, weight training was pretty much a niche activity: it was basically reserved for big dudes who wanted to be huge and/or strong, that is, the Arnold Schwarzeneggers of the world.[6] The barbell, for most people, brings to mind Olympic weightlifters, powerlifters, bodybuilders, football players, and so on. The general public saw no reason to make weight training part of a regular exercise routine. And, in fact, in a lot of other sports, building muscle was thought to actually hinder performance.[7] I barely encountered lifting weights growing up, apart from seeing the football team's dumbbells in our high school gym and noticing that hot guys in movies seemed to be very into it.

My only encounter with women lifting weights, prior to my gym-obsession awakening, was Lucy, a girl in a junior-year psych seminar, who I thought was maybe the most put-together person I had ever met. She mentioned she was heading to the gym to "do arms," and I said, "Lucy . . . doesn't that make your arms big?" "No, no, it just makes them toned," she assured me. "You should come with me; it's so fun!" I politely declined, telling her that my body, already so much larger than hers, would only bulk up from weightlifting, while her lean, toned arms probably just got even more lean and toned.

As heart disease and metabolic syndrome became larger and larger concerns for the American public, exercise became a central recommendation for promoting optimal health outcomes.[8] However, the emphasis has traditionally been placed on endurance exercise in particular. Cardio gets the heart rate up and burns a lot of calories, which obviously improves the many, many health problems associated with overconsumption and underactivity—right?

Look, *all* exercise is good for you. Getting your heart rate up is good for you. Challenging your body is good for you. There is no reason for there to be a dichotomy between cardio versus resistance training: doing a combination of the two is probably what is going to lead to the best health outcomes for everyone. But . . . since the benefits of cardio seem to be pretty well-publicized, I feel we gotta show resistance training a little extra love.

Luckily for us, research over the past few decades has been piling up exalting the benefits of resistance training when it comes to almost all the health problems that we most suffer from today. And if your physique is your main focus (which, when I was eighteen and new to college, it definitely was), resistance training is absolutely crucial. So . . . let me try to infect you all with the lifting bug.

The Calories Don't Add Up

There's no doubt that endurance exercise is a winner when it comes to calories you burn *in the workout*. When I first started getting into exercise, the calories were the only way I had of evaluating workouts. I saw the relationship between exercise and food as transactional: if I ate a 300-calorie donut, I had to do a 300-calorie run. To me, it was just adding or subtracting calories out of my daily calorie budget, and other than that, there wasn't much else to it. For this reason, running was my go-to exercise (it burned the most calories per unit time), and I absolutely hated it (because it was about nothing except said calories).

However, as we discussed in the metabolism chapter (2), it's just not that simple. Metabolism is a dynamic component of human physiology. And we know that the calorie burn from exercise does not equate to the weight loss you would expect from said calorie burn. Traditionally, our understanding of fat loss has been that one pound of fat is equivalent to ~3,500 calories. Therefore, achieving a 3,500-calorie deficit, meaning eating 3,500 calories fewer than you burn, *should* result in the scale going down a pound. But this doesn't hold true in actual experiments.[9]

In the short-term (less than sixteen weeks), randomized control trials measuring weight loss from exercise interventions have shown that participants lost 85 percent of the weight you would expect from the additional calories burned.[10] Although 85 percent is not perfect, it's not *that* bad. However, when we look at long-term randomized control trials (greater than twenty-six weeks), people lose *only* 30 percent of the weight you would expect from the extra calories burned from exercising.[11] Meaning, if you burn 3,500 calories over the course of your workouts, instead of losing one pound, like we would expect, it seems that people on average lose about one-third of a pound. The calories burned from exercise and the amount of weight lost do not seem to have a dose-dependent relationship. As we discussed in chapter 3, this is likely due to the reduced basal metabolic rate that accompanies weight loss, as well as some of the other effects associated with certain types of exercise, such as increased appetite and reduced nonexercise activities.[12]

If one of the main attractions of cardio has been its increased calorie burn, this fact alone begs the question: Why are we using calorie burn as the most important metric when it clearly is not having the effect that we think it's supposed to have? And this question: How many years of my life have I wasted running on the human equivalent of a hamster wheel while listening to the dulcet tones of Fall Out Boy? Very important questions indeed.

Calorie Burn Beyond the Workout

Instead of considering the calorie burn strictly during the workout's duration (where cardio clearly takes the cake), let's consider what happens *outside* the workout—after all, that is how you are spending 95 percent of your day, even if you're working out every day. Muscle mass can constitute up to 40 percent of your body weight. Compared to fat mass, muscle is a much more calorically expensive tissue, requiring around 5–6 calories per pound per day in untrained individuals just to maintain and repair the tissue.[13] Fat, on the other hand, requires about 2 calories per pound per day.[14] As we discussed in chapters 2 and 3, loss of muscle mass is responsible for the majority of the age-related decline we see in basal metabolic rate (BMR). As we age, we lose about 3–8 percent of muscle mass per decade after thirty, and 5–10 percent per decade after fifty. However, resistance training may have a dual effect on metabolism, besides mitigating or preventing age-related decline.

When you lift, you build muscle. And more muscle means more energy needs, even when you are sitting on your butt doing absolutely nothing. A one-kilogram increase in muscle mass may increase your daily energy needs by about 20 calories, which may not sound like a lot, but compound that over days, weeks, and years, and it makes a big difference. Also, this is not taking into account that the average woman and man can conservatively gain around one pound of muscle per month when first starting resistance training.[15]

Also, when you resistance-train, you are causing microtraumas to the muscle tissue, which then need to be repaired and remodeled. And this, of course, requires more energy. This acute effect, which can last for up to seventy-two hours after a workout, significantly increases basal metabolic rate. Studies have shown a 5 to 9 percent increase in BMR for three days, even after *just one* session of resistance training.[16] These two effects—the addition of new, metabolically active tissue and the remodeling of current muscle tissue—may result in a 100–150 calorie increase in metabolic rate *per day* from resistance training. And the coolest part is that these increases happen outside the workout, when you're chillin', not as a result of running an extra mile in your session. The effect of RT on your BMR and muscle mass are part of the reason why RT, as opposed to cardio, is such a better option when it comes to weight loss and weight-loss maintenance.[17]

Looking Good Naked

OK, let's be honest for a second. I'm writing this book for my eighteen-year-old self, and, quite honestly, my eighteen-year-old self could not give a crap about the "health" benefits of resistance training. You could've told me that muscle mass is inversely related to all-cause mortality and prevalence of metabolic syndrome,[18] and I would've just said, "Um . . . what are either of those?" You could've said resistance training has been shown to improve blood-sugar control, improve cardiovascular health, reduce resting blood pressure, improve blood lipid profiles, increase bone mineral density, improve cognition as you age, improve self-esteem, lower depression, reduce low-back pain, improve muscle function and mobility, and reverse some aging factors,[19] and I would've said, "So what?" But if you had said that resistance training and the subsequent increase in muscle mass make you look better naked, I would've been halfway down the stairs to the weight room before you'd finished your sentence.

Should looks be your main concern? No. Does chasing aesthetics sometimes lead to detrimental behaviors? Yes. But am I going to try to get you to lift weights by appealing to your vanity instead of your desire for longevity and quality of life? Abso-freakin'-lutely. I let Eddie handle all the longevity and health stuff, so I want to briefly discuss why I think, if your main concern is improving body composition, resistance training is the most crucial form of exercise for you.

Tone and Sculpt

When I was growing up, the way exercise was marketed to men and women could not have been more opposite. Men's magazines said things like "5 steps to a massive chest" or "get jacked for summer." In contrast, women's magazines said things like "the secret to toned arms" or "best ways to sculpt your legs." Recommendations for men usually went along the lines of, "Lift heavy, and often, to get big." Recommendations for women were, "Use these cute, pink dumbbells and the ThighMaster 3000 to tone up and get smaller." The implied message was clear and sometimes even outrightly stated: if you lift heavy, you'll get bulky and big—that's for men. If you lift light and high-rep, you'll get toned, smaller, more feminine muscles.

This is a total and complete crock of BS that is so nefariously false it's horrifying it still pervades fitness advertising today. There aren't different "types" of skeletal muscle you can grow. There isn't a way to tone as opposed to build, or to sculpt as opposed to grow. As far as aesthetics are concerned, the only thing that can happen to your muscles is that they can grow, a process called hypertrophy, or shrink, a process called atrophy.[20] (Note: There *are* different types of muscle fibers, but every muscle in the human body contains combinations of these different fiber types, and to see them, you would need fancy equipment in a lab.)

A similar myth is that different forms of exercise somehow produce differing types of muscle tissue. Yoga and Pilates, for example, are often marketed as activities that produce long, lean muscles. Weightlifting or sports like CrossFit supposedly produce larger, denser muscles. Again, if your body is only ever breaking down or building up muscle, there is no such thing as creating "long lean" muscles or "short dense" muscles. The way your muscles look is mostly due to the amount of fat covering the muscle and the anatomy of your body—for example, whether or not you have longer or shorter muscle bellies.

People will often point to the elite in any given discipline as proof of what excelling in that sport will make you look like. This is the logic of "I want to look like a ballerina, so I will take more barre classes." The flaw in this logic is that the reason the elite in any given sport look the way they do is because their individual body type tends to excel at that given sport. For example, the average height in the NBA is over six feet six, but we would never say, "I want to be tall, so I will play basketball."[21] We intuitively know that if we have the genes to be taller, we are much more likely to get to the higher levels of basketball. However, the pervasive myth that somehow lifting weights will make you look like a bodybuilder is still widely held today. Muscle hypertrophy, or muscle growth, is the same process that occurs in gymnasts, yogis, ballerinas, weightlifters, football players, and bodybuilders. And yet it looks different on everyone depending on how much fat you carry, which muscles you're spending more time developing, and your bone lengths and structure.

Body Recomposition: Lose Fat, Gain Muscle

When most people say they want to "get toned" or "get in better shape," they are likely referring to two processes that need to occur: fat loss and muscle gain. Gaining muscle gives your body shape and curves, and losing fat allows you to see the shape. We've discussed that fat loss, along with its implications and mechanisms, is largely a by-product of creating a calorie deficit, mostly through good nutrition. This is where the old adage "Abs are made in the kitchen" is very true. No matter how developed your abs are, you won't be able to see them unless you get to a fairly low body-fat percentage. However, there's another piece to this: we want to build the abs underneath the fat so that once body fat levels go down there are some abs to actually show.

You may have heard the phrase "muscle weighs more than fat." In classic fitness-industry fashion, this phrase is, on its face, hilariously false. One pound of muscle of course weighs exactly the same as one pound of fat, the same way one pound of feathers weighs exactly the same as one pound of rocks. However, what the phrase is (very poorly) alluding to is that muscle tissue is more dense than fat tissue.[22] One pound of muscle takes up around four-fifths of the space of a pound of fat. Which means, if you lose fat and gain muscle at equal rates (a process called "body recomposition," which is common when you first start resistance training), even if the scale doesn't move a pound, you will look leaner, more "toned," and overall less "fluffy."[23] This is why progress pictures and waist circumference are often better measures of progress than the scale: you can look completely different, even if the scale is not going down or even going up. In fact, oftentimes professional athletes or fitness models can technically be "overweight" or even "obese," according to the BMI, just because they have such high amounts of muscle mass.[24]

Another myth is "spot reduction." This is the idea that in order to lose fat in your stomach, for example, you need to work out your abs. As someone who spent countless hours doing crunches and leg raises for this very reason, I want these words to be written in the freaking sky by a plane for the whole world to see: *you cannot spot-reduce fat.*[25]

While training a specific muscle group will cause localized growth of that particular muscle (working out your arm does increase the size of your arm muscles), you cannot choose where you lose fat.[26] Working out your abs will not lower your stomach fat. Instead, your body loses fat systemically, so you basically lose a little fat everywhere. Fat distribution, as well as order of fat loss, is extremely complex and affected by a multitude of factors, including your age, gender, genetics, and so on.[27,28]

Think of fat loss like a roll of paper towels: if you really, really want to get to the center of the paper towel roll (a specific area of stubborn body fat), you can't just pull paper towels from the middle. All you can do is continue your healthy habits to the best of your abilities, and as the paper-towel roll unfolds, you'll eventually get to those center pieces . . . but not by doing crunches on your hardwood floor.

Weights Are for Boys

Along with the myths of "toning" and "spot reduction," the myth of "getting bulky" is one of the biggest things that holds women back from starting a resistance-training program or going "too hard" in the gym. On the one hand, female athletes are looked up to and idealized in our society: think of Megan Rapinoe and the US women's national soccer team, or superstar Olympians like Simone Biles. On the other hand, a commonly held fear for women in the gym is that doing the "wrong" type of exercise may lead to "excessive musculature" and looking like a female bodybuilder.[29]

One study looking at women and their attitudes toward the gym identified that the cardio area of gyms was seen to "contribute" to femininity, while lifting "detracted" from it.[30] Besides not wanting to get bulky, many women expressed that their main goal was to burn the maximum number of calories, which was perceived to be done through cardio.[31] In a study of gym-equipment use, while men and women were equally likely to have used cardio equipment, more men reported having used weight machines, and an even greater discrepancy was found in the use of free weights.[32]

As we've discussed, resistance training provides a whole host of health benefits, regardless of gender. However, RT may be of particular importance for women, the exact population that seems to be the most reluctant. For example, after menopause, women lose bone mass more quickly than men do, and resistance training can help slow this process considerably.[33] And weightlifting may act as somewhat of a buffer from psychological conditions more prevalent among female populations, such as eating disorders. EDs and their subthreshold corollaries (disordered-eating symptoms that don't fully meet diagnostic criteria) are characterized by overvaluation of body shape and size.[34] We'll talk about this more in chapter 8, but, in short, individuals with eating disorders place a disproportionate amount of their self-worth and self-esteem on their weight and body shape. And the addition of strength training, as opposed to aerobic exercise only, has been shown to significantly improve body image metrics.[35]

I find this research about women and strength training to be a mirror of my own experience, and painful to read. The pride and joy that I felt as I started to see myself get stronger and do more in the gym were profound: it was the first time I had felt ownership, love, and pride for a body that I had spent my whole life hating.

Even as my focus shifted away from constantly trying to be thinner and more toward trying to learn stuff that I thought was cool (e.g., my obsession with landing a backflip), I still found myself torn. I would scroll through Instagram watching girls do amazing things that I would *kill* to be able to do, and think, *I want to be able to do that, but I don't want to be as muscular as her.* Sometimes I think this is because I grew up in the early 2000s, when the thin, waifish supermodel body type was "in." Things *must* be different in the era of the slim-thick fit-fluencer, right? But this was clearly just wishful thinking on my part: "Why does she look like a man?" was the only response I got from my seven-year-old cousin when I showed her a video of a fitness icon doing a string of back handsprings on the beach.

Why looking like a "female bodybuilder" is such an abhorrent thought to so many women is a complicated topic, having to do with deep-rooted stereotypes of femininity and identifying as a woman. That strength and its associated physical features are seen as "masculine" even well into the twenty-first century is pretty disheartening. These are questions that need to be pondered both at the individual level and at a societal level. There are days when I see contours of my shoulder and bicep and think, *Hell, yeah, look at all my hard work!* And there are days when I see my traps in a tank top and think, *Ew, I look like a football player.* It's hard and messy and not something I'm proud to admit, but it's something I work on every time I choose not to skip upper-body day, not to shy away from the bench press, not to hold back on my weights. But for those whose main concern is their appearance, how likely is it that lifting weights will actually make you look "like a female bodybuilder"?

"I Don't Want to Look Like a Bodybuilder"

One of the things often told to women to assuage their fears of "becoming bulky" is that their biology simply does not allow for such dramatic gains in muscle mass.[36] Like many at the top of their sport, female bodybuilders are a tiny minority of the female population whose genetics likely provide an advantage with regard to muscle hypertrophy. Also, it should be said, these ladies are dedicating years and years of their lives, spending hours upon hours training with extremely high intensity, paying attention to every detail of nutrition, and sometimes using exogenous hormones to maximize all aspects of muscle growth. One study of seventy-five female bodybuilders found that about one-third reported taking illicit anabolic-androgenic steroids.[37] Thinking that "casually" going to the gym is going to produce results that take people extraordinary amounts of effort, dedication, and hard work is like saying, "If I start taking a dance class, Beyoncé may come and recruit me to be in her next music video." Bottom line is, these gals are (a) probably genetically predisposed to grow more muscle faster, (b) working their *butts off* to get the results they're getting, and (c) sometimes using steroids. Talk to your average guy who goes to the gym and is actually *trying* to gain as much muscle as possible, and they'll tell you . . . *it's freaking hard* and takes a long, long time.

However, this narrative exists in parallel with the experiences that a lot of women may have of lifting weights and noticing aesthetic changes in their bodies.[38] I know that my body does look fundamentally different than it did before I lifted weights. But, at the same time, it's nowhere near developed enough to slap on a tan and hop on stage at a bodybuilding show, despite having lifted religiously for five to six days a week for six years. So what is the genetic potential of women for building muscle? Is it different from men? Does this mean that women should train differently than men?

Men, Women, and Muscles

We all seem to intuitively think that women, on average, are weaker than men, smaller than men, and less muscular than men. But science may say something slightly different. It's true that in absolute terms, women are smaller and weaker. Specifically, women are, on average, about half as strong as men in the upper body and two-thirds as strong in the lower body.[39] The gender differences in muscle size are also significantly higher in the upper body, and this is likely because women hold a larger proportion of their lean body mass in their lower body.[40] PS: This is a very, very scientific reason for us ladies to love "leg day": we're just better at it!

However, many studies have shown that women and men actually have pretty similar potentials when it comes to relative muscle strength and size gains from early-phase resistance training.[41,42,43] I hear you saying, *"Aha!* I knew I could gain just as much muscle as men. I'm never touching a dumbbell again!" And while my massive traps may agree with you, the key word in the studies is "relative."

As a percentage of where they started off, men and women experience similar increases in strength and size, but since women start off so much smaller than men, it means, in absolute terms, they gain a lot less muscle.[44] For example, in one study where subjects trained three days a week for sixteen weeks, both males and females experienced about an 8 percent increase in relative upper-arm circumference. But in absolute terms, the men experienced about an eleven-centimeter increase in their upper-arm cross-sectional area, whereas for the women it was about seven centimeters, or about 50 percent less.[45] Other studies have reported that men may have a slight advantage in relative size gain, while women may have a slight advantage in relative strength gain. Meaning that compared to where they start, women will see a greater percent strength increase from the same training stimulus. This is likely because women start out much weaker than men, so even a small absolute gain in strength would be a greater relative gain.[46]

The idea that women are inherently weaker than men has also been shown to be misleading. Differences in muscle size and lean body mass account for around 97 percent of the strength differences observed between the sexes.[47] Meaning that the only reason women are often weaker than men is, again, because they are smaller and often have a lower-percent lean body mass and higher-percent fat mass. (This is healthy! Women's bodies actually need more fat to function properly.)[48,49] This suggests that a man and woman with the same lean body mass should actually be more or less equally strong.

What is consistent between both groups is that there is a huge variability in how people respond to training stimuli. In a study of 585 subjects going through a twelve-week progressive resistance-training program, researchers found that size changes in the cross-sectional area of the biceps ranged from -0.4 centimeters^2 to +13.6 centimeters^2 across the study. This means that some people actually had no response or maybe even *lost* size in their muscle, while others grew their biceps area by almost 14 square centimeters. Strength changes ranged from 0 percent to 250 percent: some people experienced no change, while others put more than twenty-two pounds on their one-rep max.[50] The variability in responses was found to be the same in both males and females: some people respond, and some people don't, and the majority of us fall somewhere in the middle.

All in all, this research affirms that the way any individual responds to a strength-training program is highly variable. Are some people hyper-responders? Yes (@my massive traps). Will some people have a much harder time gaining muscle? Yes. However, while men and women may possess the same potential for muscle growth in a relative sense, men do gain a lot more muscle and strength in absolute terms because they start out bigger. For example, one study found that in a nine-week training period, the men gained *more than double* the muscle volume in their quads than the women did, regardless of age.[51]

If you really are worried about gaining too much muscle, one thing you should consider is that while muscle is hard to build, it's also quick to disappear. If you just stop training a given muscle group, the muscle will quickly atrophy because it is no longer receiving a stimulus to grow.[52] We know this by looking at studies of people who have gotten injured and are subjected to periods of bed rest or limb immobilization. Prolonged disuse of a muscle (about ten to forty-two days) results in around a 0.5 percent loss of total muscle mass *per day*.[53] The rate of atrophy in free-living individuals who "stop training" may not be this dramatic, because you're still using a lot of your muscles in your daily life, even if you're not formally "training" them, albeit at a much lower intensity. But the old adage certainly holds true: use it or lose it (mostly).

Newbie Gains: Your First Few Weeks in the Gym

Now that we've tackled the idea of lifting weights, let's talk about how we actually go about the process of building muscle and getting stronger. One of the coolest parts of beginning resistance training is that when you first start, you experience a phenomenon dubbed "newbie gains." This is a period marked by rapid, consistent strength gains from workout to workout, and often periods of body recomposition (gains in lean body mass and loss of body fat simultaneously).[54]

This may seem obvious, but it's worth stating that muscle strength and cross-sectional area (muscle size) are actually highly correlated: larger muscles *really do* tend to be stronger. But when you first start resistance training, you'll likely experience a rapid increase in strength, though not due to muscle hypertrophy. In the first few weeks or months of going to the gym, you'll be hitting new personal records (PRs) every single week, putting an additional five, ten, or even more pounds on your lifts every single workout, but your muscles won't necessarily be getting any bigger.[55] PS: Getting new PRs every single week is the coolest feeling, so relish it while it's happening! This is due to the fact that a majority of the strength gains first seen when starting resistance training (in the first two to four weeks) are due to neural adaptations, not muscle hypertrophy.[56,57]

Neural adaptation is your nervous system getting better at recruiting your existing muscle fibers. The exact mechanisms are not entirely understood, but in essence, your nervous system is getting better at more fully recruiting and coordinating your muscles, even if they're not the muscles directly being trained.[58] One instance in which you can clearly see this effect is the "cross-training" or "cross-education" phenomenon. This is where training one side of your body, like your right leg, will also result in strength increases in your left leg.[59] Again, you didn't gain any muscle in your left leg, but through training your right leg, your nervous system got better at contracting existing leg muscle fibers.

Within the first few months of training, however, muscle hypertrophy becomes the dominant training adaptation and driver of strength gains. The rate at which you gain muscle and the total amount of muscle you gain are highly individual, influenced by factors like your genetics, age, and gender, but one principle is pretty universal: the longer you train, the harder it is to build muscle. In the beginning, you can follow the worst programmed exercise plan in the entire land of Instagram, and you'll still likely see pretty good progress. But as you get more advanced, proper programming and overloading become crucial to seeing continual progress in the gym.[60]

Getting Started in the Gym

When I first started lifting weights, I understood none of the science underlying muscle growth. My only sources of information were YouTube videos. I followed a body-part split (training a different body part each day), and I just tried to look the least dumb I could look while having no idea what the hell I was doing. Luckily for all of us, this guesswork and blindly stumbling our way through the first few months of the gym is entirely avoidable, because there are solid, science-based principles for how to approach resistance training that go beyond what hot YouTube girls and guys say "worked for them."

In the coming pages, I've outlined general newbie training recommendations with the goal of keeping you progressing for a long, long time. While these recommendations should hold for the average gym-goer who is looking to maximize hypertrophy and strength for time spent in the gym, that doesn't mean they're right for everybody. Your training should always be informed by your goals. So, for example, while sixty-second rest times make sense for someone just trying to get in a good workout, three-minute rest times are better for a powerlifter maximizing strength. While full-body routines make sense for a mom of two, a body-part split may make sense for a person who's been lifting for six years. The answer to what training is right for you is always going to be "it depends." But, if you're new to the gym, this is a great place to start.

Maximizing Gains

There are three main factors that tell your muscles, "It's time to grow, baby": mechanical tension, muscle damage, and metabolic stress. Understanding the difference and details of each of these is kind of beside the point, but anytime we are manipulating a training variable to better induce hypertrophy, it is likely manipulating one of these factors.

As you begin training, you will want to consider several variables that you can play around with in order to optimize progress. I thought about extensively discussing each, but who needs an explanation of the concentric versus eccentric loading of an exercise and its implications for tempo? Not me, homeys, not me. So what follows are the main principles to follow in the gym to get the best bang for your gym buck.

Intensity

Intensity, or load, may perhaps be the most important variable in your becoming-a-gym-boss tool belt. Intensity is usually expressed as a percentage of your one repetition maximum (1RM), the absolute most amount of weight you could lift once in a given exercise while still maintaining good form.[61] So if the absolute most you could squat when you first start out is one hundred pounds (this is a hypothetical number to make our math easy), lifting fifty pounds would be 50 percent of your 1RM.

In resistance training, exercises are organized by repetitions (reps) and sets (number of repetitions in a row before resting).[62] The number of reps and intensity have an inverse relationship.[63] For example, let's say I asked you to lift the *heaviest* weight you can. You squat one hundred pounds (made-up number), you can only do it one time, and it's a *struggle*. This would be high intensity, low rep. Now, if you instead squat twenty pounds, you can probably do thirty or even forty reps. This is low intensity and high rep.

Depending on what kind of adaptation you are looking for, you can manipulate intensity to varying degrees.[64] If you are most interested in getting as strong as possible, like a powerlifter, you would generally lift in a low-rep range (one to five reps per set) at a fairly high intensity (>85 percent of your 1RM). Most people interested in both strength and hypertrophy lift in the moderate range (six to twelve reps). And those most interested in endurance or conditioning generally use high-rep ranges (more than fifteen reps). It's pretty clear that when it comes to muscle hypertrophy, the low-to-moderate-rep ranges are way more effective.[65,66] Basically, you should be lifting "kinda" to "pretty" heavy to see maximal results (>65 percent of your 1RM). Especially for my ladies, who in my experience tend to underestimate their strength way more than men do, don't be afraid to actually lift a decent load when you exercise. You got this. (But be safe! I don't want any injuries on my hands.)

Volume

Volume, contrary to popular belief, is not a dial that your parents are constantly turning down on your car speaker when you're in the car together. Volume is a measure of how much work you are doing in a workout. It's computed by multiplying the number of sets, reps, and load (weight).[67] The most important thing to know about volume is that, to maximize hypertrophy, it should be increasing week to week. This is called progressive overload: you're progressively increasing the stress on your muscles, which therefore continue to give the signal to grow.[68]

No one is expecting you to bust out an abacus in the gym and start doing calculations in between sets of squats, but keeping track of how much you're doing each week is helpful. The most obvious way to increase volume is to simply increase weight from week to week. This is usually how people first start out incorporating progressive overload, because novice gym-goers get stronger so quickly. But you can also increase volume in other ways, such as increasing the number of sets, number of reps, or the time under tension (a.k.a. slowing down reps).[69]

There's no need to do crazy math, just try to increase the amount of work you do from week to week, because as the stressor increases, so does your body's adaptive response, that is, you get stronger. The key to volume is being able to balance an amount that's high enough that it is acting as a training stimulus but not so high that it is causing overtraining, at which point your body stalls or even starts regressing.[70]

Exercise Selection

There are about a million exercises, and which ones to choose and when seems like a random game of fill-in-the-blank. The important thing to know about exercise selection is that to maximize muscle hypertrophy and function, you need to vary the planes, angles, and types of movement to work each muscle in its entirety.

Exercises can be broken down into multijoint, also called compound, lifts (bench press, squats, deadlifts, overhead press), and single-joint exercises, or isolation lifts (leg extension, leg curl, tricep extensions, bicep curls). Compound lifts usually require more technique and many muscles, which means they also give you much more bang for your exercise buck.[71,72] Think of a squat versus a bicep curl. The squat is primarily a lower-body movement, but it requires stabilization from your abs, back, traps, and so on. It's estimated that a squat activates more than two hundred muscles all at once. Meanwhile, the bicep curl is just flexing your elbow, so it requires significantly less effort and significantly fewer muscles.[73]

Exercises involving multiple muscle groups or larger muscle groups have been shown to elicit greater acute hormonal responses and metabolic responses, which suggests that they are probably superior in a head-to-head comparison to isolation lifts for maximizing lean body mass. However, isolation lifts give you a chance to focus on underdeveloped muscles that may otherwise get neglected in larger movements. In general, they also require less skill and thus pose a lower risk of injury.[74] So all in all, including both compound and isolation lifts is a good idea, and varying the angles, planes, and types of exercise helps maximize your training stimulus. Remember, the exercises that are best for you are going to be those that you can perform safely and confidently with an appropriate load. Be safe!

Rest Times

"Can we start the next set now?" I hear this about a million times whenever I bring someone new to the gym. I think it's because people are so used to workouts being fitness classes or runs, where you can't stop to so much as catch your breath, let alone integrate a planned pause. "Resting" seems antithetical to "working out." But here's the dealio: if you want to maximize your workouts, you need to rest between sets in order for your muscles to be able to recover for your next set.

Studies have shown that rest times shorter than thirty seconds significantly impact performance on the following sets. However, longer rest times, while better for strength training, may reduce the amount of metabolic stress being inflicted on the muscle and thus produce less hypertrophy.[75] If you're lifting at a really high intensity and trying to get as strong as possible, taking a long rest time (about three to five minutes) is going to help maximize your strength gains. In general though, a moderate rest time (about sixty to ninety seconds) is usually best for maximizing hypertrophy along with strength.[76] Rest enough that you are performing well in all your sets, but not so long that you lose intensity and turn your workout into an Instagram stalking session

Frequency and Picking a Routine

A lot of factors go into choosing a workout routine: how much time you have, your training experience, how well you're recovering, and so on. But you don't need to be working out that much to see most of the benefits from lifting weights. Most resistance-training protocols on untrained individuals call for lifting two to three times a week, not the five to six times a week that fad exercise programs and infomercials suggest.[77] In novices, two-day-a-week programs have been shown to produce 80–90 percent of the results of more frequent programs. And once you've developed a good muscular base, studies have shown that one to two sessions per week are enough to maintain your gains.[78] Those who are more advanced may have to increase their frequency as time goes on if they want to continue progressing.

Your frequency will to some extent determine your exercise "split"—which muscle groups you are hitting during each workout. For a beginner who is going twice a week, it's probably best to do a full-body session, hitting all major muscle groups in both workouts. For an advanced lifter who is going maybe four or five times a week, dedicating specific days to your upper body and lower body, or even specific body parts, such as shoulders or back, might be a better strategy.[79] Ultimately though, it doesn't matter what science says is the "most effective" workout split if you don't like it. The best workout split is the one that gets you excited and pumped, and therefore becomes consistent. Loving your workouts should always be your most important consideration.

Another piece of good news: you don't need to be in the gym for hours. Some research actually suggests that longer workouts (more than one hour) may actually result in lowered intensity and motivation.[80] (Hmm . . . it may be time to rethink my three-hour training sessions.)

I Can't Go to the Gym Because . . .

Here are some of the excuses that stopped me from going to the gym in the past—or that I have heard from my friends when I inevitably tried to drag them along. Enjoy this little excuse buster, and may it bring you ever more PRs.

1. **I don't have enough money for a gym membership.** No prob! At-home workouts can be a great alternative for those whose finances don't allow for a gym membership. If you can afford it, getting simple accessories like resistance bands or even a single pair of dumbbells can enhance the at-home workout experience hugely. And free resources online for getting started are quite possibly endless. YouTube is your new best friend.

2. **I don't have time.** OK, as a working woman, I feel you on this one. But you *don't* need that much time. Blocking it out in your schedule, even if it's twenty minutes a day, is a great way to prioritize exercise. I treat my gym time as a daily meeting or appointment on my calendar that is just nonnegotiable. Like I literally tell coworkers, "I am unavailable at this time." I admit, this is a pretty sweet deal and one that a lot of people can't recreate given their work schedules and work circumstances. But there are ways around even the toughest schedules. I've seen people squeeze working out into lunch breaks, before or after work, or even in two solid sessions on the weekend. Or you can try to create little habit triggers around your office or house and just build a workout into your day: for example, every time I walk into my bedroom, I have to do twenty air squats. Or after

I finish a bathroom break, I have to do five push-ups. This way, there is no formal time set aside for working out, but you're applying stress to your muscles all day long.

3. **I don't know what to do.** Join the club; at first, none of us know what to do! Luckily, this is quite literally the best time to be alive when it comes to information. There are endless online videos, podcasts, articles, and posts explaining everything you need to know about exercise. It may take a little digging, but there are amazing people giving out completely free information every single day. Sorting through the snake-oil salesmen may sometimes seem intimidating, but once you practice, it becomes easier. For example, promising miraculous results, offering one-size-fits-all solutions, or speaking in absolutes are pretty consistent red flags. Somebody "looking hot" is not a credential. And somebody having the "body you want" is not the only reason you should be listening to them. Nevertheless, the truth is, *no one* starts out knowing what to do at the gym. If you can afford a few sessions with a personal trainer, that's also a great way to get started. But it's not a necessity: in my first two years of lifting, the only coaching I had was from the headphones in my ears.

4. **I'm afraid people will judge me.** This is one of the *most common* things I hear, particularly from women. It's scary doing something that makes you uncomfortable in front of complete strangers, in clothes that may make you self-conscious, especially if it's in a male-dominated area. Feeling as if you're "out of shape" or "don't belong" stops *so many people* from going to the gym. But the truth is, *nobody cares.* People are not looking at *you.* People at the gym are there to focus on *themselves.* We have a narrative in our heads that everyone is watching everything we do, when a majority of the time, people just could not give the lesser of two craps what my dumb ass is doing over at the squat rack. Everyone has been "new" to the gym. You may feel judged, embarrassed, and like you have no idea what you're

doing. In fact, I guarantee you will feel all of those things. But after a few workouts, a few months, dare I say a few weeks, you will be walking around the gym floor like you were born there. Stick it out; it's worth it.

5. **I'm afraid I'll be embarrassed.** Here is a nonexhaustive list of things that have happened to me in the gym.

   - Bra strap popped off in the middle of a squat.

   - Tripped on countless barbells, benches, and dumbbells.

   - Ran face-first into a wall. (I was bailing on a handstand . . . long story.)

   - Accidentally buckled under a bar because I didn't brace properly.

   - Jumped up to a pull-up bar, only to miss and land on my butt.

   - Been slapped in the butt, stomach, face, and crotch by resistance bands snapping out from under my feet.

   - Had my *actual butt muscles* break a hip circle when doing butt exercises.

The list goes on. Guys . . . I'm *legally blind*. I guarantee you the number of embarrassing things that have happened to me in the gym are exponentially higher than what will happen to you. You'll be embarrassed, but it will not kill you.

6. **I don't like it.** Just because resistance training is a really great form of exercise does not mean it's the only form of exercise. I would ask you to give it a fair trial, like a *real* fair trial. Decide

to dedicate two full months, going twice a week and just trying your best, and if you still really don't like it, then whatever exercise you like, that's the right exercise for you. Movement is movement. At the end of the day, you'll only be consistent with the thing you love doing. Feel free to explore all forms of resistance training. You don't have to be in a gym.

PROTEIN INTAKE: A NOTE

I know we talked all about not reducing food down to just nutrients, but I have to make a little bit of an exception for protein, because adequate protein intake is going to help you maximize strength and muscle gains in the gym. Particularly if you're working out a lot and breaking down that muscle tissue, eating enough protein is what's going to ensure that your body is going to be able to capitalize on all that hard work in the gym.

The United States–Canadian Recommended Dietary Allowance for protein intake is a modest 0.8 grams per kilogram of body weight.[81] For a 150-pound person, this would be around 54 grams of protein, the amount in a large (8-ounce) chicken breast. This is the *minimum* protein you need to keep your body properly functioning.[82]

However, over the past few decades, this number has been called into question because high-protein diets have been associated with so many benefits. Because protein is more satiating (i.e., it makes you feel more full), high-protein diets have been shown to lead to greater weight loss. Eating a higher-protein diet can also help slow down the muscle loss associated with aging (the greatest contributor to metabolic slowdown associated with getting older), and higher-protein diets help maximize muscle growth and athletic performance.[83]

So how much protein do you need? Well, of course, the answer is . . . it depends. Your level of activity, the type of exercise you're doing, your age, and even how many calories you're eating (i.e., whether or not you are in a calorie deficit) all may impact the amount of protein you need. According to the International Society of Sports Nutrition, a protein intake of 1.4–2 grams per kilogram of body weight per day is a good range for most exercising individuals.[84] For a 150-pound person (68 kilograms), that's a protein intake of 95–136 grams per day. For individuals who train and are entering a calorie deficit, even higher protein intakes are recommended to minimize the loss of muscle mass and maximize loss of fat mass over the course of the diet.[85]

A lot of these numbers can be confusing, because there's a lot of conversions in the use of kilograms, grams, and so on. Therefore, a pretty quick and, it turns out, research-backed rule of thumb is one gram of protein per pound of body weight. The old gym-bro golden rule of protein intake turns out to actually hold true! (Of course this isn't as precise, but it is a pretty good approximation.) PS: If you're at a higher body-fat level, these protein recommendations can seem insane, so to save you from having to eat a dozen eggs a day, a pretty easy rule of thumb is one gram per centimeter of height.

There is evidence to suggest that spacing protein intake throughout the day (as opposed to having it all in one sitting) is better for maximizing muscle protein synthesis[86] In other words, try to have a decent portion of protein (e.g., at least thirty grams) at every meal throughout the day to maximize the gains.

Finally, there used to be a concern about high-protein intakes and liver/kidney function because of experiments showing adverse effects on patients with kidney disease. According to a multitude of data, for healthy individuals, there are no adverse health outcomes associated with high-protein diets. The International Society of Sports Nutrition states that "no controlled scientific evidence exists indicating that increased intakes of protein pose any health risks in healthy, exercising individuals."[87] Boom. Mic drop. Go wild on the chickpeas, Greek yogurt, eggs, and chicken breasts.

The Takeaways

Types of Exercise

Exercise is a stressor, and so your body adapts. It comes in two flavors: endurance exercise (cardio), generally performed with low load for a long time, and resistance (or strength) training, generally performed with higher loads for a shorter time. In reality, a lot of exercise is a combination of these two.

Resistance Training and Fat Loss

Cardio burns more calories than resistance training *during* the workout. But because RT necessitates muscle repair and increases your muscle mass, it leads to a much higher calorie burn *outside* the workout. Because so much of the metabolic decline associated with aging is attributed to muscle loss, resistance training can be a great way to maintain your metabolic rate throughout life.

Resistance Training and Health

There's more to resistance training than looking hot. Muscle mass is inversely related to all-cause mortality and prevalence of metabolic syndrome. Resistance training has been shown to improve blood-sugar control, improve cardiovascular health, reduce resting blood pressure, improve blood lipid profiles, increase bone mineral density, improve cognition as you age, improve self-esteem, lower depression, reduce low-back pain, and improve muscle function/mobility.

Bulky vs. Toned Muscle

There aren't separate biological processes for "toning" versus "building" muscle. There aren't different exercises to get "lean" muscles versus "bulky" muscles. Your body can only either build muscle (hypertrophy) or lose muscle (atrophy). When people say "tone" or "sculpt," they likely mean build a little muscle to give shape to a body part and lose a little fat to reveal the shape underneath.

Muscle and Fat Tissue

You cannot spot-reduce fat, but you *can* spot-increase muscle. Meaning that doing crunches won't get rid of stomach fat, but it will make your abs stronger. The order in which fat comes off your body isn't really within our control and is influenced by factors like genetics and gender. Muscle is also more dense than fat (it takes up less space for the same amount of weight). So if you start working out and the scale does not budge or even goes up, that does not mean it's not working! Overall strength, endurance, or even progress pictures are a better way to see how your body is changing.

Women and Weights

The vast majority of women cannot gain as much muscle as men because they are much smaller humans and have a different hormonal profile than men. In relative terms, women are basically as strong as men. The chances of your looking like a female bodybuilder from working out are similar to the chances of you becoming a Beyoncé music-video-level backup dancer from taking a few dance classes.

Starting at the Gym

When you first start at the gym, you'll experience large, consistent gains in your strength in a period called "newbie gains." You will also likely experience body recomposition (losing body fat, increasing muscle mass). The longer you work out, the more difficult it becomes to increase muscle mass and strength.

Progressing in the Gym

The key to progressing in the gym is to increase your workload from week to week, whether that means increasing the weight, number of reps, sets, exercises, or range of motion. Specific programming variables should be based on your individual goals. For most people looking to maximize their time, two to three full body sessions a week focusing on compound movements (movements that use multiple joints) at a relatively challenging weight is enough to see the majority of the benefits from resistance training. Adequate protein intake will help you maximize strength and muscle gains.

8

Too "Fat" to Have an Eating Disorder

I feel as though, to me, the entire point of this book is *this one* chapter. It was the first thing I wrote, and it flowed out of my fingers pretty much fully written. I didn't fiddle with it or change the structure in editing. I thought of it on a long walk at one of my ten-day silent meditation retreats (more on that later) and then wrote it down the second I got home, almost verbatim.

For reasons that are hard to explain, I feel it's *the most important part, the core* of this book and, in a way, my life. I don't spend a lot of time thinking about my behaviors relating to eating and my body in the past: the three-day fasts, the hours-long treadmill sessions at 1 A.M., the torturous nights spent unable to sleep from painful binges—but when I write about them or speak about them, I feel how deeply they impacted me. Those periods of my life are difficult to revisit, and putting them down for others to read, particularly people I love, is scary and uncomfortable. I don't feel shame or regret about sharing my experience, but I feel anxious at the thought of my friends, my family, and the other people who care about me reading this. For some reason, it's easier to let those you don't know witness your lowest moments.

The incredible self-loathing and disgust I felt for my body through my teens and early twenties were such staples of my daily life that for a long time, I considered them a given. But as someone who has made it through to the other side, take it from me: it does *not* have to be. Admitting you need help is hard. Seeking treatment is hard. Giving up old patterns of thinking and behaving is hard. But you know what's harder? Living with an eating disorder. If you need support in this area, I hope this chapter gives you at least a little.

Part 1: Diets, Fasts, and Binges

The Fasts

This is too easy. Entirely too easy.

It's 7 P.M. on a Tuesday, and I lie in bed, burrowed under two comforters, a sweatshirt and sweatpants on. My body has finally started to warm up, but my hands, feet, nose, and cheeks are still icy. I pull the comforters over my face and try to breathe harder, hoping the warm air I'm exhaling will hit my face.

How could no one have noticed, I wonder.

It's been two days—*two days*—since my last meal, and neither of my parents has said a word. It shouldn't be this easy.

Even as I have the petulant thought, I know the real answer: my parents work . . . a lot. They leave before I eat breakfast and often come home after I eat dinner. They probably don't see me eat most days, let alone these past two.

But what about my lunch?!

I feel triumphant.

I knew there was something they missed. I meal-prep every single day. It's an ordeal—food scale out, five or six different vegetables everywhere, everything measured to the gram. It takes at least forty-five minutes every night. How has no one noticed the clean kitchen? The untouched food scale? The spot on the fridge shelf where my lunch container would normally be?

I picture our cramped fridge, mismatched Tupperware filled with assorted Albanian dishes—homemade kefir, meats, stews, feta cheese—all crammed into containers and piled onto plates that make up a barely contained chaos. Of course no one noticed.

Anyway, it doesn't matter. It's better this way: no explaining, no lying, and only one more day, *one more day,* until I get to eat. I get back to my favorite activity: planning the first meal.

"Juna?"

A shaft of light pierces the black room. It's my mom.

"What are you doing?" She sounds utterly confused.

I should explain: I don't ever "lie in bed." I barely even sit on my bed.

The only time I am in my bed is from 11 P.M. to 6 A.M. when I am sleeping. It must be completely bizarre seeing me in the dark, under blankets, at 7 P.M.

"Oh, nothing, just feeling a little sick," I say. "Might be coming down with something." It's funny how easily the lies came, so natural, so smooth. "Do you have a fever?" Before I can stop her, she's next to me feeling my forehead, the shaft of light now a big rectangle on my floor.

"You don't feel warm . . ." she says, taking her hand away.

No, I'm not warm. I'm cold—freezing, actually. If she had only slid her hand an inch lower, she would have felt that icy nose and those bloodless cheeks. When the body is starved, I had learned, it conserves all its energy and heat for the vital organs in the torso, leaving the extremities cold and drained.

"No, no, it's probably nothing. I'm just tired from practicing, you know."

Another easy lie. So many softballs today. . . . As if I had played a single note. I had gone to the practice rooms, going through the usual motions, then just sat on the piano bench for six hours in my puffer jacket planning: tomorrow's first meal . . . the number of hours left till food . . . the number of hours completed with no food . . . the number of calories saved . . . the number of pounds lost—so many calculations.

"Do you want some Tylenol?" my mom offers.

Will that fast-forward the next twenty-four hours?

"No," I say. "I think it's nothing. I'll get some if I need it."

"OK . . ." Sounding uncertain, she leaves the room, plunging me back into the thick, impenetrable black.

The Doctor

A few weeks later, I sit among white, white walls, white floors, white fluorescent lights—clean, clinical. *Why are hospitals always so cold?* I find myself thinking. Even the few colors around are guarded somehow, almost as if they were trying really hard to be cheerful but had given up halfway through and had settled for a much more "sensible" muted purple or off-puke yellow.

I sit on my hands to keep them warm as Dr. Li walks briskly back into the room.

Sitting at his computer, he starts scrolling and clicking.

"Yeah. . . . These don't look good. . . . You have the hormones of a menopausal woman," he says, half laughing, "or someone who's starving."

Yes, hilarious. Of course a five-foot-seven girl who weighs 170 pounds could never be starving.

"You said the last time you had a period was six months ago?"

I have no idea. It seems vaguely right . . . June or July. Who knows?

Not having a period is weirdly convenient: no tampons to buy, no timing to figure out, no PMS-ing to deal with. But no period means your hormones are fucked. And if your hormones are fucked, your weight loss is fucked. That's why I'm here.

"I think it was around six months ago," I offer noncommittally.

"Yeah. . . . We might have to put you on something." He is still clacking away at the keys.

"On something?" I'm confused. "What do you mean?"

"Well, your estrogen is so low, and it has been every single time you've come in. I'm worried about osteoporosis, especially since you exercise so much. Estrogen this low makes for very brittle bones . . . very brittle."

Osteoporosis? Isn't that something old women get? I vaguely remember some commercials: Neat, sixty-something women with stylish "put together older lady" haircuts, having what looked like engaged conversations with handsome doctors and then pictured doing yard work or folding laundry, all while the announcer proclaims *"Bone loss does not have to be permanent. Ask your doctor about such-and-such medication!"*

I'm not old. I don't even fold my laundry half the time, let alone do yard work. What the hell is going on?

"Can't I just take a calcium supplement or something?"

"It doesn't work like that." Dr. Li says this in a tone that makes it very clear that this is a stupid question.

My mind is racing. Put me "on something" meant estrogen . . . or birth control . . . ? Or both? Either way, doesn't exogenous estrogen lead to weight gain? And all those girls are always complaining about birth control making them gain weight. I cannot gain more weight.

I cannot.

Weight gain . . . or brittle bones.

Weight gain . . . or brittle bones.

I sit there, honestly not able to decide which is worse.

My stomach turns as I think about the two hundred pounds that had been on my back in the gym a couple days ago, about all the running I do around the reservoir. Can bones just break mid-squat? Can they shatter mid-run? I have no idea.

"Wait, but what's causing these test results?" I ask. I don't know why I play this game. I know the answer, the *real* answer, but I don't want that answer. I want a new one, a different one.

"Stress, just stress probably." Dr. Li still hasn't looked up.

"So what should I do?" Yikes, my tone is getting kind of shrill. How the fuck could this be from stress? We're talking about bones . . . *bones.*

I don't know what I want from him, maybe a thyroid medication? Or a Polycystic Ovarian Syndrome (PCOS) diagnosis? Something that explains the weight gain, and also gives me a pill to undo it.

"Oh, you know, take a bath . . . relax. . . . You know. . . ."

Take a bath.

Take a freaking bath?!??

I'm at the endocrinology department of Brigham and Women's Hospital, one of the best hospitals in the country, and the best I can get is a prescription for lavender L'Occitane Foaming Bath?

"I've been trying some fasting," I offer half-heartedly, trying to get his attention somehow.

"Yeah, yeah, intermittent fasting is very good." Still not looking up: "Good for health . . . weight loss . . ."

Ouch. Way to hit me right where it hurts.

"Um, yeah, I've tried like . . . a twenty-four-hour one," I try again, "and a forty-eight once." I don't dare bring up the three-day fasts. I know they sound crazy to the outside observer. But they're not *that* crazy. I mean, humans evolved not eating for weeks at a time during famines. . . . Just because modern humans eat every day doesn't mean it's normal biologically . . . right?

"Twenty-four-hour?" He finally stops typing and turns around.

"*What?* Forty-eight? What are you talking about?! No! *No, no!*" He sounds angry, and his words become louder and faster. "You can't do that! Do you know what happens when they make mice fast for eighteen hours? No period! No reproducing! Very bad!"

He seems rather in a huff now. Phew, good call on not mentioning the three-day.

"Oh . . . so . . . no fasting? At all?"

"*No.* Stop that. Don't do that. It's very dangerous for women."

He turns back around, mumbling about "Forty-eight-hour, my God" and angrily clacking the keys.

My fears confirmed, I shift my hands under my legs, a pit of dread forming in my stomach.

No fasts. . . . No fasts means no more get-out-of-jail-free cards. On the first of every month, for almost a year now, my fasts had been my way to undo the previous month's "mishaps." At first they had lasted only twenty-four hours. Of course, I told myself they were "for my health," not for weight loss. There was so much "science" to support it. I hadn't looked any of it up, per se, but people online were always talking about it. It, like, regenerates your immune system and promotes cell turnover and all that. I later found out all these studies were done on cats, not humans. Maybe some part of me knew the science was dubious, which is why I avoided looking into it.

Regardless, the twenty-four-hour fasts were almost too easy. It was dinner one day, then don't eat until dinner the next. So, I moved to forty-eight. That was a bit harder, but I didn't really mind it.

Dinner one day, no food the next, dinner the third. That one full day of no food was almost a relief. Sure, no food meant hunger. But no food also meant no planning, no stressing, no weighing, no obsessing, no thinking, no anxiety, no worrying, no weight gain, no problems. If I could get all the calories and nutrients I needed injected into my veins at the end of every day, I would. It would make my life so simple, so much . . . easier.

By this point, the binges throughout the month had started getting almost violent in their severity—painful, frequent, and unrelenting. So I bumped up my monthly "undo button" to a three-day fast, a whole seventy-two hours of just water and caffeine. And this, I had to admit, was a challenge.

It became as much about my character as the weight loss. Could I follow through? Could I control myself for these three days? Could I keep this one freaking commitment to myself? Was I too weak? Would I let myself down yet again?

All the years of weight-loss goals, of crying post-binge, swearing to myself I wouldn't do it again, even resorting to praying to a god I didn't even know existed, to "please help me stop binge eating. Please help me lose weight. Please help me stop doing this to myself."

Could I not eat for three days and actually keep one fucking promise?

It turns out yes, yes I could. For three months now, I had been able to stick to my seventy-two-hour fasts.

Although they were getting iffy. My willpower was waning. The binges were getting worse, the fasts were getting harder, and my weight was stable at best and increasing at worst.

The Binges

The fasts and binges were two sides of the same miserable coin. I fasted to make up for the binges. I binged to make up for the fasts. And they fed off of each other, growing together in strength and severity like a hideous two-headed beast.

The first time I told anyone about the binges was in senior year of college. Something had happened: a bad concert, a stressful audition—who knows what it had been?—and I was instantly in *that* headspace. The binge headspace. It had already started in the dining hall:

One bagel, two bagels, three . . . all the time "I don't eat gluten. I don't eat gluten, I don't eat gluten" playing in my head like some sadistic mantra.

One ice-cream cone, two ice-cream cones. "I don't eat ice cream. I don't eat ice cream."

Peanut butter, hot chocolate, a cup of just whipped cream—foods I would never touch with a ten-foot pole on a "normal day"—were in my mouth and swallowed before I even knew what was happening.

I stood in the dining hall, stewing in self-loathing, having run out of all the worst food I could find. Had anyone seen? Is anyone looking at me?

I went back to my room, got my coat, and left.

Food tour it is, I thought; a food tour of Harvard Square.

First stop, Starbucks, for a holiday drink and pastry.

"I don't drink calories. I don't eat pastries."

They are gone in under three minutes flat. I can't even taste it at this point, no flavors, no textures, just sweet or salty. I feel high. My cheeks are flushed, my heart pounding, I'm almost euphoric.

Next, Mike's Pastry.

"I don't eat cannolis."

Two cannolis gone.

Tacos.

A slice of pizza.

Cookies from Insomnia.

I'm not even in my body now.

Forty-five minutes later I get back to the room and slump onto the couch. There's no way to *be* in the world after a binge. No way to exist without being in excruciating pain, physically, mentally. No position that's comfortable. You can't breathe from the food that's stuffing your body. Your face is red and hot, stomach distended painfully, lips puckered from salt, throat hurting from sugar, jaw sore from chewing. Head pounding. Lying on your side hurts. Lying on your back brings the food to your throat. Lying on your stomach presses it into you. There's no position without agony. There's no second without shame and self-loathing. And the worst part: there's no one who did this to you, no one to blame, no one to be mad at besides yourself. The worst, darkest, and most bleak moments of human existence that I've ever experienced, and I made them happen.

To me.

I hate myself.

I hate myself.

I hate myself.

I squirm on our royal-purple futon. Michelle, my roommate, and I had gotten it from some seniors moving out of the quad, and my parents had driven it over in their Toyota Corolla. It was only five bucks, and it was suddenly glaringly obvious why: it was about as cushiony as the cobblestone sidewalks I had just been walking on.

I decide the most comfortable position is to be half-reclined, some-where between sitting and lying, and that's how Michelle finds me, as she comes out of her room.

"What's wrong?" she says instantly.

Again, I don't really "sit on the couch." I'm either at my desk, in a prac-tice room, at the gym, or out with friends somewhere.

There's no way to answer this question that makes any sense. I'm so tired of using euphemisms like "I'm just feeling down" or "Just really up-set with myself, you know?" This was Juna-speak for "I fucking binged again." No one knew Juna-speak besides me.

I opt for the simplest answer I can think of.

"I ate too much." It's a half moan, half whimper. It's pathetic. I sound like a child.

"It's OK, girl," she says, padding over in her slippers and patting my head.

"No, you don't understand," I moan. How to explain . . . how to explain . . . ?

"It happens to all of us!" Michelle offers helpfully. "The other day, they had pound cake in the dining hall, and I ate three pieces!"

I look at Michelle, all 105 pounds of her slim frame, her flat stomach, her nonflabby arms and thighs, and literally cannot think how to explain what the fuck just happened.

I know she's trying to make me feel better. She knows how hard I've been working recently, going to the gym first thing in the morning, not going out to eat ever, eating even cleaner, even more carefully than usual. But she really, *really* doesn't understand.

"No. No . . ." It's hard to decide what's more exhausting at this point: Do I tell her the truth and seem like an out-of-control psychopath? Or do I just pretend I ate a little too much ice cream and am having an insane overreaction. They're both just so impossibly tiring right now. And they both make me seem crazy.

"I ate cannolis . . . and pizza . . . and tacos . . . and bagels . . ." I start to list the things, leaving out half, and I can tell it's not what she thought. It's astounding to see someone who only eats vegetables at every meal, who drinks exclusively black coffee, who gets plain Greek yogurt and protein powder for breakfast start listing almost every Harvard Square eatery, all sampled in less than an hour.

It felt good to finally tell someone, even if Michelle didn't quite know what I was talking about. It lost some of its power somehow. If it could be talked about in daylight, not just in the confines of my brain, it couldn't be quite as horrible, as shameful, as I had once thought.

Getting Diagnosed

You would think that as a psychology major, I would be hypervigilant at seeing my own behavior patterns and calling them out: binge eating disorder (BED), at times bulimia nervosa, dipping into orthorexia (hyperfixation on eating "healthy") even, a constant body dysmorphia (an obsession on perceived flaws in appearance). And yet, they never seemed "bad enough" to qualify. Part of it was that I didn't want to put a label on them and make my patterns "official." Part of it was that bingeing and compensatory behaviors were so openly and commonly talked about online in the fitness space that I just thought it was part of pursuing fitness goals. But the biggest part of it was I thought that I didn't *look* like someone with an eating disorder. I wasn't anywhere close to "underweight." I barely qualified as "normal" weight. And a lot of the time, I was technically "overweight."

I remembered that on the few slides about eating disorders in my Abnormal Psych class, the professor had specifically mentioned that often people with bulimia nervosa and BED weren't underweight, but I guess the internal image of what a "proper" eating disorder should look like was too strong in my head. I was simply "too fat," in my opinion, to qualify.

The first time it became clear to me was in 2018. I sat across from Dr. Jennifer Thomas, mic and recorder in hand, interviewing her for the eating-disorders episode of our podcast. Dr. Thomas, who is the codirector of the Eating Disorders Clinical and Research Program at Massachusetts General Hospital, spoke in a soft, measured voice that instantly made me feel comfortable and calm. We were about thirty minutes into the interview when the topic of "overvaluation of shape and weight" came up.

"If you think about your self-esteem like a pie chart," Dr. Thomas explained, "and you think about all the things in your life that would have to be going well in order for you to *feel* successful, the ideal pie chart . . . would be kind of like a stock portfolio that's diversified. . . . For me, I'm a psychologist; I want my patients to be doing well. I'm a researcher; I want my research to be going well. I'm a mom; I want to be a good mom to my son. I'm a wife. . . . For individuals with eating disorders, usually those other pieces get squeezed out because they're focusing so much on their shape and weight."

I'd never heard anyone say it like that, but it perfectly encapsulated why I felt like such a failure. No matter what I had accomplished, no matter what accolades I got or goals I achieved, I was fundamentally a failure because I couldn't do the simplest thing: control my own body.

"Having an eating disorder can be kind of like a full-time job," she went on, and the meaning of her words sunk into me. How many hours, days, weeks, maybe months of my life had I spent on this one thing, this one goal? It was after that interview that I first sought formal treatment.

Part 2: Eating Disorders and Disordered Eating

The Prevalence of Eating Disorders

I want to give a brief description of the three most prevalent eating disorders. There are many other eating disorders that are not mentioned here, so if you feel like food, eating, or your preoccupation with your body is controlling your life, then from one bestie to another: please ask someone for help. (You can call the National Eating Disorders Association at 1-800-931-2237 or go to their website at www.nationaleatingdisorders.org.)

These descriptions are not meant to diagnose anyone—because, hello, I'm just some girl—but they are meant to educate and give those who need it a push to seek treatment. There were so many times when I would think about seeking help, start to google it, and then just get so overwhelmed with all the options that I would just give up. There were other times when I should've sought help, but something stopped me: "I'm too busy right now"; "I don't *actually* have a problem"; "I'm not thin enough to count"; "I don't want to make this a thing when it's not." If you're reading this and you have a pit in your stomach, or a little voice is telling you, *This might apply to you,* then that's your sign. Asking for help is the first step. There are resources at the end of this chapter to assist you.

Binge Eating Disorder

Although anorexia nervosa is perhaps the most well-known of the eating disorders, particularly to the public at large, it is not the most prevalent. The most common eating disorder is binge eating disorder (BED), affecting about 3.5 percent of women and 2 percent of men at some point in their lives.[1] This makes binge eating disorder more prevalent than anorexia nervosa and bulimia nervosa combined. Contrary to the media caricature of eating disorders, which often portrays gaunt, emaciated women, binge eating disorder is associated with severe obesity, but that does not mean you have to "be a certain weight" to have BED.[2]

So what exactly does it mean to have BED? I mean, we all overeat sometimes, right? In the past decade, the word "binge" has become a common part of our vernacular, used to describe anything from Thanksgiving dinners to accidentally eating a whole bag of chips while watching TV. But true binge eating is not the same as overeating.

Luckily for us, we have a group of people whose job involves defining things like "binge eating." Every couple of decades, the American Psychiatric Association gets together, cracks a few beers, and busts out a new edition of the *Diagnostic and Statistical Manual of Mental Disorders* (or the *DSM,* if you're in the know). The beer part may be a slight fabrication on my part . . . but the writers must be drinking something, right? Coffee? Tea? This publication describes formally recognized mental disorders and is used by psychiatrists, psychologists, hospitals, doctors, health insurance companies, and so on—all the people who need labels, basically—to clinically diagnose individuals. The *DSM-5* finally designated binge eating disorder as a distinct diagnosis in 2013.[3]

According to the most recent edition, the *DSM-5-TR,* a binge has two components: it's a discrete amount of time (less than two hours) when a person eats substantially more food than someone would normally eat in that same situation.[4] And, perhaps more importantly, it is marked by a feeling of being out of control; as in, you want to stop but you can't. This is what separates eating seconds and thirds at Thanksgiving from a binge. Those who have experienced binge eating often describe it as if they're blacked out, or unconscious, while it's happening, and then only come to afterward.

As one might guess, binge eating disorder is characterized by, well . . . frequent binges—an average of at least once per week for three months, to be exact.[5] Binge eating is often marked by eating way faster than normal, eating until you're uncomfortable physically, and eating when you're not really hungry. One crucial criteria of BED is a marked sense of distress after a binge: this can include feelings of depression, disgust at oneself, shame, or anxiety about the actual binge episode.[6]

One of the prevailing theories of the cause of binge eating disorder is that the binges serve some sort of emotion-regulation purpose.[7] "A lot of people will use binge eating in particular as a way to escape from a negative mood," says Dr. Thomas. Studies have found that individuals with BED seem to lack healthy coping strategies for negative emotions and are much more likely to suppress their emotions and ruminate (dwell on negative emotions).[8]

It's clear that negative affect plays a big role in the development of binge eating disorder. When subjects are asked to note their mood throughout the day, studies have shown that a binge is preceded by a rise in negative moods, and due to a lack of other emotion-regulation skills, those with BED engage in binge eating as a way to cope.[9] Some studies have shown that immediately following a binge, there is a decrease in negative mood, a temporary relief, before the distressful emotions of guilt, shame, or depression associated with the binge set in.[10] Thus, it's easy to see that no matter how frustrating binge eating can be in the long run, in the short run it can be incredibly reinforcing. There is also a growing body of research to suggest that binge eating disorder shares a lot of similarities with other addictive behaviors, for example, wanting to stop but not being able to or continuing to engage in a behavior despite demonstrated negative consequences. This insight may help us create more effective interventions for BED in the future.[11] (See chapter 5 for more on food addiction.)

Bulimia Nervosa

In 1979, a British psychiatrist, Gerald Russell, noted a strange behavior in thirty of his patients with anorexia nervosa. He described them as "victims of powerful and irresistible urges to overeat."[12] Due to the weight gain one might expect from such overeating, a.k.a. "the worst fears of the anorectic patient come true," Russell noted that these patients would then engage in behaviors like self-induced vomiting, use of amphetamines, or starvation in order to keep their weight below some perceived threshold. This is the first documented description of what we call today bulimia nervosa. Although Russell categorized it as a subset of anorexia nervosa, the diagnosis of bulimia nervosa most consistent with how we define it today was added to the *DSM* in 1987.[13]

Bulimia nervosa (BN) is a fairly well-known and commonly dramatized eating disorder. It is the second most prevalent, affecting approximately 1.5 percent of women and 0.5 percent of men.[14] The picture that probably comes to your mind when you think "bulimia" is someone sticking a finger down her or his throat to throw up. But, in my opinion, it's exactly reductive media narratives like this that keep people from seeking help. *I've never made myself throw up, so I don't have bulimia* was a common thought I had until I took a class in abnormal psychology sophomore year of college and found out that this is not at all a requirement of a BN diagnosis.

Like binge eating disorder, bulimia nervosa is characterized by episodes of excessive overeating, often full-out binges. But what separates it from BED is the compensatory behaviors that follow, specifically in an attempt to prevent weight gain.[15] Self-induced vomiting is one example of a "compensatory behavior," but in reality, these behaviors come in many forms: overexercising, fasting, taking laxatives or diuretics. The binge-purge cycle is particularly hard to break out of because often purging behaviors can trigger binges: if someone decides to skip meals one day to compensate for a binge, they're much more likely to binge again because they'll be famished. In this way, purges lead to binges that lead to purges, and the cycle goes on. As you can imagine, interrupting the binge-purge cycle is crucial to the treatment of BN.[16]

Individuals with bulimia nervosa tend to be normal weight or overweight, which often makes it harder for family members and friends to detect BN in them, and also makes it less likely that the individual will seek out treatment. However, BN can be an extremely dangerous mental disorder, particularly due to the health complications associated with the purging behaviors. For example, in extreme cases, self-induced vomiting can lead to electrolyte imbalance, which can cause cardiac arrhythmia, seizures, or even death.[17] Unlike in anorexia nervosa, bulimia appears to be most prevalent in Hispanic/Latino communities, followed by Black communities, and the least prevalent in non-Hispanic white communities.

Anorexia Nervosa

Many of you may be shocked to find out that anorexia nervosa, perhaps the most well-known eating disorder, is actually the least prevalent, affecting about 1 percent of women and 0.3 percent of men at some point in their lives.[18] Anorexia is characterized by taking in way less energy than you need, resulting in low body weight, an intense fear of being fat, and preoccupation with body weight and shape.[19] Individuals with anorexia also have a distorted view of their body size and shape. Anorexia may be the most well-known eating disorder because it is so incredibly physical, so visible to all: the image of anorexia is often what immediately pops into people's minds when they hear "eating disorder."

Eating disorders may seem like a "first world problem." After all, if you have anorexia, bulimia, or a binge eating disorder, you at least *have enough* food, a luxury that so many people on the planet don't have. Despite how "privileged" having these disorders may seem, they are serious and dangerous. For example, anorexia nervosa is the most lethal psychiatric disorder, with a 5.6 percent death rate and a fifty-seven-fold increase in suicidality.[20] For more than half of those diagnosed with anorexia nervosa, the illness may last for more than twenty years and is often associated with severe cardiac abnormalities, brain impairments, and early-onset bone disease (among other things).[21]

Although the prevalence of binge eating disorder, bulimia nervosa, and anorexia nervosa seems to be fueled by sociocultural factors, like internalizing the "thin ideal" and exposure to Western culture, presumed cases of anorexia nervosa have been documented for centuries across both Western and non-Western cultures.[22] In other words, anorexia nervosa may have some other biological or genetic causal factor that is separate from wanting to look like the people we see on Instagram.

Eating Disorders Don't Have a "Look"

Growing up, I felt that eating disorders were in a way glamorized by the media. The famous people I knew who had them were beautiful and thin: ballerinas, dancers, gymnasts. It was most often anorexia or bulimia, and it was always the type of people who you would look at and think, *How could these people think they're fat? They're so skinny and beautiful.* Perhaps this is why I never felt that I fit the mold or met the criteria. Binges were never mentioned. Were they too messy? Sloppy? Embarrassing? They didn't fit the mold. The only time I remember hearing about them was in an article about Princess Diana, and I felt shocked that someone so beautiful could also experience this thing that I felt was so ugly about me.

We all have an image of what eating disorders "should" look like, and because of that, many people don't seek treatment. For example, less than half of individuals with binge eating disorder and bulimia nervosa are ever treated for their disorder.[23] It's paramount to understand that an eating disorder does not have a specific weight, shape, gender, race, or sexual orientation. Eating disorders affect *people*, and if you're a person, congrats, you're eligible.

Causes and Risk Factors

As with all mental disorders, we can't pinpoint one single cause of eating disorders and say, "Aha! If you went on a diet at age thirteen, you will get an eating disorder." Wouldn't that just be so simple and easy? Instead, it's a mess of biological, genetic, environmental, and cultural influences, and the way they all tangle and interact with each other.[24] Genes and personality traits may predispose certain people to be at higher risk for developing an eating disorder, but their environments play a pivotal role as well.

Remember in chapter 1 when we talked about the history of dieting and how eating-disorder rates seem to follow whatever "body" is in vogue at the time? Well, it turns out these sociocultural effects play a pretty big role in predisposing people to developing an eating disorder. "Sometimes I wonder if there are all these narratives that get out there in society," Dr. Thomas says, "like, for example, eating disorders are all about control, and then people feel like that is what they are supposed to say." In fact, the "needing control" variable has not been corroborated by any data.[25] While most people with eating disorders do endorse using their ED as a way to control their shape and weight, they don't see it as a way to control their lives. The focus on weight and shape seems crucial to the genesis and development of EDs. Indeed, some of the greatest sociocultural contributors to eating disorders appear to be pressures for thinness, media exposure, and thin-ideal internalization.[26] We know that when non-Western countries undergo urbanization and Westernization, rates of eating disorders go up, suggesting that, yes indeed, Western culture and its obsession with a thin body is at least partially responsible.[27]

Certain personality factors are also risk factors for developing an eating disorder. Perfectionism, in particular, has been shown to be a prospective predictor of anorexia and bulimia, specifically. And it's not tough to see how: perfectionism applied to weight and body shape could easily lead to caloric restriction that gets out of hand. And bulimia nervosa could be seen as "attempting to be perfectionistic," as Thomas puts it, and then not being able to "meet those standards." For example, breaking a dietary rule leads to a binge, and then "feeling bad about it" leads to "trying to redouble your efforts." Sometimes I wonder if this common trait of perfectionism is why eating disorders seemed so incredibly prevalent at a place like Harvard, an institution where perfectionism and meticulous attention to detail are almost a prerequisite for acceptance.

Dieting also seems to be a common risk factor.[28] Many of us will diet at some point in our lives, and for most of us, it will be harmless: the majority of us will fail, shrug our shoulders, and move on. But for a subset of the population, a diet can be an incredibly powerful trigger. Some will be so "good" at the diet and so reinforced by it that it will lead to further and further cutbacks and eventually a dangerously low weight. For others, it will trigger their first binge episode due to having gone for too long being underfed. For yet others, it will trigger a binge, then a purge and re-commitment to an even stricter diet. As with many psychiatric disorders, genes load the gun, but the environment ultimately pulls the trigger.

As you can probably tell, the development of eating disorders is so complex and multifactorial that it could never be told in one simple story. Childhood trauma or abuse, parental pressure, disordered eating—all of these things put people in higher-risk categories.[29] But how a person re-sponds is completely individual and unpredictable.

People who have never experienced an eating disorder can find them hard to understand. We're all exposed to the same media environment. Why do some take the pressure to be thin so seriously that they feel the need to starve themselves, while others don't? Why would comments about my weight from my parents cause me to spiral out of control and not eat the next day, while for my sister it wouldn't cause a thing? This variability in response can make EDs hard to talk about. How can I say, "Guys, I'm really struggling; I ate half a jar of peanut butter even though I didn't want to, and now I feel sick," when my parents had actual bullets fly into their kitchen during the civil war in Albania? The individuality of how people respond to similar pressures and the shame and stigma that surround eating disorders can make them incredibly tricky to navigate.

However, while many of the factors that contribute to developing and reinforcing an ED are out of our control (genes, trauma, personality traits), there are factors we do have control over: our media consump-tion, who we follow on social media, the way we choose to talk to our-selves, and the way we let others speak to us. Even though I don't think my parents really understood, having a full-on "intervention" with them in which I explicitly said, "I don't want to ever hear a comment about my weight again," did begin to make a difference. Choosing to follow fitness influencers that have mid- and plus-sized bodies reinforces in my brain every day that all bodies are beautiful. At the end of the day, these conscious decisions are the things that make us more than just a product of our genes and environment.

Disordered Eating and Orthorexia

Just to be blunt for a second, eating disorders affect a pretty small percentage of the population. It's true, we've dedicated a substantial portion of this book to them, perhaps partially because Eddie and I are both biased by our own personal experiences, but the reality is, they are, just by numbers, rare. However, the reason I think it's so important to talk about eating disorders is because they are the extremes of a spectrum of behaviors that are substantially more common: disordered eating behaviors (DEB).

The prevalence of disordered eating behaviors varies, depending on which population you look at and your methodology. For example, rates of DEB in college students range anywhere from 10.4 percent to 31 percent, depending on how the study is conducted.[30] Regardless of the exact number, the rates of DEB are much higher than formal eating disorders. Disordered eating has a lot of the same cognitive and behavioral elements as formal eating disorders—for example, food restriction, binge eating, compensatory behaviors, overvaluing of body shape and weight, body dissatisfaction, and so on—but these behaviors are not severe enough to qualify for a formal eating disorder. For example, an individual may engage in a binge-eating episode once a month, as opposed to once a week.

What makes disordered eating so tricky is that two people could be eating the exact same things, and for one person it is "disordered eating" but for the other it's not. The lines can be blurry and awkward, not clear and crisp. Someone might be terrified of gluten because it will make them "fat" and avoid it at all costs, while another person does the same because it exacerbates symptoms of their autoimmune disease. Both individuals may refrain from cake at a birthday party, but the way they feel when saying "No thanks, I'm good" can be dramatically different.

The continuum between disordered eating and eating disorders is proof that every behavior, even positive health behaviors, taken to extremes, can be debilitating. "Orthorexia nervosa," first coined in 1997, was suggested as a separate eating-disorder category for those with an extreme fixation on healthy eating.[31] Although the term has not been officially added to the

DSM, there is an increasing interest in studying individuals who display orthorexic tendencies. Behaviors associated with orthorexia might be obsessive restriction of foods with artificial colors, sweeteners, flavorings, fat, salt, or sugar, or foods that are ultra-processed.[32]

Both as an avid health and fitness enthusiast and as a consumer of health and fitness content, I often find myself thinking, *When is something orthorexia or disordered eating versus simply "being on your health grind?"* It's why I struggle sometimes with how to present research: on the one hand, ultra-processed-food consumption is associated with a multitude of adverse health outcomes; on the other hand, does saying so encourage disordered eating, at least for that small proportion of the population that's susceptible?

Once you've recovered from an eating disorder, you can look back on that portion of your life and see how clouded your judgment was, how flawed your logic, how detrimental your behaviors. But with disordered eating, it's kind of squishy, a constant bobbing up and down. You may notice you're dipping into potentially dangerous territories, then reappraise and recalibrate to pull yourself out. I had a clinician who specialized in eating disorders at McLean Hospital in Massachusetts share that what distinguished disordered eating from healthy eating for her was how much it was impairing her patients' lives. Was their eating getting in the way of socializing? Was it causing them distress? Or was it making their lives better? Making them feel strong and energetic? As always, what's going on between the ears is the final determinant: if choosing a salad instead of a burger is making you feel full and nourished, then get that Green Goddess Leaf Bowl, baby. If you feel like you have to get a salad even though you *really* want a burger, it might be time to revisit your relationship to food and your body.

A Healthy Relationship to Food

I'd rather have somebody read the *DSM-5* to me word for word for the next hundred years than hear one more person on social media talk about their new awesome "relationship to food." It's a phrase that has become so ubiquitously used with such little explanation that it's almost ceased to mean anything, because it just "sounds good" and makes you look good to the people that follow you. A healthy relationship to food looks different for everyone, but here are some commonalities:

- **Flexibility:** You are able to adapt to different situations—restaurants, a family member's cooking, a spontaneous ice-cream trip because you happen to see a new shop open up, and so on.

- **Not following rigid rules:** It's OK to have some structure for how you eat, but you can break one of the rules without freaking out or panicking. Eating out of your routine doesn't make you irrationally distressed.

- **Hunger and fullness:** You allow yourself to eat because you're hungry and stop when you're full. However, you also allow yourself to eat because you enjoy it. Food is both a source of nourishment *and* enjoyment.

- **Thinking about food:** Thoughts of food do not dominate your day. Obviously, we can all look forward to a good meal, but the thought of your next meal isn't the only thing you're thinking about.

Treatments and Resources

Treatments for eating disorders depend on the disorder, the severity, and the person. One easy first step, if you're not sure about whether or not you have an eating disorder, is to go to www.eat-26.com and take the Eating Attitudes Test. This is a widely used, standardized self-report measure of eating-disorder-associated attitudes, symptoms, and concerns. It's free and takes fewer than five minutes. EAT-26 does not provide a definitive designation of whether or not you need professional help—that would require a mental-health professional or your doctor—but at least it can be a quick and easy preliminary measure that you can take basically on your own in a place where you feel safe and can be honest.

If you feel like you need professional guidance, consulting the National Eating Disorders Association (NEDA) is a great way to find practitioners and specialists in your area. You can find more information at www .nationaleatingdisorders.org. I highly recommend seeking out professionals who specialize in eating disorders or who have worked with individuals with eating disorders. Some individuals may need more intensive treatment at a residential facility or inpatient clinic. To get in contact with NEDA, you can use an online chat feature, or call or text the following number: 1-800-931-2237. The NEDA website provides information on when these resources are open as well as specific guidance as to what next step might be best for you.

Treatment is highly individual: For some, talking to a licensed mental-health professional is enough; for others, they may need nutritional and medical guidance as well. The most evidence-based and well-researched form of therapy for people with eating disorders is cognitive behavioral therapy (CBT). Individuals are highly encouraged to try out CBT from a trained therapist first before moving on to other forms of therapy. This type of therapy involves identifying maladaptive thoughts and challenging them in order to stop associated maladaptive behaviors.[33] For example, a common thought that individuals with eating disorders have is *I need to be skinny to be happy.* Challenging this thought might look like *Well, actually, now that I think about it, when I was at my thinnest, I was miserable. I was so anxious about not messing up my diet and exercising twice a day, I really wasn't happy at all.* Finding ways to think through deeply ingrained narratives that fuel disordered eating behaviors can be a powerful way to stop engaging in these behaviors. However, there are a multitude of treatments in addition to CBT that have been proven to be effective at treating eating disorders, and you can find out more about them on the National Eating Disorders Association website. The Academy for Eating Disorders also has a tool on their website (www.aedweb.org) that you can use to find a therapist in your area who has experience with treatment of eating disorders.

The Takeaways

- Eating disorders can affect anyone; they do not have a race, gender, or weight requirement.

- Individuals with eating disorders often place a disproportionate amount of their self-worth in their body shape or weight.

- Binge eating disorder is the most common eating disorder. It is more prevalent than anorexia nervosa and bulimia nervosa combined.

- Individuals with bulimia nervosa and binge eating disorder tend to be normal weight or overweight.

- Anorexia nervosa is the least common eating disorder and is extremely dangerous. It is the most lethal psychiatric disorder.

- There are many risk factors for developing an ED, including genetics, certain personality traits, sociocultural factors, and engaging in dieting.

- Disordered eating involves many of the same behaviors associated with eating disorders, although to a lesser degree or severity.

- A good relationship to food involves being flexible with food choices and timings, being receptive to hunger and fullness cues, enjoying your food, and seeing food as a source of nourishment.

- Treatment for eating disorders is highly individual. The most evidence-based treatment for EDs to date is cognitive behavioral therapy (CBT).

9

From a Dad

Anorexia: A Conversation with My Daughter

Note to Readers: I would like to alert our readers that some of the following discussion with my daughter Rebecca might be triggering for those struggling with disordered eating. From here on, I will be referred to as "EP" and Rebecca (or "Becca") will be "RP."

EP: Becca, first, I want to thank you for having this conversation with me. I also want to assure that you are comfortable sharing your story.

RP: I definitely feel comfortable and proud to talk about this issue with both you and the readers. I really hope that, at the very least, sharing my story can be useful to others struggling with disordered eating or eating disorders that involve restriction and overexercising. It also feels therapeutic for me to discuss my journey, reflect on my progress, and assert the goals that I have for my recovery process moving forward.

Disordered Thinking, Disordered Eating

EP: My impression is that Mom and I always did our best to provide healthy food (without going overboard, like forbidding candy and sweets) and prioritized having regular family dinners. We also wanted to give you and your brother and sister healthy respect for your bodies and encouragement to pursue some sort of exercise for fun and your health. I am curious about about how that approach set you up for developing an eating disorder. When did it start?

RP: This is a difficult question, because I don't think it began overnight, and it definitely started with my disordered thinking about food way before I began restricting. When I was a kid, I just ate whatever you gave us. But when I became a teenager, I was swimming competitively, and I became much more body conscious. When puberty struck, I struggled with how the changes in my body affected my performance in the pool. In my junior year of high school, I gained fifteen pounds. I felt very ashamed and deeply upset about this change, and I struggled to lose the weight. However, when I took Mom's suggestion to give up gluten to relieve my worsening migraines, not only did this alleviate my headaches, but I lost about seven pounds. This made me equate bread and gluten with something that automatically led to weight gain. I started to feel anxious every time I ate gluten. Then, the summer before I went off to college, we tried the Whole30 program (at your suggestion), in which we basically did an elimination diet with no grains, no processed sugar, no caffeine, and so on. I think that this diet is when I really began to demonize certain foods, starting with carbohydrates.

EP: I remember the Whole30 experiment. I like to call it "Whole13" because we only made it about thirteen days instead of the whole thirty days. I find it poignant that our attempt at clean eating led to more restriction and eventually your eating disorder.

RP: Apparently, I am not alone. This disorder has now been labeled orthorexia, which the National Eating Disorders Association (NEDA) defines as an obsession with proper or "healthful" eating that damages your well-being.[1] I definitely had the symptoms of "cutting out an increasing number of food groups (all sugar, all carbs, all dairy, all meat, all animal products)." Around that time, I also gave up meat for environmental and moral reasons. Additionally, I received other messages about eating from you and Mom that I think I internalized to the extreme. For example, you always used to say, "If you're hungry, just drink some water first," and, "Cakes and cookies at the office are poison."

E P: I object.

R P: What are you objecting to? This isn't a courtroom.

E P: True, it isn't a courtroom. But I plead guilty. I still think that ultra-processed junk food is more like a poison than food.

R P: Dad, from an eating-disorder-recovery perspective, all food is good food. I also remember really loving home-baked goods, and the first time in my life that I tried to lose weight, I started reducing my intake of all types of sweets.

E P: What happened next?

R P: When I went off to my first year at the University of St Andrews in Scotland, I was nervous about the transition to university, living in a foreign country, and making friends. I was concerned that people wouldn't like me because I was American. I remember clearly losing weight when I started morning and evening water polo workouts, lifting, and cutting out even more carbohydrates. I also became fully vegetarian and was still avoiding gluten. These behaviors were fueled by the fact that I was getting more male attention and feeling better about myself as I lost weight. I was exercising for hours a day at this point, but I still felt like I had a lot of energy and was eating full meals and snacks, particularly because I had two meals a day in the dining hall. Even so, thoughts about food and my body slowly began to take up more mind space. I never counted calories, but I was always aware of them. I was drinking more alcohol than I ever had, mostly due to peer pressure from my water polo team. I distinctly remember purposely doing extra cardio or longer workouts the days after I drank. And by spring, when a previous foot injury had healed, I was able to resume running, and I started competing in triathlons while continuing water polo training.

EP: Did our attempts at healthy eating at home set you up for your eating disorder?

RP: To be fair, there was a natural experiment going on; my brother and sister were in the same environment, and neither of them has an eating disorder. Maybe it has more to do with my perfectionism. I think I am now evolving and interrogating my emotions underlying this perfectionism and working on directing my mental energies toward other fulfilling pursuits besides food.

Demonizing Food

EP: So far it sounds like you were active in sports, getting positive attention from guys, doing well in school, but becoming increasingly preoccupied with your thoughts about food.

RP: I guess so, and I think I looked fine because I maintained my weight. I felt really good that first summer back from college, but I slowly started cutting out more foods (or decreasing them), like bread, ice cream, and most sweets, grains, and junk food, to name a few. I replaced these foods with more vegetables, of course. Food began to have more of an emotional tie to it; eating one food that I had labeled as "bad" would make me feel very anxious. Around this time, I started carrying around vegetables as snacks in my bag, usually carrots, and excessive "safe snacks." The funny thing about my eating disorder is that I worked so hard to restrict my food intake, but at the end of the day I had a fear of starving, and I always carried snacks around with me. I became afraid of going anywhere without snacks in my backpack. This behavior quickly evolved. I started compartmentalizing my meals: I would bring one rice cracker wrapped in tinfoil, put a few tablespoons of hummus into another container, vegetables in another, and some type of protein in another Tupperware. The goal was to elongate my meals so I was never completely full at any point and would not have to eat snacks, either. Or, I would *only* eat healthy snacks, no meals.

EP: This kind of reminds me of how Mom would always be sure to bring healthy snacks if we were leaving the house for almost any event. We packed a picnic for an hour at the pool, and a long car ride was a moveable feast.

RP: Maybe that's where I saw the model, but I guess I took it to the extreme.

Before I returned to St Andrews for my second year, I traveled to Hungary to take part in preseason water polo training. It was a competitive environment in which I always felt out of place. I was new to the sport and rarely earned a spot to compete. Controlling my food intake made me feel OK and adequate again in the face of this discomfort. I also started to feed off the eating disorder of two other teammates. When I started my second year, I lived in housing without a dining hall, so I ate by myself. I cooked almost every meal, but I liked the fact that I could eat whatever I wanted without judgment. However, I still felt OK; I was doing both water polo and triathlon training at this point. I remained unconcerned about my increasingly problematic relationship with food. Then, during a festival weekend at school, I fell off a table that collapsed and fractured my rib. I had no choice but to discontinue almost all the exercise and hobbies I loved to do, even playing the fiddle. Finding a comfortable position to sleep was challenging, hugs were unfathomable, and even laughing caused me an immense amount of pain. I lived way off campus, so biking to class was necessary but taxing. I became more isolated and lonely and started eating less to make up for my decreased activity. I continued to narrow what foods I thought were acceptable; the portions continued to become smaller, and vegetables became the replacement for every food I cut out. When I had potlucks with my friends, I would skip meals and eat as little as possible before these dinners.

EP: When you broke your rib, that's the time when St Andrews seemed the farthest away from Mom and me back in Boston. We talked about flying over, but it didn't seem like there was too much for us to do. I've had many patients who, when they get injured and have to stop exercising, gain weight because they just keep eating the same amount even though they are no longer as active. But you went the other way and ate even less.

RP: Not only that, but when my rib finally healed, I never replaced the calories I had cut out, even though I had resumed triathlon training (I did finally quit water polo). Another thing that propelled me to maintain a lighter weight was that I could now run faster. I had lost my period months before, but it didn't really alarm me; I told myself it was only because I was training really hard. In 2016, when I came home for winter vacation during my second year, I was substantially lighter, and Mom became alarmed. I insisted that I *wasn't* trying to lose weight. But I also certainly wasn't trying to gain any weight, either. I assured Mom that I was OK and had it under control. Then, when we went to Santa Fe, New Mexico, to visit Aunt Jane, I was offered a low-profile modeling gig for a local boutique. This opportunity only reinforced the fact that my weight was fine, that I looked good, and that if not for my lower weight, I probably wouldn't have been asked to model in the show.

EP: I remember how happy you were to do the modeling. I really don't remember hearing that you had lost your period. That is definitely a red flag that you had an eating disorder.

RP: I don't think that I was advertising it. As I said, it seemed like one less nuisance. The largely positive reinforcement I received propelled my denial to confront my unhealthy behaviors.

EP: As you tell the story now, it sounds like you were slipping down a rabbit hole and we never reached out to stop it. When did anyone set off the alarm that something was wrong?

RP: During spring break of my second year, I visited an old high school friend and former teammate in Ireland, where she was studying abroad. She confronted me about my eating habits and weight loss and confided that she struggled with anorexia in high school. She had told the team that an injury kept her from finishing practices, but it was actually her eating disorder. She told me she thought I was headed down the wrong path. One night, we went to a party at her friend's flat. "Did you notice that you were the only one who kept your jacket on during the party? You're cold because you're not eating enough." I shrugged it off at the time, but she was right: I was *always* cold, inside and outside, unless I was exercising. I told her that I had it under control, though; I had just started seeing a new Scottish therapist whom I really liked, and I had recently confided about my struggles with eating and thoughts about food. I fooled myself into believing that by just talking about it, I was working on my issues around food and I was getting better; in reality, my behaviors were slowly getting worse, and I was still exercising strenuously more than ten hours a week, minimum. Around this time, I also became close with two of my other triathlon teammates who also confided in me that they struggled with eating disorders, one of them with anorexia and the other with bulimia. They'd become key systems of support for me, and we would eat together often. However, weird unconscious competitiveness was also fueled inside of me. I couldn't run as fast as they could, but in my head, I thought I could be as thin as they were, or thinner. I'd only become aware of these dangerous thoughts and motivations months and months later.

Secretive Eating

EP: That next summer, after your second year, I was relieved that you had found a job at the summer camp just fifteen minutes from our house. I expected that you would come over for dinner all the time because I know you really don't like dining halls, but you rarely joined us.

RP: That's about the time that I was getting more secretive about my eating. I maintained my new low weight. While I wasn't competing in triathlons, I was exercising most days at the gym, swimming at the pool, or riding my bike, and I spent hours each day hauling athletic equipment around as the athletics director. I ate at the dining hall but piled my plate with mostly vegetables. I kept fooling myself to say that I was OK, but I would also avoid eating with other people as much as possible so they wouldn't judge me or think anything was wrong. Many days, when nobody was looking, I would pack up food off my plate and put it in a container or in my bag to eat later or another day. In my room, I always had a stash of safe snacks at hand. This routine of secrecy became so ingrained in me that it eventually became automatic. The more severe my behaviors became, the more secretive I became, and the more and more I ate by myself. I recall so many times over the years that I would eat meals or snacks in the bathroom, afraid of the judgment of others.

EP: Now I understand why you weren't joining us for dinner. As your dad, I respect your privacy, but I feel like I failed to adequately watch out for your well-being. Your eating disorder was clearly getting worse, and I feel sorry that I didn't see it. What happened when you went back to school?

RP: That fall, I went back to school early for preseason training as captain of the triathlon club. The training was really intense, so I had to eat more, but, looking back, it still was definitely not enough. For example, to finish off the preseason week, several teammates and I biked almost fifty miles from Glasgow to Edinburgh, in one morning. I remember so many workouts I completed with so little fuel that I am shocked I never passed out. I almost never ate full meals, just snacks. Even what I convinced myself was a full meal had nowhere near enough energy to sustain me. I hadn't touched bread in two years and was heavily restricting most food groups, particularly carbohydrates. At this point, I knew that I was losing weight, but I felt powerful and in control. I saw the scale hit a new low number but told myself that the scale was messed up. I thought, *I should probably eat some more, but I'm OK, and I don't really want to gain weight.* At this point, my stomach had also shrunk, so I became full pretty easily as well. I was probably eating well below 1,000 calories per day, even though I still never counted the calories. I had periods of brain fog but I still persevered. My body and mind became used to this state. The behaviors also had an addictive quality to them. My grades were the best they had ever been, and I was a competitive triathlete—surely I was still fine!

EP: From all appearances, everything still looked fine.

RP: When I returned home for holidays that year after an exhausting and academically challenging semester, I had lost even more weight—my lowest weight since hitting puberty. A drunk man saw me eating grapes on the plane ride home and told me I looked way too thin. I remember how appalled and concerned you and Mom were when you picked me up at the airport. I got a little freaked out when you insisted on bringing me immediately to the urgent care, where they took my blood and did an EKG. I don't think I have ever seen you so shook up. Why were you so stressed?

EP: Seeing you look so thin made me flash back to this stressful time caring for an anorexic patient. One night, while I was moonlighting at a small, private psychiatric hospital, an exceedingly thin young woman, diagnosed with anorexia nervosa, arrived for admission to the eating-disorders unit. We drew the routine labs to check her electrolytes and measured a dangerously low potassium level. Potassium is a key electrolyte that regulates the electrical conduction in your heart. If your potassium is too low, your heart can beat irregularly, leading to death. While a normal value is above 5.0, her value at 2.4 was the lowest I had ever seen. Her electrocardiogram already indicated significant changes in her heart's system of normal electrical conduction. Due to her clearly inadequate intake of nutrition, possibly worsened by losing potassium through vomiting or laxatives, this young woman was in imminent danger of coding in our small psychiatric hospital. I did not want to be responsible for a young woman dying on my watch. A 911 call got her moved rapidly to a general hospital that soon corrected her potassium level.

Diagnosis: Anorexia Nervosa

RP: When my labs and EKG came back normal, it reaffirmed my conception that things really were not that bad. But when we visited my cousins and grandparents that same weekend, the horrified looks on their faces confirmed that maybe you hadn't overreacted. But eating at this point was getting uncomfortable because of how much my stomach had shrunk. I remember that you tried having me drink Ensure, but it was vile and just made me feel like a patient, so I refused.

I guess I really had become a patient, because when we got home Mom took me to the eating-disorders treatment center, where they recommended hospitalization. They said my weight was low enough and required residential treatment. I was shocked. I bargained for the alternative of partial hospitalization (where I attended full-day treatment but slept at home), although I still thought that daily treatment was too much. I agreed to start treatment the next day. While the groups and treatment were helpful, I still struggled to gain weight in the few weeks I was there. I tried to take as long as possible to finish meals, and they would put me in another room when the planned time had elapsed and watch me until I finished every last bite on my plate or just plain refused. When I got home, I would find excuses not to stick to my meal plan and not to eat desserts. Dad, I don't fault you for not recognizing that I had an eating disorder, because I didn't see it myself until that time.

EP: I don't live with many regrets, but the decision to follow through with our plans for the family trip to Hawai'i later that month makes my list.

RP: Yes, going on that trip was against the advice of my treatment team. In hindsight, this was a terrible decision. I could not maintain eating the calories I had agreed to, especially when hiking. My treatment team told me I needed to eat 150 calories every half hour if I did hike, and I found every excuse not to eat that much. On this trip, family tensions also ran high. My sister told me, "You're not the same sister I know," and she refused to spend time with me. I realized then that my personality had changed entirely from the fun-loving, high-energy person I once was. I was highly anxious and depressed, and food consumed most of my headspace. As much as her words deeply hurt me, they also helped pull me out of my denial and gave me the motivation to get better. However, this motivation was quickly thwarted when I caught a stomach bug and lost any weight I had gained. When we returned home, I was barely more than my previous lowest weight. Despite my weight loss, I refused to return to the treatment program or to stop exercising. You and Mom finally sat me down with an ultimatum: I could return to school only if I reached 115 pounds. In the next two weeks, miraculously, I gained 5 pounds and decided to return to school, to my nutritionist's dismay. I agreed to give up being triathlon captain and all strenuous exercise, to continue to stick to my meal plan, work with my therapist in Scotland, and have weekly check-ins with my nutritionist.

EP: Were you able to recover on your own back in Scotland? Would it have been worse if you stayed home in terms of recovery?

RP: I regained my initial goal weight pretty quickly, in only a month or so. However, the speed of my weight gain scared me, especially since I was still skimping on the meal plan. Then, my weight kept going higher, soaring above my initial goal weight. I completely freaked out. Although I was eating enough to maintain a healthy weight, the majority of my disordered thoughts and behaviors remained.

You and Mom can be a bit intimidating when it comes to health and exercise. You two don't seem to have a problem eating the right foods in the right amounts. Have you always had such a good diet?

EP: Not at all. This has been a long evolution. When I was working in New York before starting medical school, I ate pizza twice a day. I had plain cheese pizza for lunch but splurged on vegetable pizza for dinner. My "pizza diet" was interspersed with a couple of juice fasts in an effort to "detoxify." Arriving at our current "healthy" eating pattern at home has not been a straight path for Mom and me. We have weathered the societal bombardment of changing diet information and fads in our effort to be healthy for ourselves and as a model for the family and our patients. We have dutifully followed the *Sesame Street* progression of the "vitamin of the day," taking vitamin C in the 1990s, vitamin E in the early 2000s, and now the popular vitamin D. We have experimented and misstepped as we swung from joining a local meat CSA (community supported agriculture) to eating a whole-food, plant-based diet. We tried the Zone Diet and fell short in our attempt at Whole30 (mentioned earlier).

RP: What about your exercise routine? I feel like the two of you are in perpetual motion, and I feel compelled to try to keep up with you. I am proud but was also a bit triggered by you guys deciding to celebrate your thirtieth anniversary by completing a Half Ironman Triathlon together.

EP: Yes, that was a long-term goal, and the seemingly endless training so that we could swim 1.2 miles, bike 56 miles, and run 13.1 miles was made doable and even fun because we trained together. The hard part was when you opted to join us in the training and the event. I remember your sister voicing her concern about you taking on this training. Looking back, I wonder if that was the best choice for someone with an eating disorder.

RP: Probably not. That was the summer of 2018, after my third year at college. While I stayed at a healthy weight, I was only trading some of my restrictive eating behaviors for overexercising (a necessity for the Half Ironman training, of course). The extra exercise allowed me to eat more without gaining even more weight, but I was definitely not in recovery yet.

Quasi Recovery

EP: You looked healthier at that time, and you were eating enough to train and finish the Half Ironman. Was that the beginning of recovery?

RP: For the next year and a half, I managed to keep my weight and added some food groups back in, but I never went all in on my recovery and was still terrified of gaining weight. I continued to restrict myself most days and rarely ate full meals. I still put food into boxes (both figuratively and literally) and restricted my carbohydrate intake. For three full years after my hospitalization, I never reached a point where eating made me feel completely full or sated. This continued restriction definitely messed up my hunger cues and damaged my metabolism. My resting metabolic rate was severely damaged, measuring at just under 1,000 calories, three and a half years after my partial hospitalization. For more than three years, I was in "quasi recovery": a period in my recovery journey in which I measurably improved from my lowest weight and was no longer in imminent danger. But I was still stuck, deeply ambivalent in many ways, and fearful of engaging in behaviors that would move my recovery forward.

EP: Did you ever relapse from your quasi recovery?

RP: At one point in my quasi recovery, I started to regress, nearing the point of relapse. At the start of COVID-19, in spring 2020, I suddenly found myself without regular work, and my training in the massage school was interrupted by the pandemic. I started eating only two small meals a day (plus more snacks) because I was sleeping in until 12 or 1 P.M. In addition, I started teaching boot-camp fitness classes online, and I spent at least an hour every day doing vigorous boot-camp workouts. I posted pictures of myself shirtless to advertise for these classes. I never weighed myself, but I certainly was at the lowest weight I had been since I had reached my goal weight two years before. I was getting positive feedback from clients in my classes who turned to me as their model of fitness.

EP: You were falling off the wagon, but you were getting more positive feedback because you had lost weight and increased your exercise.

RP: These types of cues from society are insidious. I was extolled as a health-and-fitness model throughout adolescence and young adulthood. I would often hear, "Oh, Becca, you are always so fit. You eat so well and always exercise."

EP: I remember how hard it remained for you to eat certain foods.

RP: Definitely. Around this time, during the pandemic, I also started doing exposure work (something I had put off) with my nutritionist at least once a week. I would choose a challenge food, like an egg-and-cheese bagel, and eat it during our session. She asked me how I felt before, during, and after, what thoughts and physical sensations I was experiencing. Then, after I finished, she would say, "OK, let's do it again next week." "No, I think I'm OK" was usually my first response. But it worked. I used to eat just the toppings of a pizza and throw the bread and crust away. Now I cook frozen pizzas for myself for dinner. Lately, I've been particularly working on mindfully adding sweets back into my diet. This is still a huge challenge for me. The exposure work started to bring me out of quasi-recovery land, but my fear of gaining weight, feeling full, and eating three full meals a day was still very present.

Fear of Relationships

E P : I hear your ambivalence about giving up your eating disorder. What was pushing you toward recovery?

R P : One major motivation to recover more fully from my eating disorder was to make it more possible to be in an intimate relationship. How does anyone get into a serious relationship with a problem like this?

E P : Do you feel like your eating disorder has gotten in the way of your relationships?

R P : In the summer of 2020, I started dating someone I met online. But being in an actual relationship was something I always felt nervous and wary of because I was afraid of my partner not being able to handle all my crazy food behaviors and the way they affected me every day, both mentally and physically. I ultimately ended the short relationship for a few reasons, but one of the main reasons was that I realized how much work I needed to do on my eating-disorder recovery before committing to a relationship. My fears and behaviors were still present, and even though my ex-boyfriend knew about my eating disorder, I never divulged the full extent of the issue to him.

E P : Is that about the time that you started to work at the psychiatric hospital, McLean?

R P : Yes, in fall 2020, I started a new position as a mental-health specialist in the Dissociative Disorders and Trauma unit. While stressful at times, I immediately loved the job. I really enjoyed my coworkers, the patient interaction, the feeling of purpose, and the routine of the shifts. I felt that my own experience with mental health allowed me to relate to a lot of the patients without divulging the details to them.

EP: Did you ever see patients with anorexia or other eating disorders?

RP: Yes. I worked with patients with eating disorders all the time. I could relate to them on a deep level, but I still really didn't know what to say to them to make it better or help them start recovering.

When you worked at McLean, did you see patients on the eating-disorders unit?

EP: When I consulted at McLean, I was mostly taking care of patients suffering from pain or weakness by getting them to be more active and doing more exercise. However, the eating-disorders unit seemed like a separate universe composed of "antimatter," where none of my tools or the normal laws of the universe applied. My knowledge and passion for prescribing exercise were exactly the opposite of what these patients needed. I remember feeling frustrated and impotent trying to treat patients on that unit; my quiver of usual therapeutic exercises and motivations to "get more active" were of little help or, in this case, actually harmful.

RP: When I brought a patient to that same eating-disorders residential unit, I questioned whether that might have been a better place for my treatment.

EP: So, did working at McLean help with your recovery?

RP: While I learned a ton in the hospital environment about recovery from different types of disorders and addictions, the shift work took a toll on my eating behaviors. The constant switching between early-morning and late-evening shifts made it difficult for me to find a consistent eating schedule and seemed to throw my hunger cues off more. Also, I found myself restricting even more at work, especially during the day shift. I would usually not eat breakfast or lunch and was perpetually hungry during the day. On evening shifts, I would delay eating dinner until as late as possible or subsist off snacks. No matter what, when I came home, I was *always* ravenous. However, if I did not eat enough during the day, I would be unable to fall asleep at night, or I would wake up in the middle of the night with a pit in my stomach. I started eating larger portions of food or snacks right before bed so I would not wake up hungry. This is something I still struggle with to this day.

Being in an Intimate Relationship

R P : At the end of 2020, I met and became fast friends with a coworker at McLean. We confided in each other about our individual mental-health issues. He had struggled with OCD since he was twenty years old, about the same age that I had started struggling with anorexia. He had also been hospitalized. We talked about how our thoughts manifested in our heads, realizing that our thought patterns were very similar in so many ways. Our friendship eventually progressed into a relationship. Funnily enough, I remember talking only a week or two before about how I didn't feel like I could be in a relationship because of my eating disorder, and he said the same because of his OCD. We also found that we both had names for our illnesses, the voices telling us to behave in a certain way in our heads. Mine was Bertha; his was Steve. The presence of our illnesses is so strong that sometimes it feels like we are on a double date with Bertha and Steve.

While we are very different people, our shared struggles and openness formed the basis of a strong relationship. I continued to confide in him about my thoughts and behaviors and the ways they affected me, while he did the same for his OCD. However, I was terrified of having him sleep over for the first months of our relationship because I would obsess over whether I was hungry or not and sometimes wake up at night and need to eat something. But as our trust continued to grow, I let my walls come down. We learned to read the perseveration in each other's eyes and support each other during the spurts of anxiety and fear we would both experience due to our mental illnesses. I grew to love sharing food with him. He had grown up in a family that did not prioritize healthy eating, while I had grown up with a family of doctors who were always concerned with nutrition. But I found this refreshing and healthy. I was able to help incorporate more healthy eating into his life, while he was able to challenge me and some of my rigid thoughts about food.

EP: So, wait. You're saying that if we had more junk food at home you would have been healthier?

RP: Not, necessarily, but sometimes I do wonder. . . .

EP: Did he help expose you to more foods?

RP: For sure. One night, we decided to get some ice cream together. I hadn't eaten more than a small spoonful of ice cream in four years. It probably is still the most challenging food for me. Together, we walked down Moody Street to Lizzy's ice-cream shop. I was panicking inside even before I entered the shop. But walking in, when the smells of waffle cones hit me, I felt sad. There I was, twenty-five years old, afraid to eat ice cream, while people of all ages, from two to seventy, all around me, were enjoying it with the freedom I envied. With his help, I eventually chose a flavor in size small (of course I wanted a kiddie-size, though), with a waffle cone on top. I ate as much ice cream as I could until I felt stuffed. I felt pretty terrible afterward. But we played some music and chilled out to distract me from the discomfort. However, when we tried to go to bed later that night, I started having difficulty breathing and began hyperventilating. It came in waves, but it took me almost two hours to calm down. This is the only panic attack I can ever remember having in my entire life.

Dad's Side of the Story

RP: Dad, let me ask you how my problems affected you. Where does Juna fit in with all of this?

EP: I have long been passionate about promoting exercise and healthy eating. But it wasn't until your diagnosis that I started to wrestle with the conundrum that all this focus on food and exercise might backfire and, for some, create an environment promoting eating disorders. Your illness sensitized me to the prevalence of disordered eating and how the messages out there are fundamentally screwed up. Eating the standard American diet leads most Americans to become overweight or obese. At the same time, our society is riddled with "fatphobia," so in a sense, we end up hating ourselves. The contemporary models and promoted regimens of health and fitness are often thinly veiled iterations of disordered eating. When I look at the picture of you at your lowest weight, it reminds me of Instagram influencers who receive positive attention for similar pictures supporting the ideal of thin as the beauty standard. What remains enduringly complicated in my role as a doctor is that "health" is an ultimately subjective phenomenon, one that can have disastrous effects when falsely generalized or insidiously capitalized upon. This tension is admittedly present in my work, in this book, but it compels me to be as attentive a doctor as possible. When I was introduced to Juna in the fall of 2018, as a potential cohost for a podcast from WBUR, I was perhaps in a better position to work with her to help our listeners end their "war with food."

RP: Is it easier to talk to Juna than to me about eating disorders?

EP: Juna is your age, and it is often easier to talk to a "stranger" than a loved one, particularly about really sensitive topics. When we started talking, I found our conversations to be generative and enlightening. While I would like to believe that you and your siblings seek my advice and always hang on to my every word . . . it is often easier to give advice to Juna and see her follow it.

RP: Do you think those conversations with Juna have helped you deal with my illness?

EP: I am becoming more sensitized to the messages that we are sharing in the podcast and this book so that they are hopefully less triggering of disordered eating. Hopefully, my adopting a more neutral but supportive stance is helping you in your recovery.

R P : Did you try to treat Juna?

E P : No, I am not her doctor. When I met Juna I was at first deeply unsure about what I had to offer. I am not formally trained in treating eating disorders and I felt powerless and heartbroken seeing you go through your struggles. My prior exposure to eating disorders was mystifying at best, emotionally draining, always frustrating, and terrifying at worst.

R P : Did you diagnose Juna with an eating disorder?

E P : Not formally. From the story that Juna told about her bingeing and compensatory exercising, it sure sounded like she had disordered eating at best and likely a formal diagnosis of an eating disorder. The launch of our work together in producing the first season of the podcast felt a bit like a reality-TV show as I accompanied Juna on her journey. I wondered, *When will Juna figure out that this is for real and that it applies to her? When can we move beyond the vague title of "disordered eating" toward a formally diagnosed eating disorder and get someone qualified to help her?* And yet I never assigned her the diagnosis.

As the podcast proceeded, we first addressed safer subjects: exercise, supplements, stress, and so on. Near the end of the first season, it was finally time to wrestle with eating disorders. Juna interviewed Dr. Jennifer Thomas, an eating-disorders specialist at Harvard University Health Services. While Juna may have entered the room with her microphone as the podcast cohost and producer, she left with a critical appraisal that "this applies to me." But even Juna's admission triggered my fear and self-doubt. Cast as the wise, older doctor, I was uncertain, ambivalent about how to proceed. *How am I now supposed to help her? I can't even help my own daughter. I am not an expert in this. I don't know what to think about it. This is not going to turn out well. Why doesn't she see a specialist?* And worse, I wondered whether our podcast was inadvertently encouraging her and other people's disordered eating. Was our discussion of diets causing harm?

RP: Wow, I always think that you know exactly what to say and how to say it. I didn't realize that this is so stressful for you. Where are you now?

EP: When I think about your illness and recovery, I do my best to stay compassionate and patient. I try to provide support and ask questions rather than make judgments. I am doing my best to listen deeply, and I try not to jump to providing answers or attempting to fix everything. With all that I have learned and continue to learn from you and Juna, I am now hopefully more alert and able to navigate the deluge of wayward diet and nutrition information that is causing harm to those with eating disorders and fostering a culture of disordered eating for all of us. I am also more actively questioning the paradigms of health and medical discourse in general.

Ongoing Recovery

EP: Becca, in a sense, maybe my deep dive into the food culture and disordered eating through the podcast and this book project is part of your story. Where are you now with your recovery?

RP: It remains a struggle. In the summer of 2021, I reached the highest weight of my life, more than fifty pounds greater than my lowest weight. My worst fear had come true. I had severely damaged my metabolism. I remember my partner asking me, "What is your real, deep fear about gaining weight?" I counted not just one deep fear but a cluster of fears about not being lovable, fears about what this would reflect about me and what others would think of me, and fears about not being able to control the way my body looked. Even with his reassurance, I still hated the way my body looked most days that summer. But my partner's constant support helped me reach a place of more acceptance and to continue to progress in my recovery. For the first time in three and a half years, I finally felt like I was entering true recovery.

EP: Where are you today?

RP: To this day, more than four years after the partial hospitalization, I am at a healthy weight, but I still have many of the same thoughts about demonizing food, the amount, and the times I can eat. I still struggle with my hunger cues and with skipping meals. I still get very hungry at night. I can't always trust how full I feel. I have negative thoughts about my body and body image almost every day. Restriction is still an automatic mode for me, so I have to work each and every day to resist these urges. However, I am also eating so many foods I wouldn't have touched one year ago and am finding real joy in eating again, particularly with other people.

EP: What should you and Mom and I have done differently?

RP: Looking back, I do believe I needed to hit rock bottom. I should have understood the negative health effects of losing my period and the impact of anorexia on bone density. It is an illness that kills. Ultimately, I think one essential thing is sticking through with treatment. If I could go back in time, I think having more friends who might have spoken up would have been helpful, and I should have stayed in more intensive treatment longer. I wish that I had done full residential treatment rather than a partial hospitalization and relying on my own work. Eating disorders also put a lot of stress on the family. In particular, it strained my relationship with my sister the most. Eating disorders also thrive in secrecy, so eating with others can be beneficial in both preventing and treating an eating disorder. It remains complicated. I don't know exactly what you could have done differently. You didn't restrict our food, but I think over time your feelings about eating healthier food were transmitted in one way or another.

EP: What kind of support would be best for you moving forward?

R P : Moving forward it will be helpful to have you and Mom check in with me periodically to make sure that I am doing OK, even during more emotionally difficult times. Continuing to have meals together is very helpful.

Advice for Those with Eating Disorders

E P : What is your message to others with eating disorders?

R P : Right now, recovery for me is about accepting my thoughts and not trying to engage in all of them. One of my early providers told me that my thoughts would get less intense when I began to eat more. While I do believe my view about food has changed, I still think that I have a lot of the same thoughts that I did four years ago. Food takes up an inordinate amount of my brain space, but I am better about challenging these disordered thoughts and trying my best to eat well every single day no matter what. I am also building a new kind of muscle, continuing to expose myself to foods that I previously would not have touched. Along with being OK with gaining weight, this is one of the ways to truly gain control of a restrictive eating disorder. It is also really critical to continue to interrogate the messages from society that propel disordered eating, including fatphobia.

Finding meaning and purpose in my life beyond the way my body looks and the exercise I do has been an empowering element of my recovery. I am always looking for more reasons to eat and enjoy food rather than reasons to restrict. Although I sometimes doubt how much recovery is possible from an eating disorder, I have many goals I am actively working toward in my recovery journey. While I may never have the same carefree relationship with food and my body as I did in my youth, I believe that every day I work toward my goals, I can continue to find more freedom and joy in eating and peace with my body.

10

Stress, Eating, and Weight

Whenever I get stressed, whether it's a relationship thing, a work thing, or a life event thing, there's a dark-chocolate shortage in every local Trader Joe's. Not because of a supply-chain issue or product discontinuation; it's because one local Juna Gjata becomes an all-powerful black hole of chocolate craving. You may have noticed when you're stressed that your food preferences change and you get hungrier, and you may even notice that your weight tends to correlate pretty closely with your stress levels. (If you're in the subset of the population that loses weight when stressed, unfortunately, there has been a lot less research done on your rare species. But fear not, the overall message holds true: too much stress is not good for overall health, no matter how it affects your eating!)

So . . . what is the relationship between stress, what we eat, and the scale? First, let's talk about the purpose of stress and the stress response.

We Need the Stress Response

At its core, our body's response to stressors comes back to that oh-so-familiar topic, homeostasis: our body's internal regulation of physiological states. We've seen how homeostatic mechanisms regulate our weight and energy expenditure (chapters 2 and 3), but our bodies are *constantly* adapting to both their external and internal environments. To maintain homeostasis in response to a stimulus or stressor, the body has many tools in its proverbial toolbox; for instance, it can release hormones such as cortisol and adrenaline, or regulate the autonomic nervous systems.[1]

These physiological "mediators" (like cortisol and adrenaline), as well as the changes in immune and metabolic parameters, are called allostasis, the way your body responds in order to adapt to stress.[2] This response is a good thing: it's protecting you. Imagine how crappy life would be if your body could never respond to anything: you would be at the mercy of whatever hardship you encountered in your environment, and in all likelihood, you probably wouldn't be here today. If there was an animal chasing you, you wouldn't be able to outrun it: no stress response would make you able to run away faster. If it was cold, you would freeze: no stress response would preserve heat for the vital organs. The stress response is extremely useful . . . unless it doesn't get shut off when it's supposed to.

When the body is repeatedly and chronically exposed to stress, those exact physiological mediators that are so helpful and protective in the short run start to damage the body. This wear and tear from chronic or repeated stress is called allostatic load.[3] Basically, we want our stress response to be timely *and* effective. It starts when the stressor appears, when it's not too overblown but also not too underwhelming, and then it stops when the stressor is gone. In the long term, if the stress response stays on for weeks, months, or even years, or the body overreacts or underreacts, it has downstream effects on cardiovascular, neural, metabolic, behavioral, and cellular levels. And when all these systems stop working properly, we see an association between excess stress and many health problems.

So . . . What Exactly Is This Stress Response?

On the broadest level, there are two general systems that are activated when we experience stress. The first system is called the sympathetic adrenal medullary system—this is our friend SAM. The second is the hypothalamic-pituitary-adrenal (or HPA) axis.[4] I'm gonna keep these descriptions brief because no one here signed up for a tenth-grade-biology comeback tour.

You may not know it, but you probably are intimately familiar with SAM. If I asked you to describe the stress response, SAM would be what you were describing. When we get scared or feel threatened, the brain activates the sympathetic nervous system (SNS), which sends a message to the adrenal glands, which promptly pump out a hormone called noradrenaline, which then travels around the body activating the acute stress response.[5] At the exact same time, the adrenal medulla pumps out adrenaline through the blood, which also helps prep the body for war (so to speak).[6]

You may be thinking, *Uh ... I would have never described the stress response like that. What even is noradrenaline?!* But the physical effects of SAM and its associated hormones are familiar to all of us. Your breathing quickens, your heart starts beating faster, your eyes dilate to let more light in, and digestion slows way down so that you can use your energy for more important things (like getting your patootie as far away as possible from whatever is about to kill/eat you).[7] You may know SAM by its other nickname, the "fight-or-flight" response.

The second system, the HPA axis, gets a little less love in pop culture but is just as important. OK, prepare yourself for a very, very long sentence and try to read this in one breath: The hypothalamus releases a peptide hormone into the blood, which goes to the pituitary gland, which releases *another* hormone that then goes to the adrenal cortex, which then stimulates the production of the one, the only, *cortisol!!!*[8] Yes, we have arrived at one of the most famous (and most often unfairly slandered) "evil villains" in human biology: the infamous "stress hormone" cortisol.

The function of cortisol in the context of the stress response is to increase access to energy stores and decrease inflammation. Cortisol triggers the excess energy that's stored in your liver and muscles as glycogen to be released, so it can be broken down into glucose and used by your muscle and brain to run, or fight, or hide, and so on.[9] Again, an awesome response for a short-term problem, but not an awesome response when it's all day, every day for the entire two months you're working on some big project.

Stress and Weight

Based on what we've learned so far about the physiology of the stress response, it may seem slightly counterintuitive that stress and weight gain are linked. After all, the stress response is firstly an energetically costly maneuver (it takes a lot of energy to get SAM and the HPA axis revved up), and it involves mobilizing energy stores for quick use. Shouldn't that promote weight loss?

Well, this is how a response to acute stressors is *supposed* to work, but when stressors become chronic, the effects can be very different. Chronic stress affects your weight directly: the hormones and systems that are turned on in the stress response actually facilitate fat storage.[10] But chronic stress also affects our weight *indirectly* by causing you to eat more (particularly more calorie-dense, hyper-palatable foods) and move less.[11,12] (Of course, the way you, in particular, respond to stress may be different, because we're all different. Some of you may find you lose your appetite and start pacing the floor like a madman instead, which may lead to its own problems, vis-à-vis angry downstairs neighbors.) But gaining weight when stressed is such a common problem, particularly in today's environment where we're surrounded by easy-to-access, hyperdelicious foods, that there has been a lot of research specifically dedicated to understanding it.

Let's revisit SAM and the HPA axis for a second. Chronic activation of these systems has been found to be linked to weight gain. For example, there is a well-documented association between obesity and chronic activation of the sympathetic nervous system (the "fight-or-flight" system).[13] Even before individuals exhibit signs of obesity, elevated norepinephrine levels in the blood (one of the components of SAM) actually predict subsequent weight gain.[14]

A chronically activated "fight-or-flight" response may actually desensitize fat cells or downregulate certain receptors on the fat cells so that they are less able to release fatty acids, which leads to insulin resistance.[15] Translation: Think of this as a "boy who cried wolf" situation. Your body has gotten the signal "Stressor! Stressor! *Alert!!!*" so many times (along with the associated hormonal cocktail that tells your fat cells to release their fatty acids) that eventually your fat cells just stop responding as well. So the hormones are released that are screaming, "Unleash your fatty acids," and your fat cells go, "Nah, I'm good."

Meanwhile, not only does hyperactivity of the HPA axis promote fat storage, it seems to also affect fat distribution.[16] This finding can be attributed to our good friend cortisol. Research has shown that chronically elevated cortisol particularly affects abdominal fat (the type of fat most linked to adverse health outcomes (see chapter 4). For example, when we look at lean women with a high waist-to-hip ratio (women who are lean, but have a higher distribution of fat in the stomach area) compared to lean women with a low waist-to-hip ratio, the women with more abdominial fat have much higher cortisol responses when exposed to a stressor.[17] Additionally, the women with a higher waist-to-hip ratio also don't acclimate to the stressor the way those with lower abdominal fat do; that is, even after repeated exposure to the stressor and knowing what to expect, they still show an elevated cortisol response.[18] Thus, responding to stressors with higher cortisol is linked to higher amounts of abdominal fat.

Now let's look at some of the indirect effects stress may have on our bodies. That's right, we're talking about the dark-chocolate vortex.

Stress Eating Makes Biological Sense

Yes, there actually are studies that show what we all know to be true: stress makes us more likely to overeat. Unless you are the type of person who loses your appetite when stressed . . . in which case, how can we swap? Because I can't afford to buy out the entire chocolate section every time I have a deadline. One study looking at people's self-reported "daily hassles" and eating behaviors found that increased daily hassles meant an increase of snacking on high-sugar and high-fat foods and a decrease in vegetable consumption.[19] "Daily hassles" here mean a variety of stressors: ego-threatening stressors (fear of failing a task), interpersonal stressors (getting in a fight with a friend), or even plain old work-related stressors. In this study, researchers found that work-related hassles were the type of stressor that caused the most snacking.

Even the old cliché of somebody eating out of a Ben and Jerry's pint with a spoon post-breakup may be partially driven by biology. Food, and in particular supertasty foods like cookies, chips, and so on, triggers reward pathways in our brain similar to those seen with some drugs of abuse[20] (see chapter 5). In this way, eating comfort foods is actually . . . well . . . biologically comforting, because you're getting this awesome rush of neurotransmitters associated with reward. This is why food can provide such an effective short-term way to self-sooth.

For example, in one study, researchers had half the participants watch a sad movie (*Love Story*) and the other half watch a happy movie (*Sweet Home Alabama*) while they were given a big bucket of salty, buttery popcorn. The next day, the two groups switched. After measuring their moods after each of these movies to ensure that the sad movie indeed made the subjects sad and the happy one made them happy, researchers found that the *exact same people* ate 30 percent more when they were watching the sad movie versus the happy movie.[21] In a related study, researchers also found that individuals put into a sad state also ate more M&M's, while those put in a happy state ate more of a less hedonic food: raisins.[22] This is the last time I will watch *The Notebook* with snacks anywhere in my vicinity.

Periods of high stress are also associated with lowered physical activity, which may also contribute to the association we see between stress and weight gain.[23] And, of course, it's no surprise that stress can also interfere with your gym gains. For all my fellow fitness fanatics and gym rats, yet again we are shown that what you do outside the gym is just as essential to your gains as what you do in the gym. For example, when college students went through a supervised twelve-week resistance-training program, those who reported significant life stressors didn't see the same strength gains or muscle-size gains as those who didn't report any significant stressors.[24] Maybe sometimes the best thing for your squat is to squat on this thing called a couch and only allow a bicep curl that is bringing your coffee to your mouth.

Beyond Weight

As usual, I do not want to pretend that the only thing that we should be worrying about is our eating, exercising, and weight. If we look at this big picture, your weight changing (whether you're gaining or losing) is *not* the biggest thing we should be worrying about in terms of how stress affects our body. It is simply a downstream effect of the other, potentially more harmful changes stress is causing.

Here's one straightforward example: overactivity of the SNS seems to cause high blood pressure, and I don't think I need to tell you, high blood pressure is *not good*.[25] Like, we're talking "actual structural and functional changes in your arteries" not good. Crudely put, high blood pressure can make your arteries thicker and harder (fun fact: this is called atherosclerosis), which can lead to heart attacks or stroke, among other things.

Repeated and prolonged activation of the HPA axis from chronic stress, especially in childhood and adolescence, impairs the body's ability to respond to stress appropriately later and thus increases risk of a multitude of poor health outcomes.[26,27] In other words, having to respond to a stressor over and over again in your past may actually make your body less able to respond in the future. Stress, and in particular early-childhood trauma or adversities, can even alter your gene expression (which genes are turned on and off), which is associated with a whole host of adverse health outcomes.[28]

The groundbreaking conclusion of this chapter is that too much stress is not good for us. But, as we've all experienced, stress is kind of inevitable. As Eddie said to me once, "Juna, if you want to do all the things you say you want to do, when are you ever going to truly be NOT stressed?" Thinking back on the past decade of my life, there hasn't been a single week where I wouldn't describe myself as "stressed" in some way. Oftentimes, even the things I have been most hoping for (like being able to write a book, ahem, ahem) are sources of the greatest stress. And so, "getting rid of stress," besides being unrealistic, is also not necessarily the solution we want. Sometimes stress means you're just doing a lot of cool things. A lot of the best things in life—your family, your kids, your house—come with a lot of stress. So instead of striving to eliminate it altogether, I say we learn how to better cope (and also maybe improve time management, ahem, ahem). I'm sure our bodies will highly appreciate it. (More on that in "The Takeaways.")

From the (Stressed) Doc

Stress was an experiential course in medical school. While our behaviors are paramount to our health (as we've discussed in this whole book), my medical school curriculum (nearly forty years ago) unfortunately taught very little about nutrition, exercise, or sleep. We did definitely learn of the dangers of tobacco and how to help our patients quit using it, but the curriculum on stress was taught through experience (and not all of my classmates passed).

Throughout my medical training (most specifically my year as a medical intern), I danced on the narrow edge of how much stress I could withstand and what I could do to maintain my health and my spirit. I learned to exercise when I could, to never forgo an opportunity for sleep or rest, to maintain my humor (although dark at times), and to invest in relationships with my classmates, colleagues, and family. Another lifeline was my martial arts training.

In the late 1970s, I was deeply immersed in my martial arts career and learning and practicing meditation and other internal (i.e., energy-based) practices such as baguazhang. At the same time, as a premed student, I contemplated a career in medicine as a pursuit that seemed completely distinct from my lived experience with the mind-body interface. When I read the late Dr. Herbert Benson's *New York Times* bestseller *The Relaxation Response* (1975), I understood that my experience in the karate dojo and a career in medicine were not at all at odds with each other. Indeed, my experience in lifestyle medicine is a merging of those interests and practices.

Dr. Benson's 2022 obituary reported: "In the very room at Harvard Medical School where the 'fight or flight,' or stress response, was delineated by Walter B. Cannon in the early 1900s, Dr. Benson and colleagues described its opposite. Specifically, they found that meditation reduced metabolism, rate of breathing and heart rate, and modulated brain activity. Dr. Benson labeled these changes the 'relaxation response.'"[29]

Dr. Benson graciously taught at many of our lifestyle-medicine courses, sharing his courage as a groundbreaking pioneer as well as the latest data from his lab. During one presentation, he reported dramatic data demonstrating the epigenetic benefits and the lengthening of telomeres in individuals regularly practicing ten-minute meditations twice daily. Onstage during questions and answers at the end of his talk, I shared my personal frustration with not being able to establish a regular meditation practice. Ever warmhearted, Herb gently suggested that if I couldn't regularly meditate, I should try "doing a mini." That is, a deep breath triggered by a cue. Taking his advice, to this day, whenever my computer shows a spinning circle, I am reminded to take a deep breath.

Over the years, I have been afforded the privilege of being able to progressively reduce my external stressors due to a stable occupation (that is in concert with my deeply held feelings of meaning and purpose), secure and supportive relationships with my wife and family, a stable living situation, and generally good health. I continue my work to reduce my internal stressors by exploring and trying to practice self-compassion and abandoning a drive for perfection.

The external stressors I do have are largely of my choosing. At this point in my career I am blessed with the agency to choose whether I want to give the next presentation, create a new curriculum, see more patients, or write this book. I have crafted a schedule that includes time for morning meditation (ten to fifteen minutes); regular exercise (thirty to sixty minutes per day), cooking (or at least helping in the kitchen), and sufficient sleep (about eight hours per night).

However, sometimes life gets in the way and the best-laid plans are pushed aside. As I write this section, with our manuscript submission deadline looming, I feel the stress that I remember from my internship. Ironically and poignantly, my sleep has been shortened and disrupted by writing about stress. My emails and conversations are terse and pointed. I type this with one hand while gnawing on a Fudgsicle in the other. (OK, it is already my second Fudgsicle.) I think the first one made me feel better. (Actually I ate it mindlessly so I can't remember.) I don't feel like I have the energy to go for a walk or get on my bicycle, and sitting still to rhythmically breathe for ten minutes seems like an extravagance that would take away the time to write.

I try to come up for air. I "do a mini." One deep, slow breath and conscious gratitude for all that I have (including the opportunity to be stressed by writing a book). I feel just a bit better. I sit for ten minutes doing my regular meditation, but now I'm more conscious of its calming effect as my flood of thoughts slows just a bit. I hit a block in my writing. I hear my wife calling from the kitchen for help with dinner. I stand up and enjoy the physical relief after sitting too long. Rather than asking her for the time to keep writing, I join her at the cutting board, chopping carrots, hearing about her day and receiving her wisdom, perspective, and inspiration to finish my reflection on stress.

The Takeaways

Although we often say "stress is bad," an appropriate stress response is what keeps us alive, thriving, and able to adapt to our environments. However, when the stress response does not turn off like it's supposed to, we start to experience some of the adverse health effects associated with it. The stress response is meant for the short term, which means all inessential processes, including digestion, reproduction, tissue repair, immune function—they're put on the back burner or disrupted when we perceive a threat or problem.[30] As my (Juna's) bank account can attest, optimizing for the short term does *not* make for a healthy life in the long term.

We also know that a lot of the greatest things in life are a package deal with increased stress. So in the spirit of not taking away all of life's pleasures in an attempt to eliminate all its stressors, here are some things that will help you reduce your body's stress response and make you better at coping with all of life's triumphs, trials, and tribulations.

Take a Breath, Will Ya?

Usually, we don't give a second's thought to our breathing because it just kind of happens, but maybe it's time we start. You've probably experienced that being stressed makes your breathing quick and shallow (a trademark of the "fight-or-flight" response). Well, it turns out, doing the opposite—taking slow, deep breaths deep into your stomach—may actually be one of the most potent ways we have to turn our "fight-or-flight" reaction off.[31] Taking slow, deep breaths into our belly (as opposed to chest breathing) helps expand our diaphragm, which then stimulates the vagus nerve. And do you know what the vagus nerve controls? You got it, the parasympathetic nervous system—our "rest-and-digest" mechanism.

Even relatively short breathing interventions have been shown to increase attention, decrease cortisol, and even decrease negative affect (negative emotionality)—*just by breathing!*[32] You can practice this in a group setting such as a yoga or meditation class, or you could even just look up YouTube videos for guided breathing to help you slow down. What you want to focus on is taking in air so that your belly actually expands like a balloon (no sucking in to hide your stomach, people) and then releasing the breath as slowly as possible.

Meditation: It's Not Just for Pretentious People Sharing Their Ridiculous Morning Routines

I know none of us needs another person telling us to meditate, because every Instagram "entrepreneur" has got that covered in their three-hour "Morning Routines for Success," but unfortunately, I need to add my voice to the million other pretentious pricks (darn it). Take it from someone who is constantly either working, working out, scrolling TikTok, talking on the phone, hanging with friends, or listening to a podcast: sometimes, we just need to *stop*. Meditation comes in many flavors, but at its root, it is learning to plant yourself in the present moment—not your phone, not the past, not the future, the *now*.

A couple years ago I heard someone mention on a podcast that they did a ten-day silent meditation retreat: no phones, no music, no technology, no *speaking*. As someone who literally never shuts up and talks *for a living*, it sounded like the scariest shit take I'd ever heard. So I knew I had to sign up. Two successfully completed ten-day silent retreats later, I can tell you they were the hardest but perhaps most beneficial twenty days of my life.

Meditation has been linked to so many health benefits that it would be impossible to name them all, but chief among them may be stress reduction.[33] An eight-week Mindfulness-Based Stress Reduction program in older adults was shown to not only decrease loneliness but also reduce the pro-inflammatory gene expression associated with loneliness.[34]

Mind-Body Practices (a Science-y Way to Say "Yoga")

If you can believe it, yoga is actually classified as a form of complementary and alternative medicine by the National Institutes of Health.[35] If people have been doing something for three thousand years, there must be something to it, right? Yoga comes in different flavors, but at its root, it is a practice that integrates muscular fitness and an internal focus on the self, breath, and energy. And you will be glad to hear, stretchy pants are in fact, scientifically speaking, not a requirement, though highly encouraged.

Yoga has been shown to lower stress and anxiety and improve symptoms of a whole host of mood-related disorders, including depression. Among other things, yoga has been shown to create a greater sense of well-being, make you feel relaxed, improve your self-confidence and body image (hallelujah), improve efficiency, improve interpersonal relationships, increase your attentiveness, lower irritability, and make you have a more optimistic outlook on life.[36] If that's not enough for ya, yoga can even change your gene expression. In a twelve-week intervention of breast cancer survivors with persistent cancer-related fatigue, yoga was found to reduce inflammation-related gene expression.[37] So bust out your mat, and if you think your Lululemons are great for grocery shopping, wait until you try them at yoga!

Oh, Thanks—Another Reason to Exercise!

Are we getting annoying? I swear I wouldn't keep mentioning exercise if it didn't keep popping up in the literature as an effective way to improve almost every single negative thing we deal with healthwise, but here's another one to add to the list. Exercise does indeed help manage stress (which is slightly ironic, since exercise is itself a stressor). The exact mechanisms by which exercise does this are unclear and may vary depending on the type of exercise (aerobic vs. anaerobic), but even a single bout of resistance training has been found to reduce feelings of anxiety.[38]

I think people often think of exercise as a luxury: you do it when you have the free time, when you're not swamped at work, when you're *not* stressed. But in reality, the times in our lives when we are experiencing the most stress are the times we need exercise the most. For me, exercise has become something that I prioritize no matter what I have going on, no matter how much work I have to do, no matter how much my brain is telling me it "can't fit," because I have *never* regretted a workout. It not only improves your quality of life in the long run, it's an almost instantaneous de-stressor. Next time you're stressed, check how you feel before your workout and then how you feel after. I guarantee it'll be a million times better.

Get Off Your Phone and Go Outside! It's Nice!

Research on the benefits of being outside in nature has been growing over the past decade or so, but my first real encounter with it was when I interviewed Dr. Herman Pontzer, an associate professor of evolutionary anthropology and global health at Duke University. (He conducted the studies on the Hadza tribe from chapter 2.) When I asked him about what we could learn from the Hadza tribe, to my shock, his answer was not about their entirely whole-foods based diet, or even their incredibly physically active lives, but about how they spent most of their time together outside in nature.

It can be easy to forget, but humans did not evolve in wood and concrete boxes with square holes in the sides. We evolved in nature. How the heck being in greenery is actually impacting our health needs to be further researched, but studies have shown that being in nature reduces both physical and psychological stress.[39]

Change Your Thinking

Cognitive behavioral therapy (CBT) is a form of talk therapy in which you basically identify and change maladaptive thought patterns that are leading to problematic behaviors or lowering your quality of life.[40] Some examples of maladaptive thoughts could be *If I fail this exam, I'll never graduate, and then I'll never get a job,* or *If I let down my boss, I will get fired.* Having thoughts like this is not only going to stop you from performing at your best, but it also makes for a pretty miserable existence. CBT can help you change these thoughts and the negative behaviors associated with them.

For example, one study divided college students into two groups four weeks before an exam. One group received weekly CBT instruction aimed at managing stress, and the other group did not. Researchers found that the CBT group's anxiety actually decreased in the four weeks leading up to the exam, while the control group's anxiety increased.[41] They also found lowered physiological symptoms of stress for the CBT group, and a lower cortisol response the morning of the exam.[42] Less stress before an exam just from one session a week of CBT? Sign me up. Cognitive behavioral therapy interventions can also alter the maladaptive gene expression that we've seen from adverse life events. For example, in early-stage breast cancer patients, CBT was found to reverse the proinflammatory gene expression that we so often see following a chronic stressor.[43]

11

Why You Shouldn't Sleep on Sleep

U p until about midway through college, my relationship with sleep was the following: sleep is an annoying thing that takes up my time, and if I have something due or if I want to hang out with my friends, I'll just "Venti cold-brew" my way through the following day. At my high school, people actually would *brag* about how little sleep they got, like it showed how much more you were working than other people. (You know how the cool kids are—always bragging about how much homework they're doing!) All-nighters were pretty common, especially around the end of terms and before exams.

In college, it was a similar story. But slowly, my attitude started to change. At first, it was because of my classes called the Neurobiology of Memory and the Neurobiology of Learning. It turns out getting a good night's sleep is crucial for consolidating memories and learning complex motor tasks. This was the era of my life when I was obsessed with becoming a concert pianist, which meant *a lot* of memorizing music and *a lot* of complex motor movements. So I started to take my sleep more seriously, that is, I would make sure I was getting at least six to seven hours a day.

Then, senior year of college, I took a Sleep and Circadian Rhythms class from a top sleep-medicine researcher, and my entire attitude changed. When I tell you I am *crazed* about my sleep, I mean I am *insane* about my sleep. When my family and I are all under the same roof, I walk around at 10:30 P.M. shutting off lights and devices, telling everyone to get ready for bed. I've probably used an alarm ten times in the past five years (and mostly to catch flights). I wear red glasses practically every day (to block the blue light that messes with your sleep) starting at 8 P.M. (yes, it's just as sexy as it sounds). So what follows is what I learned about sleep that has made me into the most annoying person on the planet to live with (at least after 10 P.M.).

Why We Sleep

We spend roughly a third of our lives asleep. So if we live until ninety, that's about thirty years, guys. *Thirty years of sleep.* That is a *massive* time cost. From an evolutionary perspective, sleep seems pretty dumb: you're lying there, unconscious, vulnerable, ready to be eaten at any time, not able to go forage for food. And if you do somehow wake up in time to escape whatever danger is approaching, you'd be too groggy to do more than rub your eyes before you'd be dead. For us to spend seven to nine hours a day in this state of utter incapacitation and vulnerability—it must serve an extraordinarily important purpose in our lives. So why do we sleep?

Here are just a few of the reasons that we have discovered in the past few decades:

- Sleep is absolutely essential in the encoding and storage of memories.[1] And memories are essentially how we learn.

- Partial and chronic sleep deprivation impair a huge range of cognitive functions, including memory, attention, decision-making, and vigilance.[2] The real-world implications are profound: medical residents have been shown to perform 1.5 standard deviations worse on clinical tasks when they haven't gotten sufficient sleep.[3] And 21 percent of auto crashes in which a person was killed involved a drowsy driver.[4]

- When you don't sleep enough, your negative-emotion reactivity is increased and your positive-emotion reactivity is decreased.[5] Said another way, you are much more sensitive to life stressors when you're not getting enough shut-eye.

- While you're sleeping, certain parts of the immune system seem to rev up—that is, certain inflammatory markers actually increase, preparing your immune system for the pathogens it may have to face the next day.[6] Studies have also shown that sleep improves the efficacy of vaccines.[7]

* Shorter sleep = shorter life. Sleep impacts almost every physiological system in your body, therefore it's no surprise that lack of sufficient sleep is associated with the progression of chronic disease. For example, men who sleep six hours or fewer, or nine hours or more, have 1.7 times the death rate of those sleeping seven or eight hours.[8]

* New research has found that while you sleep, your brain is performing a crucial self-cleaning task. Cerebrospinal fluid, a clear liquid that surrounds the brain and spinal cord, washes through the brain while we sleep, clearing out neurotoxins and, of particular note, the protein called beta-amyloid.[9] When these proteins build up, they form plaques in the brain, which is one of the hallmarks of Alzheimer's disease.

Honestly, the list goes on and on. Sleep affects reproductive health: men who were restricted to five hours a night for eight nights experienced the testosterone decreases seen in a decade of aging.[10] Sleep disturbances are associated with almost, if not every, mental-health disorder.[11] Just to give you a sense of how seriously we should take our sleep: the book *Guinness World Records* no longer allows sleep deprivation to be a record anymore because of the risks it poses to our health. (Keep in mind, this is a book that allows people to lie on a bed of nails while motorcycles roll over them, using them as a human bridge.)

Sleep! It's More Than Just Lying There!

One of the things that I think many people don't understand about sleep (unless you've—ahem, ahem—taken a Sleep and Circadian Rhythms class) is that it's not just about how many hours you are getting in, it's also about your overall sleep quality and circadian alignment.

Long story short, your sleep quality and your sleep timing matter just as much as your sleep quantity. Sleep can be broken down into four different stages, which we all cycle through about four to six times every night.[12] Each of these phases looks different in terms of brain activity and serves a different purpose. For example, perhaps the most "famous" sleep stage (if there could be such a thing) is rapid eye movement sleep, or REM sleep. This is characterized by, you guessed it, rapid eye movements, and it is also the phase of sleep where we do most of our dreaming.

Sleep architecture refers to the structure and organization of sleep. This is important because some things might not necessarily change sleep duration but might drastically change sleep *architecture,* which is much harder to detect for a normal person who isn't measuring their sleep performance in a lab.

The reason we should care is because a lot of the things we do in our daily lives that we may think are "helping" our sleep, such as alcohol consumption or sleeping pills, actually really mess with our sleep quality, and it's hard for us to detect that beyond just feeling tired and not performing our best throughout the day. Even low amounts of alcohol intake have been found to tamper with your sleep stages, for example, drastically lowering your amount of REM sleep in the first half of the night.[13] Sleeping pills have been shown to have minimal, if any, effects on sleep duration, but they decrease sleep quality, are associated with increased risk of death, cancer, and depression, and may promote chemical dependence.[14]

Our Internal Clock

But wait . . . there's more! Besides sleep quality, we also have our circadian alignment to think about. As kooky as it sounds, there's actually a clock in our brains called the suprachiasmatic nucleus (SCN, for short), which runs on a twenty-four-hour schedule and makes sure everything else in our bodies is also running on a twenty-four-hour schedule.[15] (PS: Obviously, I don't mean a literal clock, OK? It's just a cluster of cells, but the clock thing is way more fun, isn't it?)

"How does a group of cells even know what time it is?" I hear you asking. And the answer is, mostly through light.[16] That's right, this little cluster of cells in your brain is keeping all your body's physiology on a rhythm just based on feedback that it gets from your eyes. You have to admit, that's pretty darn cool. For most of human history, we have been exposed to light only when the sun was up, and then we were stuck in the dark—no phones, TVs, or laptops. So, it makes sense that the SCN evolved to sense these light-dark cycles and keep the rest of the body in line accordingly.

Often unnoticed by us, almost everything in our bodies runs on a tightly controlled schedule, and the SCN is responsible for keeping everything coordinated and aligned with the day-night cycle. This is all to say, timing does matter. There are consequences not only to getting less sleep than you need, or getting worse-quality sleep, but also to having sleep that is misaligned with your circadian rhythm.[17]

Sleep and Weight

In my late teens and early twenties, the research into things like dementia or heart disease, melatonin, and cortisol rhythms would have made approximately zero impression on me. Like . . . I was barely allowed to legally drink, why should I have been already worrying about chronic diseases or my circadian rhythms? However, when I started to hear about the way sleep was interfering with my fitness goals, I was *invested*. No more cramming papers in the overnight hours; I was *not* going to let bad sleep ruin all my hard work in and out of the gym. While all the stuff we've talked about thus far should provide *plenty* of reasons to prioritize sleep, here are just a few more points that may persuade those who remain unconvinced.

In research, we've seen a link between inadequate sleep and weight gain. For example, several epidemiological studies have linked insufficient sleep to a higher risk of obesity.[18] Several prospective studies have also found that in both children and adults, short sleep duration predicts weight gain and incidence of obesity.[19] And we've already discussed how even short periods of sleep restriction can cause insulin resistance in otherwise healthy individuals.[20] But is lack of sufficient sleep actually causing weight gain somehow, or is it just an association?

One of the crucial ways that sleep may impact weight is through appetite regulation. Researchers have found that even moderate reductions in sleep lead to a decrease in leptin (the hormone that makes you feel satiated), increases in ghrelin (the hormone that makes you hungry), and an increase in hunger and appetite, particularly for calorie-dense foods.[21] This is what we call a hormonal double whammy: not only are you less satisfied, but you're also hungrier. Or perhaps better yet, it's a triple whammy, because new research has shown that lack of sufficient sleep may actually make you crave less healthy food, similar to the effect we see when people use marijuana. Yes, it looks like sleep deprivation has a similar effect as "the munchies," making us crave more highly palatable, energy-dense foods through an increase in circulating endocannabinoids (types of lipids).[22]

This reminds me of so many exam weeks in college, when I would be running on two to four hours of sleep, walk into the dining hall, and book it for the waffle fries, a cult favorite from the esteemed Harvard University Dining Services. I would normally go the entire semester without even thinking about the fries, but for some reason, when I was stressed and exhausted, the smell of grease and salt was infinitely appetizing.

Something as simple as having your sleep, meal patterns, and exercise be misaligned from your body clock affects a whole host of systems that help regulate your body weight, from your insulin sensitivity, appetite, and hormone production to the function of your adrenal glands and protein concentrations in your gut that promote weight gain.[23] This may be why keeping a regular meal schedule can help promote circadian alignment.

Sleep and Fitness Goals

Lack of sufficient sleep has pretty profound effects on both weight loss and fitness efforts. One study found that higher sleep duration and better sleep quality were associated with greater fat loss.[24] And we're not talking about fractions of a pound; the researchers found that *a single* additional hour of average sleep duration over the course of the study was associated with an additional decrease of about 1.5 pounds.[25] The researchers concluded that sleep should always be taken into account when someone is looking to start a diet.

Other studies have shown that sleep plays a crucial role in the maintenance of fat-free mass (all your nonfat tissues, including muscles) during a caloric deficit. For example, restricting subjects to 5.5 hours of sleep versus 8.5 hours decreased the proportion of weight lost as fat by 55 percent and increased the proportion of weight lost as fat-free mass by 60 percent.[26] In other words, getting inadequate sleep while in a calorie deficit makes you lose less fat and lose more muscle, which, as we discussed in chapter 2, makes weight-loss maintenance a lot harder.

And finally, we don't need a study to tell you this, but, ain't nobody making optimal gains in the gym on inadequate sleep. Three consecutive nights of sleep restriction lowered maximal force production in the most effective exercises (compound, multijoint exercises, such as squats).[27] When it comes to the gym, your body's ability to adapt to the stimulus is where the gains are being made, and that happens when, you guessed it, you're recovering. Not getting enough sleep blunts your body's ability to adapt to whatever training stimulus you're throwing at it, because it increases the hormones that break down tissues (catabolic hormones) and lowers the hormones that are crucial for building muscle (anabolic hormones).[28]

So this is my appeal to those of you who don't care about chronic disease yet. Even if all you want is to progress in the gym or start making better food choices, prioritizing sleep is going to make sure that your hard work in and out of the gym is not going to waste.

From the Doc

Juna and I swear on a stack of diet books that we wrote this entire book before 10 P.M. (OK, well, definitely before 11 P.M.) My college political-philosophy professor admonished our class: "Finals are approaching, and do not put off writing your term papers until the last minute. Nothing written after midnight is worth reading." Indeed, during my early college years, I learned that joining the nightly dorm gab sessions from 11 P.M. until 1 A.M. might have improved my social life but was hurting my grades and health. Anything less than my optimal state sabotaged my ability to learn and the pleasure I took in school. I started going to bed at 11 P.M. and hitting the empty library at 8:30 A.M.

The most challenging time in my life sleepwise was during my subsequent medical training, which required me and my medical school classmates to be on call as frequently as every third night. Our work days would extend into the evening, overnight, and into the next day. While I was training to become Dr. Phillips, in the wee hours of the morning, I was closer to becoming Mr. Hyde; I lost my humor, empathy, and attention. I loved my medical school rotation in surgery but soon recognized that I was just not constitutionally able to maintain the more than eighty-hour workweeks.

When pressed with medical licensing exams, schoolwork, and clinical rotations, a young trainee's sleep suffers. For medical residents, sleep and health become commodities that are spent down in exchange for learning and caring for others. How much less sleep can I get and still perform well the next day? It is ironic that training to attend to the health of others forces students into decidedly unhealthy routines and working conditions.

Even among the health-conscious, achieving a regular sleep schedule, allowing for adequate quality and quantity of sleep, often remains elusive. Myriad factors, including irregular work schedules, raising children, and exposure to blue light, inhibit regular sleep schedules. Ironically, trying to keep up with positive health habits can reduce our time in bed. At a recent lifestyle-medicine conference, a respondent to a poll of the audience on their health habits remarked, "I am doing well with everything else besides getting enough sleep, and that's how I find the time to do all my exercising, cooking, and meditation!" Finding the proper balance is not easy, but inadequate sleep provides a shaky foundation for our overall health.

My kids will (hopefully) tell you that I try to be as generous with my time and attention as possible, to listen to their joys and challenges, giving warm, sage advice, at least until 10 P.M. Once my teeth are brushed and my pajamas are on, I start powering down in anticipation of what, I hope, will be a full, restful night of sleep. Late at night, if presented with a complicated issue requiring a thoughtful response, the best I can offer is a short answer and the suggestion that anytime tomorrow would be a much better time to talk.

When I am not seeing patients, writing books, or doing podcasts with

Juna, I devote myself to sharing lifestyle medicine with students and health-professions trainees. Medical schools "teach to the boards," meaning that their curricula are created with the intention of enabling students to pass the licensing boards. A central and enduring goal of my work in lifestyle-medicine education is to influence the medical licensing boards to include questions about nutrition, exercise, stress, and sleep.

I look forward to the day when a medical student sits bleary-eyed, late at night, reviewing board questions such as these:

Which of the following best describes the relationship between sleep and cognitive performance?

A. Partial and chronic sleep deprivation impairs a huge range of cognitive functions in addition to working, including memory, attention, decision-making, and vigilance.[29]

B. Sleep deprivation increases rigid thinking and makes it harder for you to use new information in tasks that require innovative thinking.[30]

C. Medical residents perform 1.5 standard deviations worse on clinical tasks when they haven't gotten sufficient sleep.[31]

D. People who are sleep impaired rate their performance better than those who aren't. (Yes, it's making you perform worse, but you don't even realize it.)

E. All of the above (so get some sleep).

The answer is E.

The Takeaways

There's a reason we spend a third of our lives asleep: it's absolutely crucial to our physical and mental health. You'll be healthier and happier if you get the right amount of good-quality sleep on a consistent nightly schedule. Here are some easy, science-based ways to improve your sleep.

DURING THE DAY

1. **Wake up without an alarm.** Think about this for a second: if we were all getting enough sleep, we probably wouldn't need an alarm. I know you may be thinking, *You don't understand. If I don't have an alarm, I'll sleep till noon every day!* But unless you're going to sleep at like 5 A.M., this shouldn't be the case in the long run, because the vast majority of people, when not chronically sleep deprived, should feel rested on around seven hours of sleep.[32] Your alarm does not care about which stage of sleep you're in, which can lead to you being interrupted in sleep stages that your body would never wake you up in naturally. This leads to sleep inertia—the transition from being asleep to being awake when you feel like death for fifteen to thirty minutes (i.e., you feel groggy and your brain doesn't work). Studies have shown that self-awakening not only improves alertness upon first waking, but also decreases feelings of sleepiness throughout the day, even when not getting enough sleep.[33] Aiming to set up your life in such a way that you wake up naturally will make you feel the best throughout your day. This may take some math on your part (sorry). What time do you need to be up to get ready for the day? How much time do you need in bed? (Note: I did not say sleep; I said time in bed, because chances are, you don't magically pass out the second your head hits the pillow.) How much time do you need to get ready for bed? You probably need to allot more time than you think if you want to embrace the no-alarm lifestyle.

2. **Get out in the sun.** Exposing yourself to sunlight, especially early in the morning, can help regulate your circadian rhythm and improve your sleep quality and quantity in the following night.[34] So get your butt up in the morning and go outside for a walk!

3. **Drink your coffee early.** OK, I'm not going to tell you to *not* drink coffee. (And that's definitely *not* because I myself am a coffee addict. Definitely not. Nope.) But it's true: caffeine does mess with your sleep, particularly when it's close to your bedtime. No matter how much certain people (ahem, ahem, my mom) may say, "I can have a coffee with dinner and I feel great!" Just because you fall asleep does not mean that it's not disrupting your sleep architecture and messing with your sleep stages. Caffeine has a half-life of about five hours, which means that half the caffeine you ingest is still in your system five hours later.[35] Researchers have found that having caffeine even six hours before bedtime pretty drastically impairs your sleep.[36] So if you're going to drink coffee, the earlier, the better.

4. **Exercise.** As if you needed another reason to do it . . . exercise helps improve your sleep quality and may even be an effective, nonpharmacological treatment for sleep disorders.[37]

FOR THE NIGHT

1. **Set an alarm.** Get rid of your alarms in the morning and instead make it an alarm at night to tell you it's time to start getting ready for bed. Studies have shown that going to sleep at roughly the same time every night is an important aspect of sleep hygiene (because it promotes regular circadian rhythms) and is associated with a multitude of better health outcomes.[38]

2. **Cool down.** Since our body temperature actually dips right before bedtime and reaches its all-time low during sleep, having a cooler environment may actually help us fall asleep better.[39] Ironically, taking a hot shower before bed may actually help your body start this cooling process.[40]

3. **Reduce blue light two to three hours before bedtime.** Reducing your blue-light exposure before bed helps maintain your

circadian rhythm by keeping your melatonin production on point.[41] Ideally, this would mean no phones, computers, or TV three hours before bed. But let's be honest; who's gonna actually do that? So if you still want to use screens, you can get blue-light blocking glasses. (Note: These *should* change the color of everything to look orangey-red; they're not the clear ones that only block a small portion of blue light.) Studies have shown that filtering out blue light preserves your melatonin production at night (your sleepy-time hormone).[42]

4. **Avoid food and exercise right before bed.** Vigorous exercise less than an hour before bed and eating thirty to sixty minutes before bed can both impair your sleep.[43,44]

5. **Avoid alcohol when possible.** Again, I'm not trying to be a party pooper, but while alcohol before bed may feel like it's helping because it acts as a sedative and knocks you out, it is actually really messing with your natural sleep stages.[45] On the bright side, drinking less alcohol will fit very well into your newly established "grandma" or "grandpa" persona! (WARNING: Yes, you will likely get called a grandma or grandpa by all your friends when you implement all these great new sleep-hygiene habits.)

A Final Note: Don't Ignore the Tree on Your House

With respect to sleep and stress specifically (but also . . . kind of every topic we've talked about), I want to make one final, overarching, and crucial point before we wrap up this book. I have included sections on how not taking care of specific domains of health affects our weight, eating behaviors, and gym progress. This has been my (not-so-subtle) attempt to appeal to those of you who are most motivated by reaching a fitness goal and picked up this book solely for that purpose (i.e., me for most of my life). OK, are you ready for my awesome point that I think is so important that I have made an entire section *just to say this point*?

The only reason poor sleep, high amounts of stress, or any other behavior affects our fitness goals at all is precisely because of the much more global and far-reaching effects they are having on our biological systems as a whole. To illustrate this point, my friend came up with a fantastic analogy that I am now shamelessly stealing. (No copyright, no lawsuit—am I right?)

If a tree were to fall on your house, it would have all sorts of effects on the quality of life in that house. If it were winter, it would be very cold. Perhaps you would all of a sudden have a bug infestation. Maybe the plumbing system will have gotten wrecked in the process, leaving you with no working toilet or sink. The hole in your roof would mean that anytime it rained, everything would get soaked.

The effects that poor health behaviors have on your weight are like the effects that the tree has on the temperature, the pest control, or the plumbing. Yes, it *did* get colder, but the much bigger problem is, um . . . there's a *freaking tree* that fell on your house! Getting a space heater, or five, or ten, might help make it a bit warmer, but the real root cause is still there and is still causing a whole host of other problems. Therefore, weight gain or suboptimal progress in the gym are downstream consequences of much more fundamental biological systems not working as they should. So, yes, I have used interference with fitness goals as a little extra motivation, a proverbial carrot to incentivize certain health behaviors, but always remember that removing the tree and repairing the damage is going to be much more effective than getting a million space heaters, a bunch of bug spray, hiring a plumber, and getting a crappy tarp that lets in half the rain anyway. Who wants to live in that kind of house?

At this point in the world, people get the food and exercise part, but I think a lot of the other parts, like getting enough good-quality sleep, for example, are just so unsexy and boring that they either get absurdly discounted or flat-out ignored. So whether it's sexy or not, I guess what I'm trying to say is, if there is a tree that has fallen on your house, please don't ignore it.

12

What Matters Most and Making Lasting Change

From the Doc

We started this book discussing how our metabolism works and how it is affected by caloric consumption, that is, dieting as well as overeating. We did a deep dive into what to eat, and we challenged our ingrained perceptions of our bodies and the profound and often negative influence of a society focused on the outer demonstration of health and beauty through the single metric of our weight. Movement, both cardiovascular and resistance training, was presented as one of the most critical and malleable of our health behaviors. Revealing conversations about eating disorders reminded us that the best intentions to eat well and remain active may go awry and lead to overexercising and under- or overeating. We then explored the broader aspects of other foundational self-care behaviors by focusing on the interaction of stress and sleep with our overall health and weight. It is now time to wrap this together as you plan to make sustainable changes to your health behaviors.

There are myriad apps, books, podcasts, coaches, groups, and approaches to making lifestyle changes. But before we jump to the "action" steps and reflexively resolve to "do better next time," it's important to first go through the foundational work to answer why you are trying to make a change at all. What is your underlying motivation?

The next step in optimizing your well-being and transforming your relationship with yourself and your body is to clarify your ultimate life mission and purpose by answering, "What matters most?" This step alone can be a lifesaver. "Stronger purpose in life was associated with decreased mortality" by a factor of 2.4 in a study of adults fifty years and older.[1] In this chapter, we pull it all together to review a full array of health behaviors and identify our *strengths*, that is, where our current habits most closely align with where we want to be, and our *opportunities*, where our current habits are most disparate from our goals. To guide this journey, we will use the Whole Health model.

The Whole Health model was developed to transform the clinical care given in our nation's largest integrated health-care system, the Veterans Health Administration (VA). I redirected my career to work at VA Boston in 2015 to help lead this change, described as "cultural transformation." The VA seeks to evolve from the traditional, sickness-care, reactive, episodic model of medical care to a system that provides a proactive, personalized, patient-driven experience. At the VA, part of my charge is introducing this model of care to the more than 120,000 health-professions students and trainees who come through the VA each year as part of their education. One of the most gratifying aspects of my job is witnessing the transformation of young medical and physician-assistant students who experience Whole Health for themselves and how it dramatically reorients their clinical care by placing patients at the center of care. They quickly learn to tailor their clinical recommendations to "what matters most" to the patients.

The students rapidly incorporate the importance of treating our patients as unique individuals who will make behavior changes only if it moves them closer to what matters most to them for their lives and their families. If this idea seems obvious, recognize that, outside of the VA and other early adopters of lifestyle medicine, health care remains focused on fixing what is already broken, often with pills and surgery. At the heart of lifestyle medicine and Whole Health is the recognition that the root cause of more than 80 percent of premature deaths, chronic disease, and health-care costs are simple health behaviors: physical inactivity, tobacco use, and poor nutrition.[2] Making sustainable changes in health behaviors is successful only if those new habits are in alignment with what matters most to the individual. The good news is that improved health behaviors are not just about proactively preventing an illness, such as diabetes. Rather, diet and physical-activity modification can effectively treat, and in some cases reverse, chronic illness. As a physician, I am joyously compelled by patients reporting things like, "I don't need the insulin for my diabetes now that I straightened out my diet and started exercising." But even for a condition that cannot be cured or reversed, getting in touch with what matters most and taking charge of even a small aspect of self-care can provide a deeper sense of meaning, peace, joy, and comfort.

The monumental effort of rolling out Whole Health is demonstrating impressive early results. Those patients using Whole Health decreased their opioid use three times more than those not exposed to Whole Health. Compared to those receiving conventional care, the Whole Health users reported greater improvements in perceptions of care, engagement in health care, self-care, life meaning and purpose, pain, and perceived stress.[3]

While developed for the VA, the principles of Whole Health are not exclusive to veterans or to any particular group of patients. You can use these same principles and tools to help guide yourself. Let's get started by considering what matters most to you.

I routinely ask my patients what activity they look forward to doing once they overcome the pain or injury that is limiting them. This simple question evokes the most wistful and evocative responses. One patient, who had decreased sensation in his feet with subsequent balance problems, thought for a moment about how the risk of falling was preventing him from trying to stand up on his fishing boat. "When I have my legs back, I'll go on my boat at night. That's when the magic happens." I was thrilled by his excitement and resolve. Even though I could not promise that he would reach his goal, he then engaged in his balance exercises with determination and resolve, because this was propelling him toward what he most cherished.

Another patient with knee arthritis acknowledged that her legs had become weaker when she cut back on her walking because of the pain. She pointed to her thighs and acknowledged that she had put on weight due to her reduced activity. She cut me short to explain that she was not particularly excited to follow the advice of numerous prior physicians and physical therapists to lose a few pounds and do her leg-strengthening exercises to address her knee arthritis. However, when I asked her what mattered most to her that was not happening because of the knee pain, she took a deep breath. "My granddaughter is just turning one. I want more than anything to be able to get down on the floor to play with her and to help my daughter by bathing the baby in the bathtub. Right now it just hurts too much when I bend down, and I can't easily get off the floor. She deserves a grandmother who can get around more easily." The patient then wrote her own plan of care: "Here's what I'm thinking, doc. If I do the exercises the therapist recommends and cut back on my chips and desserts, I think I might be in better shape for my granddaughter."

There is no way for me to know what matters most to my patients unless I ask.

Exercise 1. Ask Yourself: "What Matters Most to Me? What Do I Want My Health For?"

In the very first episode of our podcast, instead of asking Juna, "What's the matter with you?" I asked her, "What *matters* to you?" Her answer was focused around looking a certain way—that changing her body had been, at least in the past, the "driving factor" around all the lifestyle changes she had made. I pushed on this a bit: "Is there anything that matters more to you or goes a little deeper than that?" After a pause, she answered that she wanted to feel "happy in her body" and happy in her life. For her, looking a certain way had been equated to happiness. As we dug deeper, what became clear was that it wasn't really a certain size or weight that mattered to Juna; it was just being happy, confident, and content in her own skin. That's not a number on a scale or a size. It's, in Juna's words "effortless," a place where eating and exercising aren't sources of punishment or stress but, rather, sources of joy. It's feeling "free."

What matters most to me is to be fully present for my family; to lead a long, happy, healthy, and productive life; and to use my talents, energy, and resources to leave a legacy within medicine and beyond to help people take charge of their health and well-being. Writing this book and engaging with you, the reader, as you proceed on your journey, is fulfilling what matters most to me. Thank you.

Circle of Health and Mindful Awareness

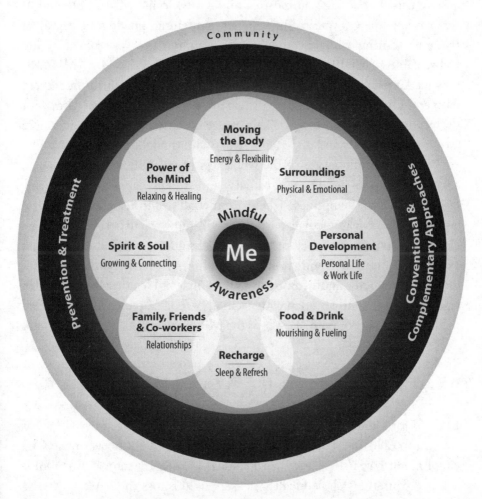

Used with permission. US Department of Veterans Affairs,
Office of Patient Centered Care and Cultural Transformation.

To guide you on this journey, let's introduce the Circle of Health.[4] At the
center of the circle is "Me." In your own circle, that would be you. This process
is all to be viewed from *your* perspective. Mindful awareness, or mindfulness,
is the skill to engage and take stock of where you are and where you would like
to be in each of the foundational health behaviors, which are represented by

the eight overlapping circles. You can cultivate mindful awareness through meditation, but you do not need to sit still for hours every day to begin to answer this: When are you most calm, focused, centered, and present? Is this while playing a musical instrument, gardening, praying, or being "in the zone" during athletic competition? "Mindfulness" was coined by Jon Kabat-Zinn in his 1994 book *Wherever You Go, There You Are*: "Mindfulness means paying attention in a particular way: on purpose, in the present moment, and nonjudgmentally."[5] There are no wrong answers. Also, your perspective and responses will likely evolve over time as you become more aware of your habits and underlying beliefs and thought patterns.

Being mindfully aware of the wholeness of your life will allow you to acknowledge your joy, peace, creativity, and fullness, as well as your suffering, unrest, and emptiness. There are myriad health benefits to mindful awareness. For our immediate purpose, it will allow you to best view the Circle of Health and take stock of your strengths and opportunities. The next exercises require you to shift your attention from the hurly-burly of constant distraction toward mindful awareness. The Circle of Health shows a series of eight areas that gently overlap with each other. For example, you might find meditation as part of both "Power of the Mind" as well as "Recharge."

Exercise 2. Complete the Personal Health Inventory

Let's go for a tour and complete the Personal Health Inventory (PHI) as we go (pp. 270-71). I will guide you through the eight areas of the Circle of Health and share my own Personal Health Inventory. This tool is adapted from the Whole Health measure used across the VA.[6]

1. Moving the Body: Energy and Flexibility

This is a more general way of thinking about all of your intentional exercise and habitual nonexercise movement. (Remember EAT and NEAT from chapter 3.) Look at the two answer columns: in the right-hand column, record on a scale of 1 being the lowest to 5 being the highest where you would like to be. Some of us (me included) live to exercise, so nothing short of a score of 5 would be an appropriate goal. The column on the left uses the same

1–5 scale to describe where you are right now. If you are doing way less than you would like to be doing, then your score might be 1 or 2. If you are feeling pretty good about getting enough physical activity, consider a score of 4 or 5. You are also invited to record why you gave yourself those numbers, and write down changes that might help you bridge the gap to reach your goal. These might include incorporating walking into your commute or other daily activities or joining an exercise class with a friend. I manage to keep physically active with a variety of different sports, and I am grading myself 5/5.

2. Family, Friends, and Co-Workers: Relationships

Although the Circle of Health starts with "Me" in the center, it is the "We" of our community that meets our need for social connection. The depth of social connection is closely related to positive health outcomes. While we are focusing on "*What* really matters," also ask yourself, "*Who* really matters?" Do you feel well supported? This may be emotional or other forms of support. How much effort do you put into increasing your social capital? How connected do you feel? I highly value my relationships and do my best to invest time and energy in a peaceful and supportive homelife. However, I score myself 4/5 because I would like to spend more time with old and new friends.

3. Recharge: Sleep and Refresh

As we discussed in chapter 11, getting adequate sleep is critical not only to managing our weight but also to so many other aspects of our health, including decreasing the incidences of hypertension, diabetes, elevated blood lipids, stroke, and heart attack. Recharging also includes taking short breaks or doing something during the day to allow you to refresh. Hopefully, we would all aspire to get enough sleep and daily breaks and score a 5 in the right-hand column. But if you have a new baby or even a new puppy at home, your sleep will be disrupted, and 5 may not be realistic. The same might hold true if your job requires late hours or overnight shifts. Assigning a number to the left-hand column reflects how much sleep you are actually getting. Over the last several years I have come to recognize that I need a lot of sleep, that is, around eight hours per night, and that I feel so much healthier, happier, clearer-thinking, and more productive when I get enough sleep. So, on a good day, I would score myself 5/5 in this category.

4. Surroundings: Physical and Emotional

We don't live in a vacuum. Our surroundings markedly impact our health and can even trigger our genetic expression (for better or worse). Surroundings can include our homes, workplaces, neighborhoods, climate and ecology, emotional surroundings, and healing environments. One of the disconcerting aspects of the COVID-19 pandemic is that previously safe and enjoyable environments—for example, being in a restaurant with friends—became potentially lethal environments to be avoided. Our surroundings also include our neighborhoods, which account for enormous health disparities in the United States for those living in underserved areas. Surroundings include the air that you breathe and access to green spaces as well. On a more personal scale, "surroundings" takes into account toxic clutter and overflowing email inboxes. While I would love to live in an uncluttered home, I don't. I need to carefully arrange my computer's camera in my hospital and home offices to not show the leaning tower of papers. However, I would like to think that I have come to some understanding and acceptance of my clutter; I score myself 2 for where I am and 3 for where I would reasonably like to be. In the right-hand column, assess your goal for yourself, and in the left-hand column, assess where you are. Do you feel as though you live and work in a healthy, supportive environment?

5. Food and Drink: Nourishing and Fueling

For many of us, this is our biggest challenge. What is a reasonable goal for your overall nutrition? How close are you to that goal? Are you feeling well-nourished but not overfed? Remember as you fill in the numbers here that this area deals with your behaviors around food and not just your weight. My family enjoys the privilege of easy access to fresh and nutritious food, which we buy and mostly prepare at home (except for ordering in or eating out about once per week). My "pandemic project" was, in part, to become more independent and confident in cooking in the kitchen. Since I'm slowly working toward an eating plan that reflects my wants and needs, I would rate myself as 5/5.

6. Personal Development: Personal Life and Work Life

How are you spending your time? Are your work and personal activities aligned with what really matters to you and brings you joy? What is the quality of your work life? Do you have autonomy, opportunities to advance, fair compensation, appropriate feedback, and manageable stress? Do you feel creative and have an avenue to express it? Have you fostered resilience in order to adapt to changing circumstances? Is reading this book part of your personal development? For some of us, engaging in lifelong learning, volunteering, and balancing our work and homelives allows us to thrive in this area. I have high aspirations in this area, but I am working on crafting the next stage of my life and career. I score myself 3/4.

7. Spirit and Soul: Growing and Connecting

For many, spirituality is really the heart of "what matters most" and perhaps gives context and meaning to suffering that we might experience, the nature of death and dying, and ultimately the meaning of life. This realm includes but also transcends religion. Spirituality can be the driving force for some or simply not that important to others. Where are you in this area? Is this of high value to you, rating a 5 in "Where I Want to Be"? Or is this of lesser importance? I belong to a faith community, which sounds like a complex way of saying that I like to go to my temple. I enjoy the annual holiday celebrations, the community, and the rituals. I have a strong sense of meaning and purpose. However, this is an area of opportunity for my growth because I aspire to be more spiritual, to "directly experience the sacred," and to be more in touch with the spirituality of nature and the cosmos.[7] I rate myself as 3/4.

8. Power of the Mind: Relaxing and Healing

This area challenges the dichotomy between the body and the mind and focuses more on the whole person. Are you able to tap into the power of your mind to heal and cope? Do you regularly use relaxation, breathing, or guided imagery? These approaches, as well as meditation, visualization, biofeedback, and hypnosis, can reduce your sympathetic "fight-or-flight" response and activate your parasympathetic "rest-and-relax" response. For those of us who stress eat, employing these skills may be very valuable. I have always found this area to be of vital importance, so my goal is a 5. However, despite extensive meditation training, it has only been in recent times that I have routinely sat each morning for my breathing and meditation. I rate myself 3/5.

Once you have completed the Personal Health Inventory, you should have numbers 1 through 5 selected in all eight areas. Circle the areas where the numbers match. In my example, I will circle Moving the Body, Food and Drink, and Recharge as 5/5, my strengths.

Personal Health Inventory

For each area of Whole Health listed here, please rate yourself on a scale of 1 (low) to 5 (high) to best represent where you are now (left) and where you would like to be (right).

Building Blocks of Health and Well-being	Where I Am Now (1–5)	Where I Want to Be (1–5)
Moving the Body: Energy and Flexibility Includes movement and physical activities like walking, dancing, gardening, sports, lifting weights, yoga, cycling, swimming, and working out in a gym.		
Family, Friends, and Co-Workers: Relationships Feeling listened to and connected to people you love and care about; the quality of your communication with family, friends, and people you work with.		
Recharge: Sleep and Refresh Getting enough rest, relaxation, and sleep.		
Surroundings: Physical and Emotional Feeling safe; having comfortable, healthy spaces where you work and live; the quality of the lighting, color, air, and water; decreasing unpleasant clutter, noises, and smells.		

Building Blocks of Health and Well-being	Where I Am Now (1–5)	Where I Want to Be (1–5)
Food and Drink: Nourishing and Fueling Eating healthy, balanced meals with plenty of fruits and vegetables each day; drinking enough water and limiting sodas, sweetened drinks, and alcohol.		
Personal Development: Personal and Work Life Learning and growing; developing abilities and talents; balancing responsibilities where you live, volunteer, and work.		
Spirit and Soul: Growing and Connecting Having a sense of purpose and meaning in your life; feeling connected to something larger than yourself; finding strength in difficult times.		
Power of the Mind: Relaxing and Healing Tapping into the power of your mind to heal and cope; using mind-body techniques such as relaxation, breathing, and guided imagery		

Adapted with permission. US Department of Veterans Affairs, Office of Patient Centered Care and Cultural Transformation.

Strengths and Opportunities

First, focus on your strengths and accomplishments. What are you most proud of right now? In the past, I didn't routinely get to sleep on time or necessarily eat consistently well. I am proud to have made, over time, small changes so that, along with exercise, those are now my areas of strength.

Second, look at where there is a difference between where you would like to be and where you are. This may represent an opportunity to evolve toward more health and happiness by potentially closing the gap. The places where there is a difference between the numbers represent my opportunities: Power of the Mind, 3/5; Spirit and Soul, 3/4; Personal Development, 3/4; Surroundings, 2/3; Family, Friends, and Co-Workers, 4/5.

What can't I change? Mindfully consider where circumstances are beyond your control. Can you be at peace knowing that an injury or illness may hamper your physical activity or that the area where you live may not have optimal open space available? Perhaps a death or divorce has ruptured your personal relationships.

Now consider what you can change and what you want to work on. Are there opportunities for you to use your strengths to support the areas where you want to and can make changes? If so, will these changes help you get closer to what matters most to you?

A patient of mine who described her faith—that is, in the Spirit and Soul category—as what matters most to her shared her frustration in the Moving the Body section because she had no safe, affordable access to places to walk or exercise on her own. She proudly described her strengths in Spirit and Soul as an active member of her church, and in Family, Friends, and Co-Workers due to her deep ties to her relatives, friends, and other members of her church. While she did not leave her apartment every day, she never missed a Sunday at church. After thinking a short while about what she could and couldn't change, she proposed that instead of getting a lift, she would begin walking to church with her neighbors each Sunday. At our next visit, she told me that she liked walking with friends so much that they started to walk to the church to volunteer a couple of times per week.

Taking Action

With a clearer (though evolving) sense of your purpose of "what matters most to you," along with a frank assessment of your strengths and opportunities, it is now time to act and proceed down your path with greater clarity or perhaps try a different path.

1. **Don't go it alone.** Behavior change is challenging, and doing it without support from your family, friends, and coworkers will likely make it even tougher. Share this change process with someone close to you who might be on the same path (and ready to make changes as well) or who is willing to support you on your journey.

2. **Think of the future.** As you chart your path, think of a goal that is worth the trip. Also, consider where you will be in your life if you don't at least try to start the journey. "A body at rest tends to stay at rest."

3. **Small changes can have big results.** As you sail across the ocean of your life, a 2 percent course correction today will chart you on a new heading in the months and years to come for arrival at a completely different place than where you were headed.

4. **Be creative and curious.** Most experiments fail, but they can all provide some insight. For example, if you are looking to join an exercise class, online or in person, keep trying out classes until you find a good fit.

5. **It's not all or nothing.** While you might have an audacious goal of getting off the couch and running a 5K race, understand that even if you just get up to a one-mile walk, you have vastly improved your fitness and are already reaping benefits from your increased physical activity.

6. **Start with the easy stuff.** As you look at your Personal Health Inventory, you'll easily see the biggest opportunities to close the gap between where you are and where you would like to be. Setting and achieving a simple goal—for example, drinking an extra glass of water each day or reaching out to old friends at least once per week—will improve your confidence and self-efficacy to next take on a bigger goal.

7. **Seek additional help.** If your budget, employer, or health plan allows, reach out to a health coach (preferably board-certified) to help you clarify and set goals and to provide accountability and support.[8]

8. **Yes, there's an app for that.** Explore the expanding options of

apps that can integrate health data (e.g., sleep, steps) and provide cues and feedback.

9. **No, thank you, I have enough apps and screen time.** Good old pen and paper and regular journaling to reflect on your purpose, plans, and progress may be perfect for you.

10. **Enjoy the journey.**

Change Is Possible . . . But It Takes Literally Forever

Juna's Box of Size-Small Crop Tops

This is something that I'm really embarrassed to share. When I was a senior in college and got really serious about fitness, I started to buy limited-edition Gymshark crop tops. These were long-sleeve shirts that stopped right above your belly button to show off a presumably flat, toned stomach. They looked exactly like the shirt that Kim Possible wore in the Disney Channel cartoon that I had been obsessed with growing up, and my biggest "When I'm skinny" fantasy was to wear these shirts.

The only thing was, I didn't buy them in my current size (medium to large, depending on the time of year), I bought them in a size small. I was *so convinced* of my inevitable "success" that I could not bear the thought of not having this "Vital Seamless Long Sleeve Crop" in the color "sand" when I had my new thin body. Of course, wearing them in my current body was out of the question.

Over the next few years, this habit continued and extended beyond crop tops. I bought size-small sports bras—keep in mind I've been at least a C cup since eighth grade (so I don't even know who *this* was meant to fool). I bought size 4 leggings. I bought size 6 dresses. No joke, I had entire outfits for my smaller self. And whenever I would get them in the mail, I would open the box, look at them in admiration, and carefully fold them to rest with their friends in a massive clear container at the top of my closet. These clothes have never been worn.

They have tags. They're brand new and beautiful. And they will likely never fit me.

I find this embarrassing for multiple reasons: (1) The fact that I so stubbornly held on to some elusive idea of something that there was *literally* no indication would ever happen is kind of pathetic. But (2) the fact that even after feeling like I had made so many strides in accepting my body— getting professional help, regaining my period and hormonal health, liking the way I looked, being proud of what my body could do—even after all that, there was still a part of me that thought, *Maybe I can do it, not in an unhealthy way, but it's possible, right?*

I have made so much progress: I've bought clothes that fit *and* make me feel good. I wear things to the gym that I would never have thought I could wear. I wore my first-ever two-piece swimsuit since age twelve only three years ago, and now I have a dozen of them. I've never been so comfortable with my body, despite being at close to the highest weight I've ever been at—substantially higher than what it was at the height of my ED. My eating is fueled by wanting to give my body the micronutrients that I deprived it of for years. My exercise is fueled by wanting to be able to do stuff that I think is cool. And yet I could not bring myself to get rid of this box of small clothes because of the tiny possibility that one day, I could wear a sand-colored crop top that was no longer sold.

Here's my problem: on my social media, in my life, to my friends, I'm determined not to reinforce dangerous methods by which to lose weight. I love getting people to see the value in health behaviors that go beyond changing the way you look. But if I've truly accepted that I don't need to be a size small, that it doesn't change anything about my worth or value, that truly all bodies are beautiful regardless of size, why the hell is there still a gigantic clear box full of limited-edition clothes in my closet? That is . . . until recently.

Not Talking for Ten Days

Because I never shut up, and find it *extremely* hard to ever chill, relax, and/ or meditate, every few years I force myself to do a ten-day silent meditation retreat. OK fine, I've done two, but I only started like four years ago, people!

Anyway, at these retreats, you spend all day with no technology, no talking, no writing, just sitting with your own thoughts. All. Freaking. Day. *For ten days.* As you can imagine, it's torture. But every time I go, I have a transformative experience.

For example, one of the main things I learned at the first retreat I went to four years ago was how much internalized disgust I felt toward specific parts of my body. I noticed I would never zip up my jackets, I would gingerly pull up my pants with my fingertips, all in an effort to never actually touch my own stomach. I was so subconsciously uncomfortable with it that my reflex, whenever my hand would come close or I passed a mirror, was to "suck in," even when I was alone. I did a million tiny actions like this all day and had *no idea.* The human brain is scary, man.

Realizations like this were common at the retreats: some subconscious thing you thought about yourself would become clear, and then you could make a conscious effort to work on it when you went back to your normal life. This for me meant touching my stomach, without judgment or emotion (easier said than done, guys, I swear), not hiding it all the time by sucking in, wearing shirts that would have previously made me uncomfortable, even posting videos online showing my body without hiding or trying to look thinner. When I arrived at the retreat two years later, the behaviors were gone, and I was proud. But something else came up.

I was in my room and telling myself that I had truly accepted my body. Yes, it was hard some days, but most days I felt fine. I was proud of the progress I had made, remembering how, only two years earlier, the fact that I would be forced to eat food that I had no control over for ten days had given me anxiety, and this time I barely thought about it. But something was bothering me. I had been calmly lying down, meditating, when I thought of the box of crop tops. I started to get agitated and restless.

I could be both, I thought. I could accept myself but still keep these clothes "just in case." Is that really so wrong? But as I lay there, trying to convince myself, I don't know what clicked, but it just became clear to me: I *have to* get rid of the crop tops. I would not be able to move on from that part of my life, from needing to be that size, if I had this box of crop tops. It was the last physical relic I had of my previous self.

So . . . the happy ending is, it only took me five years, two therapists, and twenty days of complete and utter silence while meditating to make me see that I don't need to hoard clothes that don't fit me. Guess that Ivy League education wasn't for nothing, eh?

As soon as I got home, I gathered all the clothes into a trash bag, hoisted it over my shoulder, and walked out into the backyard to our fire pit. Dumping them there, I took out my speaker. It's time for some Lizzo, a body-positive queen if I ever knew one. As the incredible vocals of Lizzo wafted through the air, I took out a lighter from our kitchen drawer, touched it to the colorful heap, and watched as it was engulfed in the triumphant flames of my newfound self-acceptance. "SCREW THE PATRIARCHY!!! SCREW THE THIN IDEAL!!!"

The End.

OK fine, that's not at all what happened. *But let me act out my innate "flair for drama"* (my therapist's words, not mine). Here's what actually happened:

I got home and brought the box over from my parents' house to my brand-new apartment in Cambridge to take photos of the clothes. I hung each piece of clothing, one by one, on a little hanger, snapping a picture of the front, the back, and its tags. In about a week, I had received a package of one hundred hot-pink plastic mailers, and my spectacular roommate handwrote little pink thank-you cards to put in each package. That's right, I sold all those teeny tiny clothes on Depop! Gotta make back at least *some* of that coin. That shit ain't cheap. Added bonus, the whole process made for some dope TikTok and Instagram vids. It may not be as cinematic as burning clothes while listening to Lizzo, but it did feel like I was letting go of something that had held me back for a really, really long time. Also, when my life is inevitably made into a Netflix TV show, can we just put in the alternate ending and not mention that it didn't happen? K, thanks.

If Information Is Useless, So Why This Book?

I can't believe we've arrived at the final section of this book. I'd like to say it's bittersweet, but honestly, I haven't had a life for six months, so straight-up, this is just sweet, like corn-syrup sweet.

On my walk, as I thought about what else I could offer, what could be missing, what final thought could make any difference, it dawned on me. This book is a source of information—reliably sourced, evidence-based information—but information nonetheless. And information, no matter how good, true, or well-explained, has a pretty bad track record. I mean, doesn't everyone *know* they *should* exercise? Doesn't everyone *know* they *should* eat more fruits and vegetables? If people acted on information, then why would we even need books like this? What is the point of finding good information if it doesn't prompt actual change?

You can imagine, this is a pretty distressing thought after dedicating six months of your life (including your very valuable nonexistent dating life!) to words on a page or screen. The truth is, information means nothing if you don't do something with it. So I realized that the last part of the book is really about *you*.

Eddie talked about the importance of knowing your *why*, and this step is crucial. Take it from my personal experience: wanting to look a certain way is not a strong enough *why*. Wanting to get back at people who wronged you with your awesome transformation is not a strong enough *why*. Being healthy today is so freaking hard, dude, it's full of so many pitfalls and distractions, you think that's going to be enough? Maybe it is for a few weeks or a few months, but a drive for aesthetics does not fuel a lifetime of taking care of your meat mobile!

The lesson I had to learn over and over again was you cannot hate your body into submission. And oftentimes, even attempting to do so costs you something much greater: your health. One of my all-time favorite fitness podcasters, Sal Di Stefano, told me in an interview, "Aesthetics are often the by-product of chasing health, but health is rarely a by-product of chasing aesthetics."

So find a better reason and you may find you also make better goals. "I want to be skinny," made the gym my prison. "I want to deadlift three hundred pounds" or "I want to land my backflip" made it my playground. And which do you think I'm more likely to go to, the prison or the playground? Hopefully, this book gives you some of the reasons health behaviors such as eating real food, moving your body, and even getting a good night's rest are about more than just getting abs.

Making It "Effortless"

The other piece of this is how to make these changes stick. Information and motivation can give you the push you need to do a behavior once, but the way behaviors become permanent is a much more complicated, difficult, and circuitous journey.

In "regular-people language," when we talk about "habits," we usually mean something that you do a lot in your daily life. In psychology, habits are defined as "actions that are triggered automatically in response to contextual cues that have been associated with their performance."[9] Basically, repeatedly performing the same action in the same context actually makes doing that action *less work* in that context. The contextual cue gets associated with the action, so when you encounter the cue, the action requires less motivation, less conscious thought. Without you really having to try, you just *do stuff.* You go to the bathroom, you wash your hands. You get into the car, you put on your seat belt. You pass the right kitchen cabinet, you get a piece of chocolate. (Don't judge me; it's a long walk back to my bedroom.)

This got me thinking: *Isn't this exactly what I described to Eddie in the first episode of our podcast?* (See the beginning of this chapter.) After getting past the "I want to be skinny" crap, I discovered that for me, being happy with myself meant that it was "effortless": my eating, my movement, my relationship with my body—it wasn't work or torture, it was just . . . habit.

Making and Breaking Habits

Habit formation happens in three phases:

1. **Initiation:** You choose the new habit and pick its associated context or cue.

2. **Learning:** You repeat the new habit over and over when you encounter this cue.

3. **Stability:** It's now "effortless."

So, in the spirit of finishing out the book with some science (since the next time I see the PubMed search engine I will be ripping out my non–fully functioning eyeballs), here are some evidence-based ways to make your new healthy habits stick.

Pick a Good Cue

Pick an obvious cue that you already encounter every day.[10] It could be a daily event, which you might phrase as: "After breakfast (cue), I meditate (behavior)," or "When I get into my office (cue), I do ten push-ups (behavior)." It could also be an object: "Every time I see my water bottle on my desk (cue), I will drink from it (behavior)." A powerful shortcut to habit formation is a concept dubbed "habit stacking," or "anchoring."[11] This consists of you stringing a new habit with an old habit you are already doing. For example, I wanted to get better about my skin-care routine, so I decided I would always cleanse my face directly after brushing my teeth. Because I never miss brushing my teeth, I began to consistently do my skin care. This almost lets your new behavior hitch a ride on the consistency of an existing habit, transferring that consistency over to your new habit.

Consistency Is Key

This should go without saying, but there's a lot of repetition involved here. The good news is, it will get easier and easier.[12] The bad news is, it does take effort, especially at first. I'm sorry to break it to everyone, but it probably takes more than 21 days (or whatever the cliché is) to build a habit. Research has shown it can take anywhere from 18 to 254 days for something to become automatic.[13] Habits like adding a glass of water are probably going to be a lot easier to add than habits like doing fifty sit-ups after breakfast. For a small habit, ten weeks is probably a pretty reasonable time frame to make something a habit.[14] Also, consistency does not just mean doing it over and over, it also means keeping the *actual behavior* consistent. Although variety is the spice of life, it is not the spice of habit formation. If you want to engrain the habit of eating more fruit, you're more likely to succeed by establishing something like "With my oatmeal (cue), I eat a banana (behavior)," rather than "With my oatmeal, I eat some sort of fruit."[15] Although picking different fruits may make things more interesting at first, it may make the habit take longer to form and require more motivation. So start with a fruit you love, stick to it for a bit, and then start branching out once it's effortless.

Start Small So You Can Go Big

Argh, I'm sorry to have to say this, but it's true: small changes are easier to make.[16] This doesn't mean your changes will stay small, but the key concept is to *start*. Research has shown that smaller changes are easier to implement and will increase self-efficacy. This means that if you're successful at making a behavior change, even if it's small, you feel like a baddie, which can give you the confidence to pursue bigger changes. (Note to Eddie: A "baddie" is a good thing.) Conversely, failing at something makes you feel like crap, and feeling like crap does not ever make you feel like doing anything good. (These are the researchers' words, not mine, obviously.)

The awesome thing is that even if you only ever make small changes, the effect will be huge. Eddie once shared a great analogy about making small changes. I am going to steal it, but, shh, do not tell him, because I want the credit. Imagine there are two ships, parallel to each other, going in the exact same direction. One ship makes a 1-degree turn. If you saw these ships, to the naked eye, they would likely still look like they were going in the exact same direction. Maybe in a couple hundred feet you would start to notice a larger gap. Now think about years down the line: you wouldn't even know that those ships were, at one point, going to the same place, just from a 1-degree change. Small changes, given time, become massive.

Make It Rewarding

You know how we've talked a lot about dopamine and how it reinforces behaviors? A lot of habits that aren't good for us—snacking on hyper-palatable foods, smoking, drinking, watching TV, and skipping the gym—are rewarding in the short term. They *feel* good, but in the long term, they screw us over. On the other hand, habits that are good for us—exercising, eating well, going to sleep early—can be boring, annoying, and even painful (*leg days*, you know the vibes). These behaviors have long-term rewards that can take weeks or months, hell, *years* to see. So what do we have to do? Use our own neurobiology to help us, of course! If you perceive a behavior as rewarding or pleasurable, you're more likely to do it, and thus it's more likely to become a habit.[17]

If you hate veggies, find a way to make them taste good. If you hate cooking, find a way to make it fun, such as doing it with a friend or working your way through a cookbook. If you don't like the gym, find awesome music you only listen to while working out. Even positive affirmations, like thinking to yourself, *Yes, I did it!!!* (no matter how corny it sounds), can help you perceive behavior as rewarding. Research has also shown that intrinsically motivated behaviors, meaning you're doing it because *you* see some benefit, not because your doctor or mom said so, are also more likely to become habits.[18]

Add Habits Before Taking Away Habits

Research has shown that people are more likely to accomplish approach-oriented goals rather than avoidance-oriented goals.[19] So something like "At lunch, I will eat one serving of vegetables" is more likely to succeed in the long run than "At lunch, I will not eat a bag of chips." You can't form a habit of *not* doing something; you can only *break* existing habits. Research shows that breaking existing habits may actually be harder than forming new ones.[20] So maybe at first, you'll have both vegetables and chips at lunch, but after a while, you'll feel like you're actually OK with just the vegetables.

Take Advantage of Friction

Friction is a tool that you can use both in forming new habits and in *breaking* old habits. Think of friction as the amount of resistance between you and accomplishing a behavior. We can see how companies use (or abuse?) friction all the time in our daily lives to get us to do what they want: Netflix starts automatically playing the next episode so you don't have time to even think about whether you want to watch it or not; Amazon has now made checking out take only one touch; and so on.

But friction need not be a source of evil; we can use it to help us. For example, in one study, researchers gave subjects stale popcorn to eat while watching a movie.[21] Those who were habitual movie-popcorn eaters ate substantially more of the popcorn than nonhabitual popcorn eaters, even though both groups reported that the popcorn was bad. Because it was their habit to eat popcorn in that context (at the movies), whether it was fresh or stale didn't matter—it was going down the hatch. When they were asked to eat with their nondominant hand, however, they ate substantially less. Because it was no longer automatic, they actually had time to think, *Hey, this popcorn is pretty bad. I don't even want this.* Even that tiny bit of friction was able to interfere with that automatic behavior.

We can reduce the friction for habits we want to add. Things like laying out your gym clothes the night before or putting the fruit bowl in the middle of the table where you can easily reach it reduce the effort that it takes you to perform the desired new habit. We can also add friction for bad habits. I've put TikTok three-folders-deep in my phone so it takes forever to get to. Eddie keeps his ice cream in a freezer in the basement (exposed!). The aim is to make behaviors we want to encourage as automatic as possible and those we want to discourage or reduce as effortful as possible.

The Takeaways

Let's talk about how we can actually make lasting change.

- Before deciding to make a lifestyle change, figure out your *why*: What matters most to you? (Hint: You'll have a higher likelihood of success if your "why" is more than looking a certain way.)

- Habits are ways that we can make new lifestyle changes easier and more permanent.

- A habit is an action that you perform automatically when you get exposed to a certain context or cue.

- A new action will be hard at first, but the more you repeat it, the easier it gets.

- It's easier to form a new habit than break an old habit. Try replacing old habits with new ones.

- Here are some ways to make forming a habit easier: make it more immediately rewarding, reduce the "friction" associated with the habit, and try pairing it with habits you already have.

Epilogue

To the Reader

From Eddie

When our beloved podcast agent, Ben Riskin, emailed us about possibly submitting a book proposal, I was busy seeing patients. I planned to call Juna at the end of the day to explain that having written two books previously, I know it's a ton of work. Also, I had my doubts about whether we had abundant material to share and whether I had enough time and energy to pursue writing a book. However, by the time I returned to my email, I was delighted and not surprised that Juna had already enthusiastically accepted for both of us and that a meeting with the publisher was already on my calendar.

To Juna: When we met, I assumed the role as a mentor helping guide you through your evolving relationship with food. But I was soon grabbing your coattails as you drove fearlessly forward. Thank you for your youthful exuberance in initiating this journey of researching and writing this book, and more so for energetically completing the work.

I was delighted and moved by the process of cowriting a book with you; I loved our back-and-forth about all sorts of topics—sleep, food, exercise, and stress. The process was much like creating an extremely lengthy long-form podcast, in which we were able to get deep into the science and our feelings about some very emotional topics, like eating. Our conversations about your eating disorder helped me subsequently broach this subject more deeply with my own daughter.

For those of you that may be wondering, Becca continues to make progress with restricting less and making better choices about food. As she noted, "I still have more thoughts about food than the average person, but it's like the volume is turned down, so it's now background noise. I still struggle with body image, but being healthy and eating all the nutrients I need is so much more important to me than restricting. I feel alive and well again, with vitality and joy."

My hope is that our work on the podcast and this book will be used by individuals to take the steps to come to peace with their weight while working to improve their health. But this transformation for individuals isn't going to happen in a vacuum. My fondest dream is that our work will also be used for medical education, so that future physicians and all health-care professionals can improve their own health and have the confidence and skills to help their patients, families, communities, and the larger health-care system.

Change is possible: In the handful of decades since the 1960s, America has been able to transform itself and shake a bad smoking habit. I really want to see a headline that American medicine has come to its senses and recognizes that our centuries-long experiment of treating our existing diseases is not working: the subject of this experiment, the American public, is getting sicker, dying sooner, and going bankrupt in the process. Yet I remain hopeful and optimistic that there is a path forward, led by intrepid young people like Juna. To you, our readers, I wish for you the blessing of good health undergirded by wise choices that bring you joy in the short term and good health in the long term. I hope to continue to make my contribution as best I can for many years to come.

From Juna

I'm going to be 100 percent honest with you guys. When we were approached to write a book, I was like *"Hell yes!!! Finally, this is the clout I've been deserving, yo!"* This was immediately followed by a year of "Good lord baby Jesus, who on God's green earth trusted me, a crop-top-collecting failed concert pianist, with this task?"

The astonishingly good news is, I finally found a use for my college degree. Thank you, Harvard, for teaching me how to read scientific papers. (Lord knows nothing else I heard in those brick buildings was even remotely applicable to literally anything in life.) The second piece of good news is that I did not have to do this alone.

There are no words to describe how helpful Eddie has been in the book-writing process. I love writing (as you can probably tell, because I never shut up), but, dear God, do I hate proofreading. This man has *painstakingly* read every single word I have written, every sarcastic parenthetical aside, every sassy chapter subheading, *countless times,* just to add commas, correct spellings, and fix fonts. His advice and ideas have sparked inspiration on the bleakest days when I felt depleted and devoid of words to write. And above all, his undying optimism has *literally* kept me going. The number of times I would call Eddie and say things like, "I don't think we can finish this," only to have him go, in his usual jovial tone, "Oh sure, it'll get done! Don't worry about it! Just plug away!" For some reason, I chose to never question him and just accepted it. If Eddie says it can be done, then it can be done. He's a doctor, right? He knows these things. Well, as has become an extremely consistent pattern, he indeed was right.

This book is, at its core, for my younger self. I wish I had it for all the times I stepped off a scale crying, or tried some stupid diet, or forced myself to run another mile on the human hamster wheel (I mean, treadmill). Weight, health, body image—these topics are so nuanced and complicated that I don't pretend for a second that everything in this book is 100 percent right. But no matter what, I do wholeheartedly believe that what we've talked about can at least help those reading it make more informed decisions, whatever their goals are.

Sometimes I feel like I occupy this weird middle ground that I don't often see represented in the media. I don't think that everyone needs to know how many calories are in everything. At the same time, I don't think that "tracking your macros" always means you have an unhealthy relationship with food. I think there are good ways and bad ways of approaching every goal. Fundamentally, I believe in the individuality and autonomy of every single person as a being capable of growth, reflection, and choice. And I feel so lucky to have experienced my life so far and to have had the opportunity to hopefully turn it into something useful. Because, lord knows, there's no other silver lining to eating five scoops of protein powder a day.

Obviously, I still wake up and have bad body-image days. I still have days when I have a lot of food at lunch and think, *Oh man, I should have less food at dinner.* I have days when I really think if I could change how much I weighed, the (XYZ) problem in my life would be fixed. But the good thing is, those days have become more and more rare. I fall into those old familiar traps less often, and when I do fall in, I know how to get out.

As freaking clichéd as it sounds, the older I get, the more I realize what really matters. (PS: I don't know why getting sappy is a symptom of getting older, but it's happening to me, too. Help.) I love making home-made bubble tea in my sister's new apartment in DC—cheese foam, crème brûlée topping, and all—and not stressing about the calories and sugar. I love my mom's homemade spanakopita, even if it has fifty pounds of butter and flaky phyllo dough. I love taking impromptu snowboarding trips to Oregon and Utah, even if it means I can't sit for the next three months and it drastically impairs my gym gains. At the end of the day, these are the things I'll remember, not what I weighed or how many calories I ate or how much I could deadlift. (OK, fine, I might remember that last one, hee-hee—355 pounds.)

Anyway, I am literally allergic to being serious for more than a few sentences, so unfortunately, I've reached my cap. Go forth, eat some food, move around, get some sleep, relax a bit, and for God's sake, please don't ever set crop tops on fire in your backyard, no matter how awesome of an ending it would make to a book!

With love,

Juna and Eddie

Acknowledgments

Eddie would like to acknowledge the passion and persistence of colleagues who have worked tirelessly to spread the wisdom of Lifestyle Medicine that serves as the foundation of this book. To Tracy Gaudet, Adam Rindfleisch, Ben Kligler, and numerous other leaders for creating and disseminating Whole Health across the VA and beyond.

To my patients, over decades of practice, who have graciously shared moments of both suffering and success. Your resiliency and creative dedication to lifestyle change is enduringly inspiring. It is a privilege to serve you and learn from you. You are my greatest teachers.

To Aliza Phillips for your energetic editing and keen insights on early drafts. To my daughter Becca for your candidness and vulnerability in sharing the challenges of your eating disorder so that others might draw inspiration.

Juna would like to profusely thank:

Eric Larson, David Armenta, and any other of my incredibly smart PhD-holding friends who took the time to patiently explain carbohydrate metabolism or other such concepts to me when I would call them on the phone crying.

My sisters, Nensi and Wendi, for both contributing their laptops to the cause of meeting deadlines on various family trips, even though this meant their accessibility settings were "all messed up" after. I know you both secretly enjoy that sexy, sexy increased contrast. Don't lie to me.

Jenna Brooks for painstakingly helping to convert all references from *APA* style to *Chicago* style. You are a saint, and that is not hyperbole.

My baby cousin Niki (also known as my personal wealth manager) for constantly asking me, "So, how much money did you make from this?" and equally my baby cousin Matilda for not caring. You both make me giggle.

Mommy, Babi, Auntie, Nena: You guys are my love, and you give me such amazing material for Eastern European family anecdotes. Keep the content coming, baby.

My friends: Michelle, Hannah, Lina, David, John, Emily, and so many others. I'm so glad you're all here with me to laugh at and lament the ridiculousness that is life. Thank you for being so patient with me, especially when I was swamped with book deadlines!

There are a whole slew of people without whom this book would not have been possible.

Firstly, thank you to our agent, Ben Riskin, and Kathy Doyle at Macmillan for originating the idea of writing a book—something that seems just as unbelievable now as it did when y'all first brought it up.

Thank you to our astute editor Elizabeth Beier for her thoughtful commentary and for saving us from ourselves. (Your knack for removing decidedly un-funny jokes is bar none.) Thank you to the entire team at St. Martin's Press for the million things they have done to make this book happen and being such a delight to work with.

Thank you to all the wonderful scientists and researchers who graciously reviewed our chapters or portions of them: Herman Pontzer, Param Dedhia, Jennifer Thomas, Katharina Vester, Wayne Westcott, Rachele Pojednic, Paul Kenny, and others. And to those who took the time to verbally clarify their research with us: Christopher Gardner, Paul MacLean, James Levine, Charles Czeisler, Daryl O'Connor, and others. Rest assured, any mistakes in this book are definitely ours, not theirs.

To our enthusiastic listeners for sharing their comments, praise, and questions that have propelled the podcast.

To our *Food, We Need to Talk* podcast team at PRX: Thanks for putting up with us when we were frazzled, sleep-deprived, and cranky due to book deadlines.

And thanks to our families for similarly putting up with us during aforementioned times of sleep-deprived-ness and crankiness.

And lastly, thank you to Carey Goldberg, our "fairy godmother," and George Hicks for introducing us and forming the fabulous O.G. team FWNTT.

Notes

1. From the Victorians to the Kardashians

1. Katharina Vester, "Regime Change: Gender, Class, and the Invention of Dieting in Post-Bellum America," *Journal of Social History* 44, no. 1 (2010): 39–70, https://www.jstor.org/stable/40802108.

2. Vester, "Regime Change."

3. Vester, "Regime Change."

4. Vester, "Regime Change."

5. Vester, "Regime Change."

6. Brett Silverstein et al., "The Role of the Mass Media in Promoting a Thin Standard of Bodily Attractiveness for Women," *Sex Roles* 14, no. 9–10 (May 1986): 519–32, https://doi.org/10.1007/BF00287452.

7. Kristen Harrison and Joanne Cantor, "The Relationship Between Media Consumption and Eating Disorders," *Journal of Communication* 47, no. 1 (March 1, 1997): 40–67, https://doi.org/10.1111/j.1460-2466.1997.tb02692.x.

8. Nia S. Mitchell et al., "Obesity: Overview of an Epidemic," *Psychiatric Clinics of North America* 34, no. 4 (December 2011): 717–32, https://doi.org/10.1016/j.psc.2011.08.005.

9. Sarah E. McComb and Jennifer S. Mills, "The Effect of Physical Appearance Perfectionism and Social Comparison to Thin-, Slim-Thick-, and Fit-Ideal Instagram Imagery on Young Women's Body Image," *Body Image* 40 (March 2022): 165–75, https://doi.org/10.1016/j.bodyim.2021.12.003.

10. McComb and Mills, "The Effect of Physical Appearance Perfectionism and Social Comparison to Thin-, Slim-Thick-, and Fit-Ideal Instagram Imagery on Young Women's Body Image."

2. Metabolism and the Physiology of Weight Loss

1. Andrea C. Buchholz and Dale A. Schoeller, "Is a Calorie a Calorie?" *American Journal of Clinical Nutrition* 79, no. 5 (May 1, 2004): 899S–906S, https://doi.org/10.1093/ajcn/79.5.899S.

2. Buchholz and Schoeller, "Is a Calorie a Calorie?"

3. Buchholz and Schoeller, "Is a Calorie a Calorie?"

4. Buchholz and Schoeller, "Is a Calorie a Calorie?"

5. Buchholz and Schoeller, "Is a Calorie a Calorie?"

6. Christian von Loeffelholz and Andreas Birkenfeld, "The Role of Non-Exercise Activity Thermogenesis in Human Obesity," in *Endotext,* ed. Kenneth R. Feingold et al. (South Dartmouth, MA: MDText.com, Inc., 2000), http://www.ncbi.nlm.nih.gov/books/NBK279077/.

7. Abdul G. Dulloo, Josiane Seydoux, and Jean Jacquet, "Adaptive Thermogenesis and Uncoupling Proteins: A Reappraisal of Their Roles in Fat Metabolism and Energy Balance," *Physiology & Behavior* 83, no. 4 (December 2004): 587–602, https://doi.org/10.1016/j.physbeh.2004.07.028.

8. Von Loeffelholz and Birkenfeld, "The Role of Non-Exercise Activity Thermogenesis in Human Obesity."

9. Dulloo, Seydoux, and Jacquet, "Adaptive Thermogenesis and Uncoupling Proteins."

10. Franesco Zurlo et al., "Skeletal Muscle Metabolism Is a Major Determinant of Resting Energy Expenditure," *Journal of Clinical Investigation* 86, no. 5 (November 1, 1990): 1423–27, https://doi.org/10.1172/JCI114857.

11. Zurlo et al., "Skeletal Muscle Metabolism Is a Major Determinant of Resting Energy Expenditure."

12. Von Loeffelholz and Birkenfeld, "The Role of Non-Exercise Activity Thermogenesis in Human Obesity."

13. Dulloo, Seydoux, and Jacquet, "Adaptive Thermogenesis and Uncoupling Proteins."

14. William T. Donahoo, James A. Levine, and Edward L. Melanson, "Variability in Energy Expenditure and Its Components," *Current Opinion in Clinical Nutrition and Metabolic Care* 7, no. 6 (November 2004): 599–605, https://doi.org/10.1097/00075197-200411000-00003.

15. Buchholz and Schoeller, "Is a Calorie a Calorie?"

16. Von Loeffelholz and Birkenfeld, "The Role of Non-Exercise Activity Thermogenesis in Human Obesity."

17. Dulloo, Seydoux, and Jacquet, "Adaptive Thermogenesis and Uncoupling Proteins."

18. Donahoo, Levine, and Melanson, "Variability in Energy Expenditure and Its Components."

19. Debra L. Blackwell and Tainya C. Clarke, "State Variation in Meeting the 2008 Federal Guidelines for Both Aerobic and Muscle-Strengthening Activities Through Leisure-Time Physical Activity Among Adults Aged 18–64: United States, 2010–2015," *National Health Statistics Reports* 112 (June 2018): 1–22, https://www.cdc.gov/nchs/data/nhsr/nhsr112.pdf.

20. Von Loeffelholz and Birkenfeld, "The Role of Non-Exercise Activity Thermogenesis in Human Obesity."

21. Dulloo, Seydoux, and Jacquet, "Adaptive Thermogenesis and Uncoupling Proteins."

22. Donahoo, Levine, and Melanson, "Variability in Energy Expenditure and Its Components."

23. Von Loeffelholz and Birkenfeld, "The Role of Non-Exercise Activity Thermogenesis in Human Obesity."

24. Dulloo, Seydoux, and Jacquet, "Adaptive Thermogenesis and Uncoupling Proteins."

25. Donahoo, Levine, and Melanson, "Variability in Energy Expenditure and Its Components."

26. J. Vina et al., "Exercise Acts as a Drug: The Pharmacological Benefits of Exercise," *British Journal of Pharmacology* 167, no. 1 (September 2012): 1–12, https://doi.org/10.1111/j.1476-5381.2012.01970.x.

27. Paul S. MacLean et al., "Regular Exercise Attenuates the Metabolic Drive to Regain Weight After Long-Term Weight Loss," *American Journal of Physiology—Regulatory, Integrative and Comparative Physiology* 297, no. 3 (September 2009): R793–802, https://doi.org/10.1152/ajpregu.00192.2009.

28. A. E. Black et al., "Human Energy Expenditure in Affluent Societies: An Analysis of 574 Doubly-Labelled Water Measurements," *European Journal of*

Clinical Nutrition 50, no. 2 (February 1996): 72–92, https://europepmc.org /article/med/8641250#abstract.

29. Black et al., "Human Energy Expenditure in Affluent Societies."

30. Black et al., "Human Energy Expenditure in Affluent Societies."

31. J. A. Levine, "Nonexercise Activity Thermogenesis—Liberating the Life-Force," *Journal of Internal Medicine* 262, no. 3 (September 2007): 273–87, https://doi.org/10.1111/j.1365-2796.2007.01842.x.

32. Levine, "Nonexercise Activity Thermogenesis."

33. Susan B. Sisson et al., "Characteristics of Step-Defined Physical Activity Categories in U.S. Adults," *American Journal of Health Promotion* 26, no. 3 (January 2012): 152–59, https://doi.org/10.4278/ajhp.100326-QUAN-95.

34. Levine, "Nonexercise Activity Thermogenesis."

35. Darcy L. Johannsen et al., "Differences in Daily Energy Expenditure in Lean and Obese Women: The Role of Posture Allocation," *Obesity* 16, no. 1 (January 2008): 34–39, https://doi.org/10.1038/oby.2007.15.

36. Isabella P. Carneiro et al., "Is Obesity Associated with Altered Energy Expenditure?" *Advances in Nutrition* 7, no. 3 (May 1, 2016): 476–87, https://doi .org/10.3945/an.115.008755.

37. Levine, "Nonexercise Activity Thermogenesis."

38. Erin Fothergill et al., "Persistent Metabolic Adaptation 6 Years After 'The Biggest Loser' Competition: Persistent Metabolic Adaptation," *Obesity* 24, no. 8 (August 2016): 1612–19, https://doi.org/10.1002/oby.21538.

39. Levine, "Nonexercise Activity Thermogenesis."

40. Levine, "Nonexercise Activity Thermogenesis."

41. Herman Pontzer et al., "Hunter-Gatherer Energetics and Human Obesity," ed. Farid F. Chehab, *PLoS ONE* 7, no. 7 (July 25, 2012): e40503, https://doi .org/10.1371/journal.pone.0040503.

42. Pontzer et al., "Hunter-Gatherer Energetics and Human Obesity."

43. D. A. Schoeller and E. van Santen, "Measurement of Energy Expenditure in Humans by Doubly Labeled Water Method," *Journal of Applied Physiology* 53, no. 4 (October 1, 1982): 955–59, https://doi.org/10.1152/jappl.1982.53 .4.955.

44. Pontzer et al., "Hunter-Gatherer Energetics and Human Obesity."

45. Dulloo, Seydoux, and Jacquet, "Adaptive Thermogenesis and Uncoupling Proteins."

46. Fothergill et al., "Persistent Metabolic Adaptation 6 Years After 'The Biggest Loser' Competition."

47. Fothergill et al., "Persistent Metabolic Adaptation 6 Years After 'The Biggest Loser' Competition."

48. Fothergill et al., "Persistent Metabolic Adaptation 6 Years After 'The Biggest Loser' Competition."

49. Fothergill et al., "Persistent Metabolic Adaptation 6 Years After 'The Biggest Loser' Competition."

50. Von Loeffelholz and Birkenfeld, "The Role of Non-Exercise Activity Thermogenesis in Human Obesity."

51. Dulloo, Seydoux, and Jacquet, "Adaptive Thermogenesis and Uncoupling Proteins."

52. Fothergill et al., "Persistent Metabolic Adaptation 6 Years After 'The Biggest Loser' Competition."

53. Paul S. MacLean et al., "Biology's Response to Dieting: The Impetus for Weight Regain," *American Journal of Physiology—Regulatory, Integrative and Comparative Physiology* 301, no. 3 (September 2011): R581–600, https://doi.org/10.1152/ajpregu.00755.2010.

54. Corby K. Martin et al., "Effect of Calorie Restriction on Resting Metabolic Rate and Spontaneous Physical Activity," *Obesity* 15, no. 12 (December 2007): 2964–73, https://doi.org/10.1038/oby.2007.354.

55. Pontzer et al., "Hunter-Gatherer Energetics and Human Obesity."

56. Kevin D. Hall, "Energy Compensation and Metabolic Adaptation: 'The Biggest Loser' Study Reinterpreted," *Obesity* 30, no. 1 (January 2022): 11–13, https://doi.org/10.1002/oby.23308.

57. Herman Pontzer et al., "Constrained Total Energy Expenditure and Metabolic Adaptation to Physical Activity in Adult Humans," *Current Biology* 26, no. 3 (February 8, 2016): 410–17, https://doi.org/10.1016/j.cub.2015.12.046.

58. Robert Ross and Ian Janssen, "Physical Activity, Total and Regional Obesity: Dose-Response Considerations," *Medicine and Science in Sports and Exercise* 33

(June 1, 2001): S521–27, discussion S528, https://doi.org/10.1097/00005768 -200106001-00023.

59. Hall, "Energy Compensation and Metabolic Adaptation."

60. Pontzer et al., "Constrained Total Energy Expenditure and Metabolic Adaptation to Physical Activity in Adult Humans."

61. Hall, "Energy Compensation and Metabolic Adaptation."

62. Vincent Careau et al., "Energy Compensation and Adiposity in Humans," *Current Biology* 31, no. 20 (October 2021): 4659–66.e2, https://doi.org/10 .1016/j.cub.2021.08.016.

63. Hall, "Energy Compensation and Metabolic Adaptation."

64. Pontzer et al., "Constrained Total Energy Expenditure and Metabolic Adaptation to Physical Activity in Adult Humans."

65. Herman Pontzer, "Energy Constraint as a Novel Mechanism Linking Exercise and Health," *Physiology* 33, no. 6 (November 1, 2018): 384–93, https: //doi.org/10.1152/physiol.00027.2018.

66. Pontzer, "Energy Constraint as a Novel Mechanism Linking Exercise and Health."

67. Pontzer, "Energy Constraint as a Novel Mechanism Linking Exercise and Health."

68. Pontzer, "Energy Constraint as a Novel Mechanism Linking Exercise and Health."

69. Pontzer, "Energy Constraint as a Novel Mechanism Linking Exercise and Health."

70. Anthony Hackney et al., "Endurance Exercise Training and Male Sexual Libido," *Medicine & Science in Sports & Exercise* 49 (February 1, 2017): 1, https: //doi.org/10.1249/MSS.0000000000001235.

71. Pontzer, "Energy Constraint as a Novel Mechanism Linking Exercise and Health."

72. Herman Pontzer, "Constrained Total Energy Expenditure and the Evolutionary Biology of Energy Balance," *Exercise and Sport Sciences Reviews* 43, no. 3 (July 2015): 110–16, https://doi.org/10.1249/JES.00000000000 00048.

73. Pontzer, "Constrained Total Energy Expenditure and the Evolutionary Biology of Energy Balance."

74. James A. Levine, Norman L. Eberhardt, and Michael D. Jensen, "Role of Nonexercise Activity Thermogenesis in Resistance to Fat Gain in Humans," *Science* 283, no. 5399 (January 8, 1999): 212–14, https://doi.org/10.1126/science.283.5399.212.

75. Claude Bouchard et al., "The Response to Long-Term Overfeeding in Identical Twins," *New England Journal of Medicine* 322, no. 21 (May 24, 1990): 1477–82, https://doi.org/10.1056/NEJM199005243222101.

76. Bouchard et al., "The Response to Long-Term Overfeeding in Identical Twins."

77. Bouchard et al., "The Response to Long-Term Overfeeding in Identical Twins."

78. Levine, Eberhardt, and Jensen, "Role of Nonexercise Activity Thermogenesis in Resistance to Fat Gain in Humans."

79. John W. Apolzan et al., "Effects of Weight Gain Induced by Controlled Overfeeding on Physical Activity," *American Journal of Physiology—Endocrinology and Metabolism* 307, no. 11 (December 1, 2014): E1030–37, https://doi.org/10.1152/ajpendo.00386.2014.

80. Apolzan et al., "Effects of Weight Gain Induced by Controlled Overfeeding on Physical Activity."

81. Eric T. Trexler, Abbie E. Smith-Ryan, and Layne E. Norton, "Metabolic Adaptation to Weight Loss: Implications for the Athlete," *Journal of the International Society of Sports Nutrition* 11, no. 1 (August 15, 2014): 7, https://doi.org/10.1186/1550-2783-11-7.

82. Trexler, Smith-Ryan, and Norton, "Metabolic Adaptation to Weight Loss: Implications for the Athlete."

83. Pontzer et al., "Constrained Total Energy Expenditure and Metabolic Adaptation to Physical Activity in Adult Humans."

84. Pontzer, "Energy Constraint as a Novel Mechanism Linking Exercise and Health."

85. Hall, "Energy Compensation and Metabolic Adaptation."

86. Herman Pontzer et al., "Daily Energy Expenditure through the Human Life Course," *Science* 373, no. 6556 (August 13, 2021): 808–12, https://doi.org/10.1126/science.abe5017.

87. Pontzer et al., "Daily Energy Expenditure through the Human Life Course."

88. Pontzer et al., "Daily Energy Expenditure through the Human Life Course."

89. Pontzer et al., "Daily Energy Expenditure through the Human Life Course."

90. Pontzer et al., "Daily Energy Expenditure through the Human Life Course."

91. Todd M. Manini, "Energy Expenditure and Aging," *Ageing Research Reviews* 9, no. 1 (January 2010): 1–11, https://doi.org/10.1016/j.arr.2009.08.002.

92. Manini, "Energy Expenditure and Aging."

93. Manini, "Energy Expenditure and Aging."

94. Mark D. Peterson, Ananda Sen, and Paul M. Gordon, "Influence of Resistance Exercise on Lean Body Mass in Aging Adults: A Meta-Analysis," *Medicine & Science in Sports & Exercise* 43, no. 2 (February 2011): 249–58, https://doi.org/10.1249/MSS.0b013e3181eb6265.

95. Manini, "Energy Expenditure and Aging."

96. Pontzer et al., "Daily Energy Expenditure through the Human Life Course."

3. Why All Diets Work . . . Then Don't

1. Eurídice Martínez Steele et al., "Ultra-Processed Foods and Added Sugars in the US Diet: Evidence from a Nationally Representative Cross-Sectional Study," *BMJ Open* 6, no. 3 (January 2016): e009892, https://doi.org/10.1136/bmjopen-2015-009892.

2. Zhilei Shan et al., "Trends in Dietary Carbohydrate, Protein, and Fat Intake and Diet Quality Among US Adults, 1999–2016," *JAMA* 322, no. 12 (September 24, 2019): 1178, https://doi.org/10.1001/jama.2019.13771.

3. John R. Speakman and Catherine Hambly, "Starving for Life: What Animal Studies Can and Cannot Tell Us About the Use of Caloric Restriction to Prolong Human Lifespan," *The Journal of Nutrition* 137, no. 4 (April 1, 2007): 1078–86, https://doi.org/10.1093/jn/137.4.1078.

4. Corey A. Rynders et al., "Effectiveness of Intermittent Fasting and Time-Restricted Feeding Compared to Continuous Energy Restriction for Weight Loss," *Nutrients* 11, no. 10 (October 14, 2019): 2442, https://doi.org/10.3390/nu11102442.

5. Kevin D. Hall et al., "Energy Expenditure and Body Composition Changes After an Isocaloric Ketogenic Diet in Overweight and Obese Men," *The*

American Journal of Clinical Nutrition 104, no. 2 (August 2016): 324–33, https://doi.org/10.3945/ajcn.116.133561.

6.   Rynders et al., "Effectiveness of Intermittent Fasting and Time-Restricted Feeding Compared to Continuous Energy Restriction for Weight Loss."

7.   Douglas Paddon-Jones et al., "Protein, Weight Management, and Satiety," *American Journal of Clinical Nutrition* 87, no. 5 (May 1, 2008): 1558S–61S, https://doi.org/10.1093/ajcn/87.5.1558S.

8.   Jennie Macdiarmid and John Blundell, "Assessing Dietary Intake: Who, What and Why of Under-Reporting," *Nutrition Research Reviews* 11, no. 2 (December 1998): 231–53, https://doi.org/10.1079/NRR19980017.

9.   Hall et al., "Energy Expenditure and Body Composition Changes After an Isocaloric Ketogenic Diet in Overweight and Obese Men."

10.   Christopher D. Gardner et al., "Effect of Low-Fat vs. Low-Carbohydrate Diet on 12-Month Weight Loss in Overweight Adults and the Association with Genotype Pattern or Insulin Secretion: The DIETFITS Randomized Clinical Trial," *JAMA* 319, no. 7 (February 20, 2018): 667, https://doi.org/10.1001/jama.2018.0245.

11.   Gardner et al., "Effect of Low-Fat vs. Low-Carbohydrate Diet on 12-Month Weight Loss in Overweight Adults and the Association with Genotype Pattern or Insulin Secretion."

12.   Dylan A. Lowe et al., "Effects of Time-Restricted Eating on Weight Loss and Other Metabolic Parameters in Women and Men with Overweight and Obesity: The TREAT Randomized Clinical Trial," *JAMA Internal Medicine* 180, no. 11 (November 1, 2020): 1491, https://doi.org/10.1001/jamainternmed.2020.4153.

13.   James W. Anderson et al., "Long-Term Weight-Loss Maintenance: A Meta-Analysis of US Studies," *American Journal of Clinical Nutrition* 74, no. 5 (November 1, 2001): 579–84, https://doi.org/10.1093/ajcn/74.5.579.

14.   Michael R. Lowe et al., "Dieting and Restrained Eating as Prospective Predictors of Weight Gain," *Frontiers in Psychology* 4 (2013), https://doi.org/10.3389/fpsyg.2013.00577.

15.   A. G. Dulloo et al., "How Dieting Makes the Lean Fatter: From a Perspective of Body Composition Autoregulation through Adipostats and Protein-stats Awaiting Discovery," *Obesity Reviews* 16 (February 2015): 25–35, https://doi.org/10.1111/obr.12253.

16.   Eric Stice et al., "Naturalistic Weight-Reduction Efforts Prospectively
      Predict Growth in Relative Weight and Onset of Obesity Among Female
      Adolescents.," *Journal of Consulting and Clinical Psychology* 67, no. 6 (1999):
      967–74, https://doi.org/10.1037/0022-006X.67.6.967.

17.   Maarit Korkeila et al., "Weight-Loss Attempts and Risk of Major Weight
      Gain: A Prospective Study in Finnish Adults," *American Journal of Clinical
      Nutrition* 70, no. 6 (December 1, 1999): 965–75, https://doi.org/10.1093/ajcn
      /70.6.965.

18.   Dulloo et al., "How Dieting Makes the Lean Fatter."

19.   Korkeila et al., "Weight-Loss Attempts and Risk of Major Weight Gain."

20.   K. H. Pietiläinen et al., "Does Dieting Make You Fat? A Twin Study," *Inter-
      national Journal of Obesity* 36, no. 3 (March 2012): 456–64, https://doi.org/10
      .1038/ijo.2011.160.

21.   S. E. Saarni et al., "Weight Cycling of Athletes and Subsequent Weight Gain
      in Middleage," *International Journal of Obesity* 30, no. 11 (November 2006):
      1639–44, https://doi.org/10.1038/sj.ijo.0803325.

22.   Ancel Keys et al., *The Biology of Human Starvation*, 2 vols. (Minneapolis: Uni-
      versity of Minnesota Press, 1950).

23.   Keys et al., *The Biology of Human Starvation.*

24.   B. Nindl et al., "Physical Performance and Metabolic Recovery Among Lean,
      Healthy Men Following a Prolonged Energy Deficit," *International Journal of
      Sports Medicine* 18, no. 5 (July 1997): 317–24, https://doi.org/10.1055/s-2007
      -972640.

25.   Paul S. MacLean et al., "Biology's Response to Dieting: The Impetus for
      Weight Regain," *American Journal of Physiology—Regulatory, Integrative and
      Comparative Physiology* 301, no. 3 (September 2011): R581–600, https://doi
      .org/10.1152/ajpregu.00755.2010.

26.   John R. Speakman et al., "Set Points, Settling Points and Some Alternative
      Models: Theoretical Options to Understand How Genes and Environments
      Combine to Regulate Body Adiposity," *Disease Models & Mechanisms* 4, no. 6
      (November 1, 2011): 733–45, https://doi.org/10.1242/dmm.008698.

27.   Korin Miller, "Charlize Theron: Gaining 50 Lbs. Was 'Depressing,'" *Yahoo!
      News*, April 19, 2018, https://sg.news.yahoo.com/charlize-theron-gaining-50
      -lbs-190200780.html?guccounter=1.

28. MacLean et al., "Biology's Response to Dieting."

29. Speakman et al., "Set Points, Settling Points and Some Alternative Models."

30. MacLean et al., "Biology's Response to Dieting."

31. MacLean et al., "Biology's Response to Dieting."

32. Paul S. MacLean et al., "The Role for Adipose Tissue in Weight Regain After Weight Loss," *Obesity Reviews* 16, no. S1 (February 2015): 45–54, https://doi.org/10.1111/obr.12255.

33. Karin G. Stenkula and Charlotte Erlanson-Albertsson, "Adipose Cell Size: Importance in Health and Disease," *American Journal of Physiology—Regulatory, Integrative and Comparative Physiology* 315, no. 2 (August 1, 2018): R284–95, https://doi.org/10.1152/ajpregu.00257.2017.

34. Rexford S. Ahima, "Revisiting Leptin's Role in Obesity and Weight Loss," *Journal of Clinical Investigation*, June 1, 2008, JCI36284, https://doi.org/10.1172/JCI36284.

35. Ahima, "Revisiting Leptin's Role in Obesity and Weight Loss."

36. Kevin D. Hall and Scott Kahan, "Maintenance of Lost Weight and Long-Term Management of Obesity," *Medical Clinics of North America* 102, no. 1 (January 2018): 183–97, https://doi.org/10.1016/j.mcna.2017.08.012.

37. Ahima, "Revisiting Leptin's Role in Obesity and Weight Loss."

38. MacLean et al., "Biology's Response to Dieting."

39. Ahima, "Revisiting Leptin's Role in Obesity and Weight Loss."

40. MacLean et al., "Biology's Response to Dieting."

41. MacLean et al., "Biology's Response to Dieting."

42. Erin Fothergill et al., "Persistent Metabolic Adaptation 6 Years After 'The Biggest Loser' Competition," *Obesity* 24, no. 8 (August 2016): 1612–19, https://doi.org/10.1002/oby.21538.

43. Herman Pontzer et al., "Hunter-Gatherer Energetics and Human Obesity," ed. Farid F. Chehab, *PLoS ONE* 7, no. 7 (July 25, 2012): e40503, https://doi.org/10.1371/journal.pone.0040503.

44. MacLean et al., "Biology's Response to Dieting."

45. MacLean et al., "Biology's Response to Dieting."

46. MacLean et al., "Biology's Response to Dieting."

47. Anderson et al., "Long-Term Weight-Loss Maintenance."

48. MacLean et al., "Biology's Response to Dieting."

49. MacLean et al., "Biology's Response to Dieting."

50. MacLean et al., "The Role for Adipose Tissue in Weight Regain After Weight Loss."

51. MacLean et al., "The Role for Adipose Tissue in Weight Regain After Weight Loss."

52. MacLean et al., "Biology's Response to Dieting."

53. MacLean et al., "The Role for Adipose Tissue in Weight Regain After Weight Loss."

54. MacLean et al., "The Role for Adipose Tissue in Weight Regain After Weight Loss."

55. MacLean et al., "The Role for Adipose Tissue in Weight Regain After Weight Loss."

56. Donna H. Ryan and Sarah Ryan Yockey, "Weight Loss and Improvement in Comorbidity: Differences at 5%, 10%, 15%, and Over," *Current Obesity Reports* 6, no. 2 (June 2017): 187–94, https://doi.org/10.1007/s13679-017-0262-y.

57. R. M. Foright et al., "Is Regular Exercise an Effective Strategy for Weight Loss Maintenance?" *Physiology & Behavior* 188 (May 2018): 86–93, https://doi.org/10.1016/j.physbeh.2018.01.025.

58. Victoria A. Catenacci et al., "Physical Activity Patterns in the National Weight Control Registry," *Obesity* 16, no. 1 (January 2008): 153–61, https://doi.org/10.1038/oby.2007.6.

59. US Department of Health and Human Services, *Physical Activity Guidelines for Americans*, 2nd ed. (2018), https://health.gov/our-work/nutrition-physical-activity/physical-activity-guidelines/current-guidelines.

60. Rena R. Wing and Suzanne Phelan, "Long-Term Weight Loss Maintenance," *American Journal of Clinical Nutrition* 82, no. 1 (July 1, 2005): 222S–25S, https://doi.org/10.1093/ajcn/82.1.222S.

61. Meghan L. Butryn et al., "Consistent Self-Monitoring of Weight: A Key Component of Successful Weight Loss Maintenance," *Obesity* 15, no. 12 (December 2007): 3091–96, https://doi.org/10.1038/oby.2007.368.

62. C. M. Goldstein et al., "Successful Weight Loss Maintainers Use Health-Tracking Smartphone Applications More Than a Nationally Representative Sample: Comparison of the National Weight Control Registry to Pew Tracking for Health: Technology Use in Weight Maintainers," *Obesity Science & Practice* 3, no. 2 (June 2017): 117–26, https://doi.org/10.1002/osp4.102.

63. C. R. Pacanowski, J. A. Linde, and D. Neumark-Sztainer, "Self-Weighing: Helpful or Harmful for Psychological Well-Being? A Review of the Literature," *Current Obesity Reports* 4, no. 1 (March 2015): 65–72, https://doi.org/10.1007/s13679-015-0142-2.

64. Wing and Phelan, "Long-Term Weight Loss Maintenance."

65. Inês Santos et al., "Weight Control Behaviors of Highly Successful Weight Loss Maintainers: The Portuguese Weight Control Registry," *Journal of Behavioral Medicine* 40, no. 2 (April 2017): 366–71, https://doi.org/10.1007/s10865-016-9786-y.

66. Santos et al., "Weight Control Behaviors of Highly Successful Weight Loss Maintainers."

67. Wing and Phelan, "Long-Term Weight Loss Maintenance."

68. Santos et al., "Weight Control Behaviors of Highly Successful Weight Loss Maintainers."

69. Sonja Ohsiek and Mary Williams, "Psychological Factors Influencing Weight Loss Maintenance: An Integrative Literature Review," *Journal of the American Academy of Nurse Practitioners* 23, no. 11 (November 2011): 592–601, https://doi.org/10.1111/j.1745-7599.2011.00647.x.

70. Ohsiek and Williams, "Psychological Factors Influencing Weight Loss Maintenance."

71. Ohsiek and Williams, "Psychological Factors Influencing Weight Loss Maintenance."

72. James O. Hill et al., "The National Weight Control Registry: Is It Useful in Helping Deal with Our Obesity Epidemic?," *Journal of Nutrition Education and Behavior* 37, no. 4 (July 2005): 206–10, https://doi.org/10.1016/S1499-4046(06)60248-0.

4. Weight and Health

1. Vojtech Hainer and Irena Aldhoon-Hainerová, "Obesity Paradox Does Exist," *Diabetes Care* 36, supp. 2 (August 1, 2013): S276–81, https://doi.org/10.2337/dcS13-2023.

2. Ahmad Jayedi et al., "Central Fatness and Risk of All Cause Mortality: Systematic Review and Dose-Response Meta-Analysis of 72 Prospective Cohort Studies," *BMJ*, September 23, 2020, m3324, https://doi.org/10.1136/bmj.m3324.

3. Mi-Jeong Lee, Yuanyuan Wu, and Susan K. Fried, "Adipose Tissue Heterogeneity: Implication of Depot Differences in Adipose Tissue for Obesity Complications," *Molecular Aspects of Medicine* 34, no. 1 (February 2013): 1–11, https://doi.org/10.1016/j.mam.2012.10.001.

4. Amy Berrington de Gonzalez et al., "Body-Mass Index and Mortality Among 1.46 Million White Adults," *New England Journal of Medicine* 363, no. 23 (December 2, 2010): 2211–19, https://doi.org/10.1056/NEJMoa1000367.

5. Steven H. Woolf and Heidi Schoomaker, "Life Expectancy and Mortality Rates in the United States, 1959–2017," *JAMA* 322, no. 20 (November 26, 2019): 1996, https://doi.org/10.1001/jama.2019.16932.

6. Ali H. Mokdad, "Actual Causes of Death in the United States, 2000," *JAMA* 291, no. 10 (March 10, 2004): 1238, https://doi.org/10.1001/jama.291.10.1238.

7. Ali H. Mokdad et al., "Correction: Actual Causes of Death in the United States, 2000," *JAMA* 293, no. 3 (2005): 293–94, https://doi.org/doi:10.1001/jama.293.3.293/.

8. Mokdad et al., "Correction."

9. Ray Moynihan, "Obesity Task Force Linked to WHO Takes 'Millions' from Drug Firms," *BMJ* 332, no. 7555 (June 17, 2006): 1412.2, https://doi.org/10.1136/bmj.332.7555.1412-a.

10. Katherine M. Flegal et al., "Excess Deaths Associated with Underweight, Overweight, and Obesity," *JAMA* 293, no. 15 (April 20, 2005): 1861–67, https://doi.org/10.1001/jama.293.15.1861.

11. Katherine M. Flegal et al., "Association of All-Cause Mortality with Overweight and Obesity Using Standard Body Mass Index Categories: A Systematic Review and Meta-Analysis," *JAMA* 309, no. 1 (January 2, 2013): 71, https://doi.org/10.1001/jama.2012.113905.

12. Berrington de Gonzalez et al., "Body-Mass Index and Mortality Among 1.46 Million White Adults."

13. Hainer and Aldhoon-Hainerová, "Obesity Paradox Does Exist."

14. Hainer and Aldhoon-Hainerová, "Obesity Paradox Does Exist."

15. Hainer and Aldhoon-Hainerová, "Obesity Paradox Does Exist."

16. Jayedi et al., "Central Fatness and Risk of All Cause Mortality."

17. Antigone Oreopoulos et al., "Association Between Direct Measures of Body Composition and Prognostic Factors in Chronic Heart Failure," *Mayo Clinic Proceedings* 85, no. 7 (July 2010): 609–17, https://doi.org/10.4065/mcp.2010.0103.

18. Oreopoulos et al., "Association Between Direct Measures of Body Composition and Prognostic Factors in Chronic Heart Failure."

19. Hainer and Aldhoon-Hainerová, "Obesity Paradox Does Exist."

20. S. Goya Wannamethee et al., "Decreased Muscle Mass and Increased Central Adiposity Are Independently Related to Mortality in Older Men," *American Journal of Clinical Nutrition* 86, no. 5 (November 1, 2007): 1339–46, https://doi.org/10.1093/ajcn/86.5.1339.

21. Wannamethee et al., "Decreased Muscle Mass and Increased Central Adiposity Are Independently Related to Mortality in Older Men."

22. Lorenzo Maria Donini et al., "Obesity or BMI Paradox? Beneath the Tip of the Iceberg," *Frontiers in Nutrition* 7 (2020), https://doi.org/10.3389/fnut.2020.00053.

23. Donini et al., "Obesity or BMI Paradox? Beneath the Tip of the Iceberg."

24. Dagfinn Aune et al., "BMI and All Cause Mortality: Systematic Review and Non-Linear Dose-Response Meta-Analysis of 230 Cohort Studies with 3.74 Million Deaths Among 30.3 Million Participants," *BMJ*, May 4, 2016, i2156, https://doi.org/10.1136/bmj.i2156.

25. Shunsuke Edakubo and Kiyohide Fushimi, "Mortality and Risk Assessment for Anorexia Nervosa in Acute-Care Hospitals: A Nationwide Administrative Database Analysis," *BMC Psychiatry* 20, no. 1 (December 2020): 19, https://doi.org/10.1186/s12888-020-2433-8.

26. Michael R. Lowe et al., "Dieting and Restrained Eating as Prospective Predictors of Weight Gain," *Frontiers in Psychology* 4 (2013), https://doi.org/10.3389/fpsyg.2013.00577.

27. A. G. Dulloo et al., "How Dieting Makes the Lean Fatter: From a Perspective of Body Composition Autoregulation through Adipostats and Proteinstats Awaiting Discovery," *Obesity Reviews* 16 (February 2015): 25–35, https://doi .org/10.1111/obr.12253.

28. J.-P. Montani et al., "Weight Cycling During Growth and Beyond as a Risk Factor for Later Cardiovascular Diseases: The 'Repeated Overshoot' Theory," *International Journal of Obesity* 30, no. S4 (December 2006): S58–66, https: //doi.org/10.1038/sj.ijo.0803520.

29. Jayedi et al., "Central Fatness and Risk of All Cause Mortality."

30. Surapon Tangvarasittichai, Suthap Pongthaisong, and Orathai Tangvarasit-tichai, "Tumor Necrosis Factor-A, Interleukin-6, C-Reactive Protein Levels and Insulin Resistance Associated with Type 2 Diabetes in Abdominal Obe-sity Women," *Indian Journal of Clinical Biochemistry* 31, no. 1 (January 2016): 68–74, https://doi.org/10.1007/s12291-015-0514-0.

31. Stephan Wueest et al., "Mesenteric Fat Lipolysis Mediates Obesity-Associated Hepatic Steatosis and Insulin Resistance," *Diabetes* 65, no. 1 (January 1, 2016): 140–48, https://doi.org/10.2337/db15-0941.

32. Kristoffer Jensen Kolnes et al., "Effect of Exercise Training on Fat Loss—Energetic Perspectives and the Role of Improved Adipose Tissue Function and Body Fat Distribution," *Frontiers in Physiology* 12 (September 24, 2021): 737709, https://doi.org/10.3389/fphys.2021.737709.

33. Kolnes et al., "Effect of Exercise Training on Fat Loss."

34. Sylvie Franckhauser et al., "Increased Fatty Acid Re-Esterification by PEPCK Overexpression in Adipose Tissue Leads to Obesity Without Insu-lin Resistance," *Diabetes* 51, no. 3 (March 2002): 624–30, https://doi.org/10 .2337/diabetes.51.3.624.

35. Donna H. Ryan and Sarah Ryan Yockey, "Weight Loss and Improvement in Comorbidity: Differences at 5%, 10%, 15%, and Over," *Current Obesity Reports* 6, no. 2 (June 2017): 187–94, https://doi.org/10.1007/s13679-017-0262-y.

36. Rebecca M. Puhl and Kelly M. King, "Weight Discrimination and Bully-ing," *Best Practice & Research Clinical Endocrinology & Metabolism* 27, no. 2 (April 2013): 117–27, https://doi.org/10.1016/j.beem.2012.12.002.

37. Puhl and King, "Weight Discrimination and Bullying."

38. Mark L. Hatzenbuehler, Katherine M. Keyes, and Deborah S. Hasin, "Associations Between Perceived Weight Discrimination and the Prevalence of Psychiatric Disorders in the General Population," *Obesity* 17, no. 11 (November 2009): 2033–39, https://doi.org/10.1038/oby.2009.131.

39. Puhl and King, "Weight Discrimination and Bullying."

40. Rebecca M. Puhl and Kelly D. Brownell, "Confronting and Coping with Weight Stigma: An Investigation of Overweight and Obese Adults," *Obesity* 14, no. 10 (October 2006): 1802–15, https://doi.org/10.1038/oby.2006.208.

41. Natasha A. Schvey, Rebecca M. Puhl, and Kelly D. Brownell, "The Impact of Weight Stigma on Caloric Consumption," *Obesity* 19, no. 10 (October 2011): 1957–62, https://doi.org/10.1038/oby.2011.204.

42. Lenny R. Vartanian and Jacqueline G. Shaprow, "Effects of Weight Stigma on Exercise Motivation and Behavior: A Preliminary Investigation Among College-Aged Females," *Journal of Health Psychology* 13, no. 1 (January 2008): 131–38, https://doi.org/10.1177/1359105307084318.

43. Puhl and King, "Weight Discrimination and Bullying."

44. Marla E. Eisenberg, Dianne Neumark-Sztainer, and Mary Story, "Associations of Weight-Based Teasing and Emotional Well-Being Among Adolescents," *Archives of Pediatrics & Adolescent Medicine* 157, no. 8 (August 1, 2003): 733, https://doi.org/10.1001/archpedi.157.8.733.

45. Eisenberg, Neumark-Sztainer, and Story, "Associations of Weight-Based Teasing and Emotional Well-Being Among Adolescents."

46. Eisenberg, Neumark-Sztainer, and Story, "Associations of Weight-Based Teasing and Emotional Well-Being Among Adolescents."

47. Danice K. Eaton et al., "Associations of Body Mass Index and Perceived Weight with Suicide Ideation and Suicide Attempts Among US High School Students," *Archives of Pediatrics & Adolescent Medicine* 159, no. 6 (June 1, 2005): 513, https://doi.org/10.1001/archpedi.159.6.513.

48. Jeanne Walsh Pierce and Jane Wardle, "Cause and Effect Beliefs and Self-Esteem of Overweight Children," *Journal of Child Psychology and Psychiatry* 38, no. 6 (September 1997): 645–50, https://doi.org/10.1111/j.1469-7610.1997.tb01691.x.

49. Heather P. Libbey et al., "Teasing, Disordered Eating Behaviors, and Psychological Morbidities Among Overweight Adolescents," *Obesity* 16, special issue:

Weight Bias: New Science on a Significant Social Problem, no. S2 (November 2008): S24–29, https://doi.org/10.1038/oby.2008.455.

50. Frank Q. Nuttall, "Body Mass Index: Obesity, BMI, and Health: A Critical Review," *Nutrition Today* 50, no. 3 (May 2015): 117–28, https://doi.org/10.1097/NT.0000000000000092.

51. Nuttall, "Body Mass Index: Obesity, BMI, and Health."

52. Thomas T. Samaras, Harold Elrick, and Lowell H. Storms, "Is Height Related to Longevity?" *Life Sciences* 72, no. 16 (March 2003): 1781–802, https://doi.org/10.1016/S0024-3205(02)02503-1.

53. Elizabeth Cohen and Anne McDermott, "Who's Fat? New Definition Adopted," CNN Interactive, June 17, 1998, http://www.cnn.com/HEALTH/9806/17/weight.guidelines/.

54. Nuttall, "Body Mass Index: Obesity, BMI, and Health."

55. Oreopoulos et al., "Association Between Direct Measures of Body Composition and Prognostic Factors in Chronic Heart Failure."

56. Nuttall, "Body Mass Index: Obesity, BMI, and Health."

57. Samaras, Elrick, and Storms, "Is Height Related to Longevity?"

58. Nuttall, "Body Mass Index: Obesity, BMI, and Health."

59. Nuttall, "Body Mass Index: Obesity, BMI, and Health."

60. Lee, Wu, and Fried, "Adipose Tissue Heterogeneity."

61. Rishi Caleyachetty et al., "Ethnicity-Specific BMI Cutoffs for Obesity Based on Type 2 Diabetes Risk in England: A Population-Based Cohort Study," *The Lancet—Diabetes & Endocrinology* 9, no. 7 (July 2021): 419–26, https://doi.org/10.1016/S2213-8587(21)00088-7.

62. Christy Harrison, *Anti-Diet: Reclaim Your Time, Money, Well-Being, and Happiness Through Intuitive Eating* (New York: Little, Brown Spark, 2019).

5. What to Eat

1. Gerald M. Oppenheimer and I. Daniel Benrubi, "McGovern's Senate Select Committee on Nutrition and Human Needs Versus the Meat Industry on the Diet-Heart Question (1976–1977)," *American Journal of Public*

Health 104, no. 1 (January 2014): 59–69, https://doi.org/10.2105/AJPH .2013.301464.

2. Select Committee on Nutrition and Human Needs, United States Senate, "Dietary Goals for the United States," February 1977, 13, https://naldc.nal .usda.gov/download/1758834/PDF.

3. Select Committee on Nutrition and Human Needs, United States Senate, "Dietary Goals for the United States," 2nd ed., December 1977, 4, https: //naldc.nal.usda.gov/download/1759572/PDF.

4. Michael Pollan, *In Defense of Food: An Eater's Manifesto* (New York: Penguin, 2009).

5. Pollan, *In Defense of Food.*

6. Oppenheimer and Benrubi, "McGovern's Senate Select Committee on Nutrition and Human Needs."

7. Nita G. Forouhi et al., "Dietary Fat and Cardiometabolic Health: Evidence, Controversies, and Consensus for Guidance," *BMJ*, June 13, 2018, k2139, https://doi.org/10.1136/bmj.k2139.

8. Forouhi et al., "Dietary Fat and Cardiometabolic Health."

9. Forouhi et al., "Dietary Fat and Cardiometabolic Health."

10. Frank B. Hu, JoAnn E. Manson, and Walter C. Willett, "Types of Dietary Fat and Risk of Coronary Heart Disease: A Critical Review," *Journal of the American College of Nutrition* 20, no. 1 (February 1, 2001): 5–19, https://doi .org/10.1080/07315724.2001.10719008.

11. Hu, Manson, and Willett, "Types of Dietary Fat and Risk of Coronary Heart Disease."

12. Oppenheimer and Benrubi, "McGovern's Senate Select Committee on Nutrition and Human Needs."

13. Eurídice Martínez Steele et al., "Ultra-Processed Foods and Added Sugars in the US Diet: Evidence from a Nationally Representative Cross-Sectional Study," *BMJ Open* 6, no. 3 (January 2016): e009892, https://doi.org/10.1136 /bmjopen-2015-009892.

14. Tanya L. Blasbalg et al., "Changes in Consumption of Omega-3 and Omega-6 Fatty Acids in the United States During the 20th Century," *American Journal*

of Clinical Nutrition 93, no. 5 (May 2011): 950–62, https://doi.org/10.3945
/ajcn.110.006643.

15. Lee S. Gross et al., "Increased Consumption of Refined Carbohydrates and
the Epidemic of Type 2 Diabetes in the United States: An Ecologic Assessment," *American Journal of Clinical Nutrition* 79, no. 5 (May 1, 2004): 774–79,
https://doi.org/10.1093/ajcn/79.5.774.

16. Blasbalg et al., "Changes in Consumption of Omega-3 and Omega-6 Fatty
Acids in the United States During the 20th Century."

17. Fred A. Kummerow, "The Negative Effects of Hydrogenated Trans Fats and
What to Do About Them," *Atherosclerosis* 205, no. 2 (August 1, 2009): 458–
65, https://doi.org/10.1016/j.atherosclerosis.2009.03.009.

18. David J. McClements, "Reduced-Fat Foods: The Complex Science of Developing
Diet-Based Strategies for Tackling Overweight and Obesity," *Advances in Nutrition* 6, no. 3 (May 2015): 338S–52S, https://doi.org/10.3945/an.114.006999.

19. Gross et al., "Increased Consumption of Refined Carbohydrates and the Epidemic of Type 2 Diabetes in the United States."

20. Gross et al., "Increased Consumption of Refined Carbohydrates and the Epidemic of Type 2 Diabetes in the United States."

21. Gross et al., "Increased Consumption of Refined Carbohydrates and the Epidemic of Type 2 Diabetes in the United States."

22. Michael Pollan, *The Omnivore's Dilemma: A Natural History of Four Meals*
(New York: Penguin, 2007).

23. Blasbalg et al., "Changes in Consumption of Omega-3 and Omega-6 Fatty
Acids in the United States During the 20th Century."

24. Pollan, *In Defense of Food*.

25. Gross et al., "Increased Consumption of Refined Carbohydrates and the
Epidemic of Type 2 Diabetes in the United States."

26. Hu, Manson, and Willett, "Types of Dietary Fat and Risk of Coronary Heart
Disease."

27. Hu, Manson, and Willett, "Types of Dietary Fat and Risk of Coronary Heart
Disease."

28. Hu, Manson, and Willett, "Types of Dietary Fat and Risk of Coronary Heart
Disease."

29. Pollan, *In Defense of Food.*

30. Forouhi et al., "Dietary Fat and Cardiometabolic Health."

31. Pollan, *In Defense of Food.*

32. Forouhi et al., "Dietary Fat and Cardiometabolic Health."

33. Forouhi et al., "Dietary Fat and Cardiometabolic Health."

34. Forouhi et al., "Dietary Fat and Cardiometabolic Health."

35. Russell J. de Souza et al., "Intake of Saturated and Trans Unsaturated Fatty Acids and Risk of All Cause Mortality, Cardiovascular Disease, and Type 2 Diabetes: Systematic Review and Meta-Analysis of Observational Studies," *BMJ* 351 (August 12, 2015): h3978, https://doi.org/10.1136/bmj.h3978.

36. De Souza et al., "Intake of Saturated and Trans Unsaturated Fatty Acids and Risk of All Cause Mortality, Cardiovascular Disease, and Type 2 Diabetes."

37. Hu, Manson, and Willett, "Types of Dietary Fat and Risk of Coronary Heart Disease."

38. Hu, Manson, and Willett, "Types of Dietary Fat and Risk of Coronary Heart Disease."

39. Christopher E. Ramsden et al., "Re-Evaluation of the Traditional Diet-Heart Hypothesis: Analysis of Recovered Data from Minnesota Coronary Experiment (1968–73)," *BMJ* 353 (April 12, 2016): i1246, https://doi.org/10.1136/bmj.i1246.

40. Ramsden et al., "Re-Evaluation of the Traditional Diet-Heart Hypothesis."

41. Ramsden et al., "Re-Evaluation of the Traditional Diet-Heart Hypothesis."

42. C. E. Ramsden et al., "Use of Dietary Linoleic Acid for Secondary Prevention of Coronary Heart Disease and Death: Evaluation of Recovered Data from the Sydney Diet Heart Study and Updated Meta-Analysis," *BMJ* 346 (February 4, 2013): e8707, https://doi.org/10.1136/bmj.e8707.

43. Ramsden et al., "Use of Dietary Linoleic Acid for Secondary Prevention of Coronary Heart Disease and Death."

44. G. A. Rose, W. B. Thomson, and R. T. Williams, "Corn Oil in Treatment of Ischaemic Heart Disease," *British Medical Journal* 1, no. 5449 (June 12, 1965): 1531–33, https://www.ncbi.nlm.nih.gov/pmc/articles/PMC2166702/.

45.   Ramsden et al., "Re-Evaluation of the Traditional Diet-Heart Hypothesis."

46.   Earl S. Ford et al., "Explaining the Decrease in U.S. Deaths from Coronary Disease, 1980–2000," *New England Journal of Medicine* 356, no. 23 (June 7, 2007): 2388–98, https://doi.org/10.1056/NEJMsa053935.

47.   Ford et al., "Explaining the Decrease in U.S. Deaths from Coronary Disease, 1980–2000."

48.   Pollan, *In Defense of Food.*

49.   Hu, Manson, and Willett, "Types of Dietary Fat and Risk of Coronary Heart Disease."

50.   Pollan, *In Defense of Food.*

51.   Pollan, *In Defense of Food.*

52.   Steele et al., "Ultra-Processed Foods and Added Sugars in the US Diet."

53.   Michael J Gibney, "Ultra-Processed Foods: Definitions and Policy Issues," *Current Developments in Nutrition* 3, no. 2 (February 1, 2019): nzy077, https://doi.org/10.1093/cdn/nzy077.

54.   Laure Schnabel et al., "Association Between Ultraprocessed Food Consumption and Risk of Mortality Among Middle-Aged Adults in France," *JAMA Internal Medicine* 179, no. 4 (April 1, 2019): 490–98, https://doi.org/10.1001/jamainternmed.2018.7289.

55.   Thibault Fiolet et al., "Consumption of Ultra-Processed Foods and Cancer Risk: Results from NutriNet-Santé Prospective Cohort," *BMJ* 360 (February 14, 2018): k322, https://doi.org/10.1136/bmj.k322.

56.   Raquel de Deus Mendonça et al., "Ultraprocessed Food Consumption and Risk of Overweight and Obesity: The University of Navarra Follow-Up (SUN) Cohort Study," *American Journal of Clinical Nutrition* 104, no. 5 (November 1, 2016): 1433–40, https://doi.org/10.3945/ajcn.116.135004.

57.   Xiaojia Chen et al., "Consumption of Ultra-Processed Foods and Health Outcomes: A Systematic Review of Epidemiological Studies," *Nutrition Journal* 19, no. 1 (August 20, 2020): 86, https://doi.org/10.1186/s12937-020-00604-1.

58.   Gross et al., "Increased Consumption of Refined Carbohydrates and the Epidemic of Type 2 Diabetes in the United States."

59.   Kevin D. Hall et al., "Ultra-Processed Diets Cause Excess Calorie Intake and Weight Gain: An Inpatient Randomized Controlled Trial of *Ad Libitum*

Food Intake," *Cell Metabolism* 30, no. 1 (July 2, 2019): 67–77.e3, https://doi .org/10.1016/j.cmet.2019.05.008.

60. Hall et al., "Ultra-Processed Diets Cause Excess Calorie Intake and Weight Gain."

61. Paul M. Johnson and Paul J. Kenny, "Addiction-like Reward Dysfunction and Compulsive Eating in Obese Rats: Role for Dopamine D2 Receptors," *Nature Neuroscience* 13, no. 5 (May 2010): 635–41, https://doi.org/10.1038/nn.2519.

62. Erica M. Schulte, Nicole M. Avena, and Ashley N. Gearhardt, "Which Foods May Be Addictive?: The Roles of Processing, Fat Content, and Glycemic Load," *PLOS ONE* 10, no. 2 (February 18, 2015): e0117959, https://doi .org/10.1371/journal.pone.0117959.

63. Johnson and Kenny, "Addiction-like Reward Dysfunction and Compulsive Eating in Obese Rats."

64. Johnson and Kenny, "Addiction-like Reward Dysfunction and Compulsive Eating in Obese Rats."

65. Paul C. Fletcher and Paul J. Kenny, "Food Addiction: A Valid Concept?," *Neuropsychopharmacology* 43, no. 13 (December 2018): 2506–13, https://doi .org/10.1038/s41386-018-0203-9.

66. Fletcher and Kenny, "Food Addiction."

67. Jennifer M. Poti, Bianca Braga, and Bo Qin, "Ultra-Processed Food Intake and Obesity: What Really Matters for Health—Processing or Nutrient Content?" *Current Obesity Reports* 6, no. 4 (December 2017): 420–31, https://doi .org/10.1007/s13679-017-0285-4.

68. Poti, Braga, and Qin, "Ultra-Processed Food Intake and Obesity."

69. Dana M. Small and Alexandra G. DiFeliceantonio, "Processed Foods and Food Reward," *Science* 363, no. 6425 (January 25, 2019): 346–47, https://doi .org/10.1126/science.aav0556.

70. Small and DiFeliceantonio, "Processed Foods and Food Reward."

71. C. Peter Herman et al., "Mechanisms Underlying the Portion-Size Effect," *Physiology & Behavior* 144 (May 2015): 129–36, https://doi.org/10.1016/j .physbeh.2015.03.025.

72. Brian Wansink and Pierre Chandon, "Can 'Low-Fat' Nutrition Labels Lead to Obesity?" *Journal of Marketing Research* 43, no. 4 (November 2006): 605–17, https://doi.org/10.1509/jmkr.43.4.605.

73. Wansink and Chandon, "Can 'Low-Fat' Nutrition Labels Lead to Obesity?"

74. Gross et al., "Increased Consumption of Refined Carbohydrates and the Epidemic of Type 2 Diabetes in the United States."

75. Wansink and Chandon, "Can 'Low-Fat' Nutrition Labels Lead to Obesity?"

76. Michael Mink et al., "Nutritional Imbalance Endorsed by Televised Food Advertisements," *Journal of the American Dietetic Association* 110, no. 6 (June 1, 2010): 904–10, https://doi.org/10.1016/j.jada.2010.03.020.

77. Frederick J. Zimmerman and Sandhya V. Shimoga, "The Effects of Food Advertising and Cognitive Load on Food Choices," *BMC Public Health* 14, no. 1 (April 10, 2014): 342, https://doi.org/10.1186/1471-2458-14-342.

78. Jennifer L. Harris, John A. Bargh, and Kelly D. Brownell, "Priming Effects of Television Food Advertising on Eating Behavior," *Health Psychology* (July 2009): 404–13, https://doi.org/10.1037/a0014399.

79. Poti, Braga, and Qin, "Ultra-Processed Food Intake and Obesity."

80. Poti, Braga, and Qin, "Ultra-Processed Food Intake and Obesity."

81. Maria Laura da Costa Louzada et al., "Impact of Ultra-Processed Foods on Micronutrient Content in the Brazilian Diet," *Revista de Saúde Pública* 49 (August 7, 2015), https://doi.org/10.1590/S0034-8910.2015049006211.

82. Da Costa Louzada et al., "Impact of Ultra-Processed Foods on Micronutrient Content in the Brazilian Diet."

83. Da Costa Louzada et al., "Impact of Ultra-Processed Foods on Micronutrient Content in the Brazilian Diet."

84. Maria Laura da Costa Louzada et al., "Ultra-Processed Foods and the Nutritional Dietary Profile in Brazil," *Revista de Saúde Pública* 49 (2015), https://doi.org/10.1590/S0034-8910.2015049006132.

85. Da Costa Louzada et al., "Impact of Ultra-Processed Foods on Micronutrient Content in the Brazilian Diet."

86. Jean-Claude Moubarac et al., "Consumption of Ultra-Processed Foods Predicts Diet Quality in Canada," *Appetite* 108 (January 1, 2017): 512–20, https://doi.org/10.1016/j.appet.2016.11.006.

87. Poti, Braga, and Qin, "Ultra-Processed Food Intake and Obesity."

88. Fredrik Rosqvist et al., "Potential Role of Milk Fat Globule Membrane in

Modulating Plasma Lipoproteins, Gene Expression, and Cholesterol Metabolism in Humans: A Randomized Study," *American Journal of Clinical Nutrition* 102, no. 1 (July 1, 2015): 20–30, https://doi.org/10.3945/ajcn.115.107045.

89. Noori S. Al-Waili, "Natural Honey Lowers Plasma Glucose, C-Reactive Protein, Homocysteine, and Blood Lipids in Healthy, Diabetic, and Hyperlipidemic Subjects: Comparison with Dextrose and Sucrose," *Journal of Medicinal Food* 7, no. 1 (April 2004): 100–107, https://doi.org/10.1089/109662004322984789.

90. Emma L. Feeney et al., "Dairy Matrix Effects: Response to Consumption of Dairy Fat Differs When Eaten Within the Cheese Matrix—a Randomized Controlled Trial," *American Journal of Clinical Nutrition* 108, no. 4 (October 1, 2018): 667–74, https://doi.org/10.1093/ajcn/nqy146.

91. Select Committee on Nutrition and Human Needs, United States Senate, "Dietary Goals for the United States."

92. Select Committee on Nutrition and Human Needs, United States Senate, "Dietary Goals for the United States."

93. Lars T. Fadnes et al., "Estimating Impact of Food Choices on Life Expectancy: A Modeling Study," *PLOS Medicine* 19, no. 2 (February 8, 2022): e1003889, https://doi.org/10.1371/journal.pmed.1003889.

94. Scott Kahan and JoAnn E. Manson, "Nutrition Counseling in Clinical Practice: How Clinicians Can Do Better," *JAMA* 318, no. 12 (September 26, 2017): 1101, https://doi.org/10.1001/jama.2017.10434.

95. Colin D. Rehm et al., "Dietary Intake Among US Adults, 1999–2012," *JAMA* 315, no. 23 (June 21, 2016): 2542–53, https://doi.org/10.1001/jama.2016.7491.

96. Julia A. Wolfson and Sara N. Bleich, "Is Cooking at Home Associated with Better Diet Quality or Weight-Loss Intention?" *Public Health Nutrition* 18, no. 8 (June 2015): 1397–406, https://doi.org/10.1017/S1368980014001943.

97. Susanna Mills et al., "Health and Social Determinants and Outcomes of Home Cooking: A Systematic Review of Observational Studies," *Appetite* 111 (April 1, 2017): 116–34, https://doi.org/10.1016/j.appet.2016.12.022.

98. *Lays Potato Chips 1967: Betcha Can't Eat Just One (Bert Lahr)*, YouTube, 2021, https://www.youtube.com/watch?v=lPdK-W0G7bM.

99. Dariush Mozaffarian, "Dietary and Policy Priorities for Cardiovascular Disease, Diabetes, and Obesity: A Comprehensive Review," *Circulation* 133, no. 2

(January 12, 2016): 187–225, https://doi.org/10.1161/CIRCULATIONAHA .115.018585.

100. D. Mozaffarian and S. Capewell, "United Nations' Dietary Policies to Prevent Cardiovascular Disease," *BMJ* 343 (September 14, 2011): d5747, https://doi .org/10.1136/bmj.d5747.

101. Rani Polak et al., "Health-Related Culinary Education: A Summary of Representative Emerging Programs for Health Professionals and Patients," *Global Advances in Health and Medicine* 5, no. 1 (January 2016): 61–68, https: //doi.org/10.7453/gahmj.2015.128.

102. Rani Polak, "CHEF Coaching: Translating Nutritional Science into Practical Tools," *Alternative and Complementary Therapies* 23, no. 3 (June 2017): 87–89, https://doi.org/10.1089/act.2017.29110.rpo.

103. "Medical Schools," CulinaryMedicine.org, accessed August 24, 2022, https: //culinarymedicine.org/culinary-medicine-partner-schools/partner-medical -schools/.

104. Walter Willett et al., "Food in the Anthropocene: The EAT–*Lancet* Commission on Healthy Diets from Sustainable Food Systems," *The Lancet* 393, no. 10170 (February 2, 2019): 447–92, https://doi.org/10.1016/S0140-6736(18)31788-4.

105. Willett et al., "Food in the Anthropocene."

106. Willett et al., "Food in the Anthropocene."

107. Dariush Mozaffarian and David S. Ludwig, "Dietary Guidelines in the 21st Century—A Time for Food," *JAMA* 304, no. 6 (August 11, 2010): 681, https: //doi.org/10.1001/jama.2010.1116.

108. Eric O. Verger et al., "Dietary Diversity Indicators and Their Associations with Dietary Adequacy and Health Outcomes: A Systematic Scoping Review," *Advances in Nutrition* 12, no. 5 (October 1, 2021): 1659–72, https://doi .org/10.1093/advances/nmab009.

109. Susanna Mills et al., "Frequency of Eating Home Cooked Meals and Potential Benefits for Diet and Health: Cross-Sectional Analysis of a Population-Based Cohort Study," *International Journal of Behavioral Nutrition and Physical Activity* 14 (August 17, 2017): 109, https://doi.org/10.1186/s12966-017-0567-y.

110. Pauline Ducrot et al., "Meal Planning Is Associated with Food Variety, Diet Quality and Body Weight Status in a Large Sample of French Adults," *Inter-*

national Journal of Behavioral Nutrition and Physical Activity 14 (February 2, 2017): 12, https://doi.org/10.1186/s12966-017-0461-7.

111. Denise de Ridder and Marleen Gillebaart, "How Food Overconsumption Has Hijacked Our Notions About Eating as a Pleasurable Activity," *Current Opinion in Psychology* 46 (August 1, 2022): 101324, https://doi.org/10.1016/j.copsyc.2022.101324.

112. Janet M. Warren, Nicola Smith, and Margaret Ashwell, "A Structured Literature Review on the Role of Mindfulness, Mindful Eating and Intuitive Eating in Changing Eating Behaviours: Effectiveness and Associated Potential Mechanisms," *Nutrition Research Reviews* 30, no. 2 (December 2017): 272–83, https://doi.org/10.1017/S0954422417000154.

6. Exercise: The Magic Pill

1. C. J. Caspersen, K. E. Powell, and G. M. Christenson, "Physical Activity, Exercise, and Physical Fitness: Definitions and Distinctions for Health-Related Research," *Public Health Reports* 100, no. 2 (1985): 126–31, https://www.ncbi.nlm.nih.gov/pmc/articles/PMC1424733/.

2. Caspersen, Powell, and Christenson, "Physical Activity, Exercise, and Physical Fitness."

3. Rachel Persinger et al., "Consistency of the Talk Test for Exercise Prescription," *Medicine and Science in Sports and Exercise* 36, no. 9 (September 2004): 1632–36, https://pubmed.ncbi.nlm.nih.gov/15354048/.

4. US Department of Health and Human Services, *Physical Activity Guidelines for Americans,* 2nd ed., 2018, https://health.gov/our-work/nutrition-physical-activity/physical-activity-guidelines/current-guidelines.

5. Centers for Disease Control and Prevention, "FastStats," Exercise or Physical Activity, June 11, 2021, https://www.cdc.gov/nchs/fastats/exercise.htm.

6. US Department of Health and Human Services, *2008 Physical Activity Guidelines for Americans,* 2008, https://health.gov/our-work/nutrition-physical-activity/physical-activity-guidelines/previous-guidelines/2008-physical-activity-guidelines.

7. Victoria A. Catenacci et al., "Physical Activity Patterns in the National Weight Control Registry," *Obesity* 16, no. 1 (January 2008): 153–61, https://doi.org/10.1038/oby.2007.6.

8. US Department of Health and Human Services, *2008 Physical Activity Guidelines for Americans.*

9. "Rx for Health Series," *Exercise Is Medicine* (blog), accessed August 26, 2022, https://www.exerciseismedicine.org/eim-in-action/health-care/resources/rx -for-health-series/.

10. Wayne L. Westcott et al., "Prescribing Physical Activity: Applying the ACSM Protocols for Exercise Type, Intensity, and Duration Across 3 Training Frequencies," *Physician and Sportsmedicine* 37, no. 2 (June 2009): 51–58, https://doi.org/10.3810/psm.2009.06.1709.

11. Robert R. Wolfe, "The Underappreciated Role of Muscle in Health and Disease," *American Journal of Clinical Nutrition* 84, no. 3 (December 1, 2006): 475–82, https://doi.org/10.1093/ajcn/84.3.475.

12. Barbara Strasser and Wolfgang Schobersberger, "Evidence for Resistance Training as a Treatment Therapy in Obesity," *Journal of Obesity* 2011 (August 10, 2010): e482564, https://doi.org/10.1155/2011/482564.

13. Timothy Heden et al., "One-Set Resistance Training Elevates Energy Expenditure for 72 H Similar to Three Sets," *European Journal of Applied Physiology* 111, no. 3 (March 1, 2011): 477–84, https://doi.org/10.1007/s00421-010 -1666-5.

14. William J. Kraemer, Nicholas A. Ratamess, and Duncan N. French, "Resistance Training for Health and Performance," *Current Sports Medicine Reports* 1, no. 3 (May 1, 2002): 165–71, https://doi.org/10.1007/s11932 -002-0017-7.

15. Wolfgang Kemmler et al., "Exercise Effects on Fitness and Bone Mineral Density in Early Postmenopausal Women: 1-Year EFOPS Results," *Medicine and Science in Sports and Exercise* 34, no. 12 (December 1, 2002): 2115–23, https://doi.org/10.1097/00005768-200212000-00038.

16. Maria Fiataraone Singh et al., "ACSM Guidelines for Strength Training: Featured Download," American College of Sports Medicine, accessed October 21, 2022, https://www.acsm.org/search-results/all-blog-posts/certification -blog/acsm-certified-blog/2019/07/31/acsm-guidelines-for-strength-training -featured-download.

17. Michael R. Esco, "ACSM Information on . . . Resistance Training for Health and Fitness" (American College of Sports Medicine, n.d.), https: //www.prescriptiontogetactive.com/static/pdfs/resistance-training-ACSM .pdf.

18. Carolina O. C. Werle, Brian Wansink, and Collin R. Payne, "Is It Fun or
     Exercise? The Framing of Physical Activity Biases Subsequent Snacking,"
     Marketing Letters 26, no. 4 (December 1, 2015): 691–702, https://doi.org/10
     .1007/s11002-014-9301-6.

19. US Department of Health and Human Services, *2008 Physical Activity
     Guidelines for Americans.*

20. US Department of Health and Human Services, *2008 Physical Activity
     Guidelines for Americans.*

21. Michelle L. Segar, Jacquelynne S. Eccles, and Caroline R. Richardson,
     "Rebranding Exercise: Closing the Gap Between Values and Behavior,"
     International Journal of Behavioral Nutrition and Physical Activity 8, no. 1
     (August 31, 2011): 94, https://doi.org/10.1186/1479-5868-8-94.

22. US Department of Health and Human Services, *2008 Physical Activity
     Guidelines for Americans.*

7. A Love Letter to the Gym

1.   David C. Hughes, Stian Ellefsen, and Keith Baar, "Adaptations to Endur-
     ance and Strength Training," *Cold Spring Harbor Perspectives in Medicine* 8,
     no. 6 (June 1, 2018): a029769, https://doi.org/10.1101/cshperspect.a029769.

2.   Hughes, Ellefsen, and Baar, "Adaptations to Endurance and Strength Training."

3.   Hughes, Ellefsen, and Baar, "Adaptations to Endurance and Strength Training."

4.   Hughes, Ellefsen, and Baar, "Adaptations to Endurance and Strength Training."

5.   Hughes, Ellefsen, and Baar, "Adaptations to Endurance and Strength Training."

6.   Wayne L. Westcott, "Resistance Training Is Medicine: Effects of Strength
     Training on Health," *Current Sports Medicine Reports* 11, no. 4 (August 2012):
     209–16, https://doi.org/10.1249/JSR.0b013e31825dabb8.

7.   Westcott, "Resistance Training Is Medicine."

8.   Westcott, "Resistance Training Is Medicine."

9.   Diana M. Thomas et al., "Time to Correctly Predict the Amount of Weight
     Loss with Dieting," *Journal of the Academy of Nutrition and Dietetics* 114, no. 6
     (June 2014): 857–61, https://doi.org/10.1016/j.jand.2014.02.003.

10. Robert Ross and Ian Janssen, "Physical Activity, Total and Regional Obesity:
     Dose-Response Considerations," *Medicine and Science in Sports and Exercise*

33, no. 6, supp. (June 2001): S521–27, https://doi.org/10.1097/00005768
-200106001-00023.

11.   Ross and Janssen, "Physical Activity, Total and Regional Obesity."

12.   Edward L. Melanson et al., "Resistance to Exercise-Induced Weight Loss:
       Compensatory Behavioral Adaptations," *Medicine and Science in Sports and
       Exercise* 45, no. 8 (August 2013): 1600–9, https://doi.org/10.1249/MSS
       .0b013e31828ba942.

13.   Westcott, "Resistance Training Is Medicine."

14.   ZiMian Wang et al., "Evaluation of Specific Metabolic Rates of Major Organs
       and Tissues: Comparison Between Nonobese and Obese Women," *Obesity*
       20, no. 1 (January 2012): 95–100, https://doi.org/10.1038/oby.2011.256.

15.   Westcott, "Resistance Training Is Medicine."

16.   Westcott, "Resistance Training Is Medicine."

17.   Barbara Strasser and Wolfgang Schobersberger, "Evidence for Resistance
       Training as a Treatment Therapy in Obesity," *Journal of Obesity* 2011 (August
       10, 2010): e482564, https://doi.org/10.1155/2011/482564.

18.   Strasser and Schobersberger, "Evidence for Resistance Training as a Treatment
       Therapy in Obesity."

19.   Westcott, "Resistance Training Is Medicine."

20.   Brad J. Schoenfeld, "The Mechanisms of Muscle Hypertrophy and Their
       Application to Resistance Training," *Journal of Strength and Conditioning
       Research* 24, no. 10 (October 2010): 2857–72, https://doi.org/10.1519/JSC
       .0b013e3181e840f3.

21.   Rūtenis Paulauskas et al., "Basketball Game-Related Statistics That Discrim-
       inate Between European Players Competing in the NBA and in the Euro-
       league," *Journal of Human Kinetics* 65, no. 1 (December 31, 2018): 225–33,
       https://doi.org/10.2478/hukin-2018-0030.

22.   Barry M. Prior et al., "Muscularity and the Density of the Fat-Free Mass in
       Athletes," *Journal of Applied Physiology* 90, no. 4 (April 2001): 1523–31, https:
       //doi.org/10.1152/jappl.2001.90.4.1523.

23.   Christopher Barakat et al., "Body Recomposition: Can Trained Individuals
       Build Muscle and Lose Fat at the Same Time?," *Strength & Conditioning*

Journal 42, no. 5 (October 2020): 7–21, https://doi.org/10.1519/SSC .0000000000000584.

24. Joshua J. Ode et al., "Body Mass Index as a Predictor of Percent Fat in College Athletes and Nonathletes," *Medicine & Science in Sports & Exercise* 39, no. 3 (March 2007): 403–9, https://doi.org/10.1249/01.mss.0000247008.19127.3e.

25. Rodrigo Ramírez-Campillo et al., "Regional Fat Changes Induced by Localized Muscle Endurance Resistance Training," *Journal of Strength and Conditioning Research* 27, no. 8 (August 2013): 2219–24, https://doi.org/10.1519 /JSC.0b013e31827e8681.

26. Sachin S. Vispute et al., "The Effect of Abdominal Exercise on Abdominal Fat," *Journal of Strength and Conditioning Research* 25, no. 9 (September 2011): 2559–64, https://doi.org/10.1519/JSC.0b013e3181fb4a46.

27. Ellen Blaak, "Gender Differences in Fat Metabolism," *Current Opinion in Clinical Nutrition & Metabolic Care* 4, no. 6 (November 2001): 499–502, https://journals.lww.com/co-clinicalnutrition/Abstract/2001/11000/Gender _differences_in_fat_metabolism.6.aspx.

28. M. C. Zillikens et al., "Sex-Specific Genetic Effects Influence Variation in Body Composition," *Diabetologia* 51, no. 12 (December 1, 2008): 2233–41, https://doi.org/10.1007/s00125-008-1163-0.

29. Shari L. Dworkin, "Holding Back: Negotiating the Glass Ceiling on Women's Muscular Strength," *Sociological Perspective* 44, no. 3 (2001): 333–50, https: //doi.org/10.1525/sop.2001.44.3.333.

30. Dworkin, "Holding Back."

31. Dworkin, "Holding Back."

32. Jessica Salvatore and Jeanne Marecek, "Gender in the Gym: Evaluation Concerns as Barriers to Women's Weight Lifting," *Sex Roles* 63, no. 7 (October 1, 2010): 556–67, https://doi.org/10.1007/s11199-010-9800-8.

33. Salvatore and Marecek, "Gender in the Gym."

34. Salvatore and Marecek, "Gender in the Gym."

35. Ruth N. Henry, Mark H. Anshel, and Timothy Michael, "Effects of Aerobic and Circuit Training on Fitness and Body Image Among Women," *RedOrbit*, December 2, 2006, https://www.redorbit.com/news/health/752154/effects _of_aerobic_and_circuit_training_on_fitness_and_body/.

36. Dworkin, "Holding Back."

37. Amanda J. Gruber and Harrison G. Pope Jr., "Psychiatric and Medical Effects of Anabolic-Androgenic Steroid Use in Women," *Psychotherapy and Psychosomatics* 69, no. 1 (2000): 19–26, https://doi.org/10.1159/000012362.

38. Dworkin, "Holding Back."

39. A. E. J. Miller et al., "Gender Differences in Strength and Muscle Fiber Characteristics," *European Journal of Applied Physiology and Occupational Physiology* 66, no. 3 (March 1, 1993): 254–62, https://doi.org/10.1007/BF00235103.

40. Miller et al., "Gender Differences in Strength and Muscle Fiber Characteristics."

41. K. J. Cureton et al., "Muscle Hypertrophy in Men and Women," *Medicine and Science in Sports and Exercise* 20, no. 4 (August 1, 1988): 338–44, https://doi.org/10.1249/00005768-198808000-00003.

42. R. S. Staron et al., "Skeletal Muscle Adaptations During Early Phase of Heavy-Resistance Training in Men and Women," *Journal of Applied Physiology* 76, no. 3 (March 1, 1994): 1247–55, https://doi.org/10.1152/jappl.1994.76.3.1247.

43. Monica J. Hubal et al., "Variability in Muscle Size and Strength Gain After Unilateral Resistance Training," *Medicine & Science in Sports & Exercise* 37, no. 6 (June 2005): 964–72, https://journals.lww.com/acsm-msse/Fulltext/2005/06000/Variability_in_Muscle_Size_and_Strength_Gain_after.10.aspx.

44. Cureton et al., "Muscle Hypertrophy in Men and Women."

45. Cureton et al., "Muscle Hypertrophy in Men and Women."

46. Hubal et al., "Variability in Muscle Size and Strength Gain After Unilateral Resistance Training."

47. Phillip Bishop, Kirk Cureton, and Mitchell Collins, "Sex Difference in Muscular Strength in Equally-Trained Men and Women," *Ergonomics* 30, no. 4 (April 1987): 675–87, https://doi.org/10.1080/00140138708969760.

48. Blaak, "Gender Differences in Fat Metabolism."

49. Bishop, Cureton, and Collins, "Sex Difference in Muscular Strength in Equally-Trained Men and Women."

50. Hubal et al., "Variability in Muscle Size and Strength Gain After Unilateral Resistance Training."

51. Frederick M. Ivey et al., "Effects of Age, Gender, and Myostatin Genotype on the Hypertrophic Response to Heavy Resistance Strength Training," *Journals of Gerontology: Series A* 55, no. 11 (November 1, 2000): M641–48, https://doi.org/10.1093/gerona/55.11.M641.

52. Benjamin T. Wall, Marlou L. Dirks, and Luc J. C. van Loon, "Skeletal Muscle Atrophy During Short-Term Disuse: Implications for Age-Related Sarcopenia," *Ageing Research Reviews* 12, no. 4 (September 1, 2013): 898–906, https://doi.org/10.1016/j.arr.2013.07.003.

53. Wall, Dirks, and van Loon, "Skeletal Muscle Atrophy During Short-Term Disuse."

54. Barakat et al., "Body Recomposition."

55. Schoenfeld, "The Mechanisms of Muscle Hypertrophy and Their Application to Resistance Training."

56. Schoenfeld, "The Mechanisms of Muscle Hypertrophy and Their Application to Resistance Training."

57. Jakob Škarabot et al., "The Knowns and Unknowns of Neural Adaptations to Resistance Training," *European Journal of Applied Physiology* 121, no. 3 (March 1, 2021): 675–85, https://doi.org/10.1007/s00421-020-04567-3.

58. Škarabot et al., "The Knowns and Unknowns of Neural Adaptations to Resistance Training."

59. Škarabot et al., "The Knowns and Unknowns of Neural Adaptations to Resistance Training."

60. Schoenfeld, "The Mechanisms of Muscle Hypertrophy and Their Application to Resistance Training."

61. Schoenfeld, "The Mechanisms of Muscle Hypertrophy and Their Application to Resistance Training."

62. Schoenfeld, "The Mechanisms of Muscle Hypertrophy and Their Application to Resistance Training."

63. William J. Kraemer and Nicholas A. Ratamess, "Fundamentals of Resistance Training: Progression and Exercise Prescription," *Medicine & Science in Sports & Exercise* 36, no. 4 (April 2004): 674–88, https://doi.org/10.1249/01.MSS.0000121945.36635.61.

64. Kraemer and Ratamess, "Fundamentals of Resistance Training."

65.   Schoenfeld, "The Mechanisms of Muscle Hypertrophy and Their Application to Resistance Training."

66.   Kraemer and Ratamess, "Fundamentals of Resistance Training."

67.   Schoenfeld, "The Mechanisms of Muscle Hypertrophy and Their Application to Resistance Training."

68.   Kraemer and Ratamess, "Fundamentals of Resistance Training."

69.   Kraemer and Ratamess, "Fundamentals of Resistance Training."

70.   Kraemer and Ratamess, "Fundamentals of Resistance Training."

71.   Schoenfeld, "The Mechanisms of Muscle Hypertrophy and Their Application to Resistance Training."

72.   Kraemer and Ratamess, "Fundamentals of Resistance Training."

73.   Schoenfeld, "The Mechanisms of Muscle Hypertrophy and Their Application to Resistance Training."

74.   Kraemer and Ratamess, "Fundamentals of Resistance Training."

75.   Schoenfeld, "The Mechanisms of Muscle Hypertrophy and Their Application to Resistance Training."

76.   Kraemer and Ratamess, "Fundamentals of Resistance Training."

77.   S. P. Bird, K. M. Tarpenning, and Frank Marino, "Designing Resistance Training Programmes to Enhance Muscular Fitness: A Review of the Acute Programme Variables," *Sports Medicine* 35 (January 1, 2005): 841.

78.   Bird, Tarpenning, and Marino, "Designing Resistance Training Programmes to Enhance Muscular Fitness."

79.   Bird, Tarpenning, and Marino, "Designing Resistance Training Programmes to Enhance Muscular Fitness."

80.   Schoenfeld, "The Mechanisms of Muscle Hypertrophy and Their Application to Resistance Training."

81.   Stuart M. Phillips, Stéphanie Chevalier, and Heather J. Leidy, "Protein 'Requirements' Beyond the RDA: Implications for Optimizing Health," *Applied Physiology, Nutrition, and Metabolism* 41, no. 5 (May 2016): 565–72, https://doi.org/10.1139/apnm-2015-0550.

82.   Phillips, Chevalier, and Leidy, "Protein 'Requirements' Beyond the RDA."

83. Phillips, Chevalier, and Leidy, "Protein 'Requirements' Beyond the RDA."

84. Ralf Jäger et al., "International Society of Sports Nutrition Position Stand: Protein and Exercise," *Journal of the International Society of Sports Nutrition* 14, no. 1 (June 20, 2017): 20, https://doi.org/10.1186/s12970-017-0177-8.

85. Eric R. Helms et al., "A Systematic Review of Dietary Protein During Caloric Restriction in Resistance Trained Lean Athletes: A Case for Higher Intakes," *International Journal of Sport Nutrition and Exercise Metabolism* 24, no. 2 (April 2014): 127–38, https://doi.org/10.1123/ijsnem.2013-0054.

86. Jäger et al., "International Society of Sports Nutrition Position Stand."

87. Jäger et al., "International Society of Sports Nutrition Position Stand."

8. Too "Fat" to Have an Eating Disorder

1. James I. Hudson et al., "The Prevalence and Correlates of Eating Disorders in the National Comorbidity Survey Replication," *Biological Psychiatry* 61, no. 3 (February 2007): 348–58, https://doi.org/10.1016/j.biopsych.2006.03.040.

2. Hudson et al., "The Prevalence and Correlates of Eating Disorders in the National Comorbidity Survey Replication."

3. American Psychiatric Association, *Diagnostic and Statistical Manual of Mental Disorders,* 5th ed., text revision (*DSM-5-TR*) (Washington, DC: American Psychiatric Association Publishing, 2022), https://doi.org/10.1176/appi .books.9780890425787.

4. APA, *DSM-5-TR.*

5. APA, *DSM-5-TR.*

6. APA, *DSM-5-TR.*

7. Alexandra Dingemans, Unna Danner, and Melissa Parks, "Emotion Regulation in Binge Eating Disorder: A Review," *Nutrients* 9, no. 11 (November 22, 2017): 1274, https://doi.org/10.3390/nu9111274.

8. Dingemans, Danner, and Parks, "Emotion Regulation in Binge Eating Disorder."

9. Dingemans, Danner, and Parks, "Emotion Regulation in Binge Eating Disorder."

10. Dingemans, Danner, and Parks, "Emotion Regulation in Binge Eating Disorder."

11. Ashley N. Gearhardt, Marney A. White, and Marc N. Potenza, "Binge Eating Disorder and Food Addiction," *Current Drug Abuse Reviews* 4, no. 3 (September 1, 2011): 201–7, https://doi.org/10.2174/1874473711104030201.

12. Marigold Castillo and Eric Weiselberg, "Bulimia Nervosa/Purging Disorder," *Current Problems in Pediatric and Adolescent Health Care* 47, no. 4 (April 2017): 85–94, https://doi.org/10.1016/j.cppeds.2017.02.004.

13. Castillo and Weiselberg, "Bulimia Nervosa/Purging Disorder."

14. Hudson et al., "The Prevalence and Correlates of Eating Disorders in the National Comorbidity Survey Replication."

15. APA, *DSM-5-TR*.

16. Castillo and Weiselberg, "Bulimia Nervosa/Purging Disorder."

17. Castillo and Weiselberg, "Bulimia Nervosa/Purging Disorder."

18. Hudson et al., "The Prevalence and Correlates of Eating Disorders in the National Comorbidity Survey Replication."

19. APA, *DSM-5-TR*.

20. Stuart B. Murray et al., "Treatment Outcomes for Anorexia Nervosa: A Systematic Review and Meta-Analysis of Randomized-Controlled Trials— CORRIGENDUM," *Psychological Medicine* 49, no. 4 (March 2019): 701–4, https://doi.org/10.1017/S0033291718003185.

21. Murray et al., "Treatment Outcomes for Anorexia Nervosa."

22. Pamela K. Keel and Kelly L. Klump, "Are Eating Disorders Culture-Bound Syndromes? Implications for Conceptualizing Their Etiology," *Psychological Bulletin* 129, no. 5 (2003): 747–69, https://doi.org/10.1037/0033-2909.129 .5.747.

23. Hudson et al., "The Prevalence and Correlates of Eating Disorders in the National Comorbidity Survey Replication."

24. Kristen M. Culbert, Sarah E. Racine, and Kelly L. Klump, "Research Review: What We Have Learned About the Causes of Eating Disorders—A Synthesis of Sociocultural, Psychological, and Biological Research," *Journal of Child Psychology and Psychiatry* 56, no. 11 (November 2015): 1141–64, https://doi.org/10.1111/jcpp.12441.

25. Helen B. Murray et al., "Are Eating Disorders 'All About Control?' The Elusive Psychopathology of Nonfat Phobic Presentations," *International Journal*

of Eating Disorders 50, no. 11 (November 2017): 1306–12, https://doi.org/10.1002/eat.22779.

26. Culbert, Racine, and Klump, "Research Review: What We Have Learned About the Causes of Eating Disorders."

27. Mariko Makino, Koji Tsuboi, and Lorraine Dennerstein, "Prevalence of Eating Disorders: A Comparison of Western and Non-Western Countries," *MedGenMed* (*Medscape General Medicine*) 6, no. 3 (September 27, 2004): 49, https://pubmed.ncbi.nlm.nih.gov/15520673/.

28. Culbert, Racine, and Klump, "Research Review: What We Have Learned About the Causes of Eating Disorders."

29. Culbert, Racine, and Klump, "Research Review: What We Have Learned About the Causes of Eating Disorders."

30. Ana Paula de Matos et al., "Prevalence of Disordered Eating Behaviors and Associated Factors in Brazilian University Students," *Nutrition and Health* 27, no. 2 (June 2021): 231–41, https://doi.org/10.1177/0260106020971136.

31. Antoni Niedzielski and Natalia Kaźmierczak-Wojtaś, "Prevalence of Orthorexia Nervosa and Its Diagnostic Tools—A Literature Review," *International Journal of Environmental Research and Public Health* 18, no. 10 (May 20, 2021): 5488, https://doi.org/10.3390/ijerph18105488.

32. Niedzielski and Kaźmierczak-Wojtaś, "Prevalence of Orthorexia Nervosa and Its Diagnostic Tools."

33. Rebecca Murphy et al., "Cognitive Behavioral Therapy for Eating Disorders," *Psychiatric Clinics of North America* 33, no. 3 (September 2010): 611–27, https://doi.org/10.1016/j.psc.2010.04.004.

9. From a Dad

1. "Orthorexia," National Eating Disorders Association, accessed August 29, 2022, https://www.nationaleatingdisorders.org/learn/by-eating-disorder/other/orthorexia.

10. Stress, Eating, and Weight

1. Daryl B. O'Connor, Julian F. Thayer, and Kavita Vedhara, "Stress and Health: A Review of Psychobiological Processes," *Annual Review of Psychology* 72, no. 1 (January 4, 2021): 663–88, https://doi.org/10.1146/annurev-psych-062520-122331.

2.   O'Connor, Thayer, and Vedhara, "Stress and Health."

3.   Bruce S. McEwen, "Allostasis and Allostatic Load: Implications for Neuro-psychopharmacology," *Neuropsychopharmacology* 22, no. 2 (February 1, 2000): 108–24, https://doi.org/10.1016/S0893-133X(99)00129-3.

4.   O'Connor, Thayer, and Vedhara, "Stress and Health."

5.   O'Connor, Thayer, and Vedhara, "Stress and Health."

6.   O'Connor, Thayer, and Vedhara, "Stress and Health."

7.   O'Connor, Thayer, and Vedhara, "Stress and Health."

8.   O'Connor, Thayer, and Vedhara, "Stress and Health."

9.   O'Connor, Thayer, and Vedhara, "Stress and Health."

10. Karen A. Scott, Susan J. Melhorn, and Randall R. Sakai, "Effects of Chronic Social Stress on Obesity," *Current Obesity Reports* 1, no. 1 (March 1, 2012): 16–25, https://doi.org/10.1007/s13679-011-0006-3.

11. Scott, Melhorn, and Sakai, "Effects of Chronic Social Stress on Obesity."

12. Matthew A. Stults-Kolehmainen and Rajita Sinha, "The Effects of Stress on Physical Activity and Exercise," *Sports Medicine* 44, no. 1 (January 2014): 81–121, https://doi.org/10.1007/s40279-013-0090-5.

13. Scott, Melhorn, and Sakai, "Effects of Chronic Social Stress on Obesity."

14. Kazuko Masuo et al., "Serum Uric Acid and Plasma Norepinephrine Con-centrations Predict Subsequent Weight Gain and Blood Pressure Elevation," *Hypertension* 42, no. 4 (October 2003): 474–80, https://doi.org/10.1161/01 .HYP.0000091371.53502.D3.

15. Scott, Melhorn, and Sakai, "Effects of Chronic Social Stress on Obesity."

16. Scott, Melhorn, and Sakai, "Effects of Chronic Social Stress on Obesity."

17. Elissa S. Epel et al., "Stress and Body Shape: Stress-Induced Cortisol Se-cretion Is Consistently Greater Among Women with Central Fat," *Psychoso-matic Medicine* 62, no. 5 (October 2000): 623–32, https://journals.lww.com /psychosomaticmedicine/Abstract/2000/09000/Stress_and_Body_Shape __Stress_Induced_Cortisol.5.aspx.

18. Epel et al., "Stress and Body Shape."

19. Daryl B. O'Connor et al., "Effects of Daily Hassles and Eating Style on Eating Behavior," *Health Psychology* 27, no. 1, supp. (2008): S20–31, https://doi.org/10.1037/0278-6133.27.1.S20.

20. Y. H. C. Yau and M. N. Potenza, "Stress and Eating Behaviors," *Minerva Endocrinologica* 38, no. 3 (September 2013): 255–67.

21. Nitika Garg, Brian Wansink, and J. Jeffrey Inman, "The Influence of Incidental Affect on Consumers' Food Intake," *Journal of Marketing* 71, no. 1 (January 1, 2007): 194–206, https://doi.org/10.1509/jmkg.71.1.194.

22. Garg, Wansink, and Inman, "The Influence of Incidental Affect on Consumers' Food Intake."

23. Stults-Kolehmainen and Sinha, "The Effects of Stress on Physical Activity and Exercise."

24. John B. Bartholomew et al., "Strength Gains After Resistance Training: The Effect of Stressful, Negative Life Events," *Journal of Strength and Conditioning Research* 22, no. 4 (July 2008): 1215–21, https://doi.org/10.1519/JSC.0b013e318173d0bf.

25. James P. Fisher, Colin N. Young, and Paul J. Fadel, "Central Sympathetic Overactivity: Maladies and Mechanisms," *Autonomic Neuroscience: Basic & Clinical* 148, no. 1–2 (June 15, 2009): 5–15, https://doi.org/10.1016/j.autneu.2009.02.003.

26. Ioana Maria Bunea, Aurora Szentágotai-Tătar, and Andrei C. Miu, "Early-Life Adversity and Cortisol Response to Social Stress: A Meta-Analysis," *Translational Psychiatry* 7, no. 12 (December 11, 2017): 1–8, https://doi.org/10.1038/s41398-017-0032-3.

27. Eva Fries et al., "A New View on Hypocortisolism," *Psychoneuroendocrinology* 30, special issue, *Stress, Sensitisation and Somatisation: A Special Issue in Honour of Holger Ursin*, no. 10 (November 1, 2005): 1010–16, https://doi.org/10.1016/j.psyneuen.2005.04.006.

28. Steven W. Cole, "Social Regulation of Human Gene Expression: Mechanisms and Implications for Public Health," *American Journal of Public Health* 103, supp., no. S1 (October 2013): S84–92, https://doi.org/10.2105/AJPH.2012.301183.

29. See https://bensonhenryinstitute.org/the-passing-of-herbert-benson-md/.

30. O'Connor, Thayer, and Vedhara, "Stress and Health."

31. Roderik J. S. Gerritsen and Guido P. H. Band, "Breath of Life: The Respiratory Vagal Stimulation Model of Contemplative Activity," *Frontiers in Human Neuroscience* 12 (October 9, 2018): 397, https://doi.org/10.3389/fnhum.2018 .00397.

32. Xiao Ma et al., "The Effect of Diaphragmatic Breathing on Attention, Negative Affect and Stress in Healthy Adults," *Frontiers in Psychology* 8 (June 6, 2017): 874, https://doi.org/10.3389/fpsyg.2017.00874.

33. Hari Sharma, "Meditation: Process and Effects," *Ayu* 36, no. 3 (2015): 233–37, https://doi.org/10.4103/0974-8520.182756.

34. J. David Creswell et al., "Mindfulness-Based Stress Reduction Training Reduces Loneliness and Pro-Inflammatory Gene Expression in Older Adults: A Small Randomized Controlled Trial," *Brain, Behavior, and Immunity* 26, no. 7 (October 1, 2012): 1095–1101, https://doi.org/10.1016/j .bbi.2012.07.006.

35. Catherine Woodyard, "Exploring the Therapeutic Effects of Yoga and Its Ability to Increase Quality of Life," *International Journal of Yoga* 4, no. 2 (2011): 49–54, https://doi.org/10.4103/0973-6131.85485.

36. Woodyard, "Exploring the Therapeutic Effects of Yoga and Its Ability to Increase Quality of Life."

37. Julienne E. Bower et al., "Yoga Reduces Inflammatory Signaling in Fatigued Breast Cancer Survivors: A Randomized Controlled Trial," *Psychoneuroendocrinology* 43 (May 1, 2014): 20–29, https://doi.org/10.1016/j.psyneuen.2014.01.019.

38. Justin C. Strickland and Mark A. Smith, "The Anxiolytic Effects of Resistance Exercise," *Frontiers in Psychology* 5 (July 10, 2014): 753, https://doi.org /10.3389/fpsyg.2014.00753.

39. Alan Ewert and Yun Chang, "Levels of Nature and Stress Response," *Behavioral Sciences* 8, no. 5 (May 17, 2018): 49, https://doi.org/10.3390/bs8050049.

40. Beth Fordham et al., "The Evidence for Cognitive Behavioural Therapy in Any Condition, Population or Context: A Meta-Review of Systematic Reviews and Panoramic Meta-Analysis," *Psychological Medicine* 51, no. 1 (January 2021): 21–29, https://doi.org/10.1017/S0033291720005292.

41. J. Gaab et al., "Psychoneuroendocrine Effects of Cognitive-Behavioral Stress Management in a Naturalistic Setting—A Randomized Controlled Trial,"

Psychoneuroendocrinology 31, no. 4 (May 2006): 428–38, https://doi.org/10
.1016/j.psyneuen.2005.10.005.

42.   Gaab et al., "Psychoneuroendocrine Effects of Cognitive-Behavioral Stress
Management in a Naturalistic Setting."

43.   Michael H. Antoni et al., "Cognitive-Behavioral Stress Management Re-
verses Anxiety-Related Leukocyte Transcriptional Dynamics," *Biological
Psychiatry*, 71, no. 4 (February 15, 2012): 366–72, https://doi.org/10.1016/j
.biopsych.2011.10.007.

11. Why You Shouldn't Sleep on Sleep

1.   Susanne Diekelmann and Jan Born, "The Memory Function of Sleep," *Nature
Reviews Neuroscience* 11, no. 2 (February 2010): 114–26, https://doi.org/10
.1038/nrn2762.

2.   Paula Alhola and Päivi Polo-Kantola, "Sleep Deprivation: Impact on Cognitive
Performance," *Neuropsychiatric Disease and Treatment* 3, no. 5 (2007): 553–67.

3.   Ingrid Philibert, "Sleep Loss and Performance in Residents and Nonphysicians: A Meta-Analytic Examination," *Sleep* 28, no. 11 (November 2005):
1392–402, https://doi.org/10.1093/sleep/28.11.1392.

4.   Brian Christopher Tefft, "Prevalence of Motor Vehicle Crashes Involving
Drowsy Drivers, United States, 1999–2008," *Accident Analysis & Prevention*
45 (March 2012): 180–86, https://doi.org/10.1016/j.aap.2011.05.028.

5.   Marie Vandekerckhove and Yu-lin Wang, "Emotion, Emotion Regulation
and Sleep: An Intimate Relationship," *AIMS Neuroscience* 5, no. 1 (December
1, 2017): 1–17, https://doi.org/10.3934/Neuroscience.2018.1.1.

6.   Michael R. Irwin, "Sleep and Inflammation: Partners in Sickness and in
Health," *Nature Reviews Immunology* 19, no. 11 (November 2019): 702–15,
https://doi.org/10.1038/s41577-019-0190-z.

7.   Petra Zimmermann and Nigel Curtis, "Factors That Influence the Immune
Response to Vaccination," *Clinical Microbiology Reviews* 32, no. 2 (March 13,
2019): e00084–18, https://doi.org/10.1128/CMR.00084-18.

8.   Michiaki Nagai, Satoshi Hoshide, and Kazuomi Kario, "Sleep Duration as a
Risk Factor for Cardiovascular Disease—A Review of the Recent Literature,"
Current Cardiology Reviews 6, no. 1 (February 1, 2010): 54–61, https://doi.org
/10.2174/157340310790231635.

9. Lulu Xie et al., "Sleep Drives Metabolite Clearance from the Adult Brain," *Science* 342, no. 6156 (October 18, 2013): https://doi.org/10.1126/science.1241224.

10. Rachel Leproult and Eve Van Cauter, "Effect of 1 Week of Sleep Restriction on Testosterone Levels in Young Healthy Men," *JAMA* 305, no. 21 (June 1, 2011): 2173–74, https://doi.org/10.1001/jama.2011.710.

11. Alexander J. Scott, Thomas L. Webb, and Georgina Rowse, "Does Improving Sleep Lead to Better Mental Health? A Protocol for a Meta-Analytic Review of Randomised Controlled Trials," *BMJ Open* 7, no. 9 (September 18, 2017): e016873, https://doi.org/10.1136/bmjopen-2017-016873.

12. Aakash K. Patel, Vamsi Reddy, and John F. Araujo, "Physiology, Sleep Stages," in *StatPearls* (Treasure Island, FL: StatPearls Publishing, 2022), http://www.ncbi.nlm.nih.gov/books/NBK526132/.

13. Ian M. Colrain, Christian L. Nicholas, and Fiona C. Baker, "Alcohol and the Sleeping Brain," *Handbook of Clinical Neurology* 125 (2014): 415–31, https://doi.org/10.1016/B978-0-444-62619-6.00024-0.

14. Daniel F. Kripke, "Hypnotic Drug Risks of Mortality, Infection, Depression, and Cancer: But Lack of Benefit," *F1000Research* 5 (November 12, 2018): 918, https://doi.org/10.12688/f1000research.8729.3.

15. Patricia J. Sollars and Gary E. Pickard, "The Neurobiology of Circadian Rhythms," *Psychiatric Clinics of North America* 38, no. 4 (December 2015): 645–65, https://doi.org/10.1016/j.psc.2015.07.003.

16. Sollars and Pickard, "The Neurobiology of Circadian Rhythms."

17. Kenneth P. Wright Jr. et al., "Sleep and Wakefulness Out of Phase with Internal Biological Time Impairs Learning in Humans," *Journal of Cognitive Neuroscience* 18, no. 4 (April 1, 2006): 508–21, https://doi.org/10.1162/jocn.2006.18.4.508.

18. Erin C. Hanlon et al., "Sleep Restriction Enhances the Daily Rhythm of Circulating Levels of Endocannabinoid 2-Arachidonoylglycerol," *Sleep* 39, no. 3 (March 1, 2016): 653–64, https://doi.org/10.5665/sleep.5546.

19. Hanlon et al., "Sleep Restriction Enhances the Daily Rhythm of Circulating Levels of Endocannabinoid 2-Arachidonoylglycerol."

20. Kristen L. Knutson, "Impact of Sleep and Sleep Loss on Glucose Homeostasis and Appetite Regulation," *Sleep Medicine Clinics* 2, no. 2 (June 2007): 187–97, https://doi.org/10.1016/j.jsmc.2007.03.004.

21. Karine Spiegel et al., "Brief Communication: Sleep Curtailment in Healthy Young Men Is Associated with Decreased Leptin Levels, Elevated Ghrelin Levels, and Increased Hunger and Appetite," *Annals of Internal Medicine* 141, no. 11 (December 7, 2004): 846–50, https://doi.org/10.7326/0003-4819-141 -11-200412070-00008.

22. Hanlon et al., "Sleep Restriction Enhances the Daily Rhythm of Circulating Levels of Endocannabinoid 2-Arachidonoylglycerol."

23. Margriet S. Westerterp-Plantenga, "Sleep, Circadian Rhythm and Body Weight: Parallel Developments," *Proceedings of the Nutrition Society* 75, no. 4 (November 2016): 431–39, https://doi.org/10.1017/S0029665116000227.

24. Jean-Philippe Chaput and Angelo Tremblay, "Sleeping Habits Predict the Magnitude of Fat Loss in Adults Exposed to Moderate Caloric Restriction," *Obesity Facts* 5, no. 4 (2012): 561–66, https://doi.org/10.1159/000342054.

25. Chaput and Tremblay, "Sleeping Habits Predict the Magnitude of Fat Loss in Adults Exposed to Moderate Caloric Restriction."

26. Arlet V. Nedeltcheva et al., "Insufficient Sleep Undermines Dietary Efforts to Reduce Adiposity," *Annals of Internal Medicine* 153, no. 7 (October 5, 2010): 435–41, https://doi.org/10.7326/0003-4819-153-7-201010050-00006.

27. Olivia E. Knowles et al., "Inadequate Sleep and Muscle Strength: Implications for Resistance Training," *Journal of Science and Medicine in Sport* 21, no. 9 (September 1, 2018): 959–68, https://doi.org/10.1016/j.jsams.2018.01.012.

28. Knowles et al., "Inadequate Sleep and Muscle Strength."

29. Alhola and Polo-Kantola, "Sleep Deprivation: Impact on Cognitive Performance."

30. Alhola and Polo-Kantola, "Sleep Deprivation: Impact on Cognitive Performance."

31. Philibert, "Sleep Loss and Performance in Residents and Nonphysicians."

32. Nathaniel F. Watson et al., "Recommended Amount of Sleep for a Healthy Adult: A Joint Consensus Statement of the American Academy of Sleep Medicine and Sleep Research Society," *Sleep* 38, no. 6 (June 1, 2015): 843–44, https://doi.org/10.5665/sleep.4716.

33. Hiroki Ikeda et al., "Self-Awakening Improves Alertness in the Morning and During the Day After Partial Sleep Deprivation," *Journal of Sleep Research* 23, no. 6 (December 2014): 673–80, https://doi.org/10.1111/jsr.12176.

34. Emma J. Wams et al., "Linking Light Exposure and Subsequent Sleep: A Field Polysomnography Study in Humans," *Sleep* 40, no. 12 (December 1, 2017): zsx165, https://doi.org/10.1093/sleep/zsx165.

35. Institute of Medicine (US) Committee on Military Nutrition Research, *Pharmacology of Caffeine, Caffeine for the Sustainment of Mental Task Performance: Formulations for Military Operations* (Washington, DC: National Academies Press, 2001), https://www.ncbi.nlm.nih.gov/books/NBK223808/.

36. Christopher Drake et al., "Caffeine Effects on Sleep Taken 0, 3, or 6 Hours Before Going to Bed," *Journal of Clinical Sleep Medicine* 9, no. 11 (November 15, 2013): 1195–200, https://doi.org/10.5664/jcsm.3170.

37. Christopher E. Kline, "The Bidirectional Relationship Between Exercise and Sleep: Implications for Exercise Adherence and Sleep Improvement," *American Journal of Lifestyle Medicine* 8, no. 6 (2014): 375–79, https://doi.org/10.1177/1559827614544437.

38. Jean-Philippe Chaput et al., "Sleep Timing, Sleep Consistency, and Health in Adults: A Systematic Review," *Applied Physiology, Nutrition, and Metabolism* 45, no. 10 (supp. 2) (October 2020): S232–47, https://doi.org/10.1139/apnm-2020-0032.

39. Edward C. Harding, Nicholas P. Franks, and William Wisden, "The Temperature Dependence of Sleep," *Frontiers in Neuroscience* 13 (April 24, 2019): 336, https://doi.org/10.3389/fnins.2019.00336.

40. Shahab Haghayegh et al., "Before-Bedtime Passive Body Heating by Warm Shower or Bath to Improve Sleep: A Systematic Review and Meta-Analysis," *Sleep Medicine Reviews* 46 (August 2019): 124–35, https://doi.org/10.1016/j.smrv.2019.04.008.

41. Christine Blume, Corrado Garbazza, and Manuel Spitschan, "Effects of Light on Human Circadian Rhythms, Sleep and Mood," *Somnologie* 23, no. 3 (September 2019): 147–56, https://doi.org/10.1007/s11818-019-00215-x.

42. Leonid Kayumov et al., "Blocking Low-Wavelength Light Prevents Nocturnal Melatonin Suppression with No Adverse Effect on Performance During Simulated Shift Work," *Journal of Clinical Endocrinology & Metabolism* 90, no. 5 (May 1, 2005): 2755–61, https://doi.org/10.1210/jc.2004-2062.

43. Jan Stutz, Remo Eiholzer, and Christina M. Spengler, "Effects of Evening Exercise on Sleep in Healthy Participants: A Systematic Review and Meta-Analysis," *Sports Medicine* 49, no. 2 (February 2019): 269–87, https://doi.org/10.1007/s40279-018-1015-0.

44. Cibele Aparecida Crispim et al., "Relationship Between Food Intake and Sleep Pattern in Healthy Individuals," *Journal of Clinical Sleep Medicine* 07, no. 6 (December 15, 2011): 659–64, https://doi.org/10.5664/jcsm.1476.

45. Colrain, Nicholas, and Baker, "Alcohol and the Sleeping Brain."

12. What Matters Most and Making Lasting Change

1. Aliya Alimujiang et al., "Association Between Life Purpose and Mortality Among US Adults Older Than 50 Years," *JAMA Network Open* 2, no. 5 (May 24, 2019): e194270, https://doi.org/10.1001/jamanetworkopen.2019 .4270.

2. Edward M. Phillips, Elizabeth P. Frates, and David J. Park, "Lifestyle Medicine," *Physical Medicine and Rehabilitation Clinics of North America* 31, no. 4 (November 2020): 515–26, https://doi.org/10.1016/j.pmr.2020.07.006.

3. Barbara G. Bokhour et al., "From Patient Outcomes to System Change: Evaluating the Impact of VHA's Implementation of the Whole Health System of Care," *Health Services Research* 57, no. S1 (June 2022): 53–65, https://doi.org /10.1111/1475-6773.13938.

4. US Department of Veterans Affairs, "The Circle of Health—Whole Health," last updated September 23, 2022, https://www.va.gov/WHOLEHEALTH /circle-of-health/index.asp.

5. Jon Kabat-Zinn, *Wherever You Go, There You Are: Mindfulness Meditation in Everyday Life* (New York: Hachette Books, 2009).

6. US Department of Veterans Affairs, "Whole Health: Personal Health Inventory," last updated September 28, 2022, https://www.va.gov/WHOLE HEALTH/docs/PHI-long-May22-fillable-508.pdf.

7. Roger Walsh, *Essential Spirituality: The 7 Central Practices to Awaken Heart and Mind* (New York: Wiley, 2000).

8. "National Board for Health and Wellness Coaching," NBHWC, accessed August 26, 2022, https://nbhwc.org/.

9. Benjamin Gardner, Phillippa Lally, and Jane Wardle, "Making Health Habitual: The Psychology of 'Habit-Formation' and General Practice," *British Journal of General Practice* 62, no. 605 (December 2012): 664–66, https://doi .org/10.3399/bjgp12X659466.

10. Gardner, Lally, and Wardle, "Making Health Habitual."

11. James Clear, *Atomic Habits: An Easy & Proven Way to Build Good Habits &
     Break Bad Ones* (New York: Penguin, 2018).

12. Gardner, Lally, and Wardle, "Making Health Habitual."

13. Phillippa Lally et al., "How Are Habits Formed: Modelling Habit Formation
     in the Real World," *European Journal of Social Psychology* 40, no. 6 (October
     2010): 998–1009, https://doi.org/10.1002/ejsp.674.

14. Gardner, Lally, and Wardle, "Making Health Habitual."

15. Gardner, Lally, and Wardle, "Making Health Habitual."

16. Gardner, Lally, and Wardle, "Making Health Habitual."

17. Gaby Judah et al., "Exploratory Study of the Impact of Perceived Reward on
     Habit Formation," *BMC Psychology* 6, no. 1 (December 2018): 62, https://doi
     .org/10.1186/s40359-018-0270-z.

18. Judah et al., "Exploratory Study of the Impact of Perceived Reward on Habit
     Formation."

19. Martin Oscarsson et al., "A Large-Scale Experiment on New Year's Reso-
     lutions: Approach-Oriented Goals Are More Successful Than Avoidance-
     Oriented Goals," ed. Justin C. Brown, *PLOS ONE* 15, no. 12 (December 9,
     2020): e0234097, https://doi.org/10.1371/journal.pone.0234097.

20. Gardner, Lally, and Wardle, "Making Health Habitual."

21. David T. Neal et al., "The Pull of the Past: When Do Habits Persist Despite
     Conflict with Motives?" *Personality and Social Psychology Bulletin* 37, no. 11
     (November 2011): 1428–37, https://doi.org/10.1177/0146167211419863.

INDEX